The Psychiatric Evaluation in Clinical Practice

The Psychiatric Evaluation in Clinical Practice

Roger A. MacKinnon, M.D.
Professor of Clinical Psychiatry
Columbia University
College of Physicians and Surgeons
Training and Supervising Analyst
Columbia University Center for
Psychoanalytic Training and Research
New York, New York

Stuart C. Yudofsky, M.D.
Associate Professor of Clinical Psychiatry
Columbia University
College of Physicians and Surgeons
Director of Psychiatry
Allegheny General Hospital
Pittsburgh, Pennsylvania

J. B. LIPPINCOTT COMPANY
Philadelphia London Mexico City
New York St. Louis São Paulo Sydney

Sponsoring Editor: Delois Patterson
Manuscript Editor: Virginia M. Barishek
Indexer: Barbara Littlewood
Design Director: Tracy Baldwin
Designer: Don Shenkle
Production Supervisor: Kathleen Dunn
Production Coordinator: George V. Gordon
Compositor: Bi-Comp, Incorporated
Printer/Binder: R. R. Donnelley & Sons Company

6   5   4   3   2   1

Library of Congress Cataloging-in-Publication Data

MacKinnon, Roger A.
  The psychiatric evaluation in clinical practice.

  Includes bibliographies and index.
  1. Psychodiagnostics.   I. Yudofsky, Stuart C.
II. Title: [DNLM: 1. Interview, Psychological—methods.
2. Mental Disorders—diagnosis.   3. Physical Examination—
methods.   4. Psychiatric Status Rating Scales.   5. Psychological Tests—methods.   WM 141 M158pa]
RC469.M345   1986   616.89'075   86-2749
ISBN   0-397-50688-0

The authors and publisher have exerted every effort to ensure that drug selection and dosage set forth in this text are in accord with current recommendations and practice at the time of publication. However, in view of ongoing research, changes in government regulations, and the constant flow of information relating to drug therapy and drug reactions, the reader is urged to check the package insert for each drug for any change in indications and dosage and for added warnings and precautions. This is particularly important when the recommended agent is a new or infrequently employed drug.

Foreword

The practice of psychiatry has changed markedly over the past few decades. The almost exclusive dominance of psychodynamic and psychoanalytic models that characterized the major academic centers in the 1950s has been transformed by scientific advances, new patterns of clinical care, and new methods of diagnosis and treatment. Descriptive, developmental, biologic, social, and neuropsychological approaches have broadened and enriched the clinician's strategies. Operational diagnostic criteria and reliable (and in some cases demonstrably valid) categories have increased the value and power of clinical diagnosis. Psychometric and laboratory procedures are more elegant, specific, and informative while less burdensome or invasive than in the past. Finally, new treatments mean that clinical assessment makes a difference to the patient and to the ultimate outcome.

In some psychiatric centers the new themes in psychiatry have replaced the old. The excitement associated with new discoveries makes this easy to understand. However, in the best setting, the most important features of dynamic psychiatry have been preserved and have made contributions to our growing knowledge of descriptive, developmental, biologic, and social psychiatry. The complete modern psychiatrist evaluating a patient with depression, panic disorder, borderline personality, or dyslexia has many tools at his disposal and many frameworks within which to conceptualize the problem. The clinician who is skilled at one, but not knowledgeable of the others, will not be able to provide his patient with optimal care. Psychodynamic considerations are always relevant and often essential, but are seldom sufficient in modern psychiatry.

Doctors MacKinnon and Yudofsky are master clinicians and master teachers of clinical psychiatry. One is a psychoanalyst with a special interest in personality and how it shapes the psychiatric interview; the other is a neuropsychiatrist who has done pioneering research on brain disorders and their psychopathologic sequelae. Their collaboration epitomizes the essence of contemporary psychiatry. Their book is designed for students who want to combine the best of the old with the most effective and useful of the new. The psychiatrist who understands transference and resistance will have a decided advantage in evaluating a patient with Alzheimer's disease, just as the psychiatrist who knows the role of the dexamethasone suppression test will be better able to advise a patient with a masochistic personality disorder. Knowledge of modern diagnosis will be essential for both if they are to communicate effectively with colleagues. The student who has studied this book will have made an important step toward each of these goals.

Doctors MacKinnon and Yudofsky have gone further. They have described and discussed the role of laboratory procedures, psychometric tests, rating scales, and structured interviews, with illustrations and examples of each, in terms that will be most useful to the clinician. They have used clinical vignettes and illustrations throughout. The reader will have no doubt that this is a book by and for doctors who see patients regularly.

Finally, they have gone beyond the observation, collection, and description of the clinical data. They discuss the principles of a case formulation, and provide us with several detailed and rich examples of psychodynamic case formulations, modeling the way in which a modern psychiatrist integrates clinical information with an understanding of psychiatric theory in a format that is of practical assistance in caring for patients. This is one of the unique and most valuable features of this volume.

The learning of clinical psychiatry requires clinical settings, patients, teachers, and exposure to the knowledge and ideas of the field. Nothing can substitute for the settings, patients, and teachers, but this text is certainly one of the finest introductions to the basic knowledge the psychiatrist will want at his side as he approaches his patients. The field is indebted to Doctors MacKinnon and Yudofsky not only for the comprehensive scope of their work, but for the elegance of its presentation as well.

Robert Michels, M.D.

Preface

Although the fundamental clinical skills utilized to perform a modern psychiatric evaluation remain constant, the data base in psychiatry has broadened significantly over the past 30 years. For example, new knowledge of genetic and familial aspects of psychiatric illness has added increased relevance to the family history; the research of Mahler, Piaget, and other developmental psychologists has opened new areas of inquiry regarding the patient's childhood; the increased understanding of character disorders has necessitated specific questioning about the nature of the patient's object relations; the sharper, more objective clinical diagnostic criteria have led to the need for a more precise mental status examination; the rapid growth of data concerning the biological aspects of mental illness has made the physiological, endocrinological, and neurohormonal evaluation of the psychiatric inpatient almost a routine necessity; and the effective new somatic treatments of psychiatric illnesses have increased the importance of laboratory testing in the assessment of clinical response. The data base in psychiatry also has been broadened significantly by novel electrodiagnostic and imaging techniques such as PET, MRI, BEAM, and cerebral blood flow testing, all now widely available to provide objective information to assist in diagnosis. Discrete neuropathological or neurophysiological syndromes such as sleep disorders, psychiatric symptoms associated with temporal lobe epilepsy, and cognitive and mood changes in multiple sclerosis are now better understood and have opened up new areas for evaluation.

We have chosen to write about these basic skills, because we find that teacher and student enthusiasm about the expanding frontiers of psychiatry often leads to insufficient classroom time being devoted to the beginner's mastery of the methodology of conducting a comprehensive and valid psychiatric evaluation. Further, the basic skills of taking a psychiatric history or performing a mental status examination cannot be learned adequately solely by watching more experienced colleagues interview patients (although videotape, which can be used to demonstrate important issues such as the difference between restricted affect and mild depression, may be a useful tool).

Once the data that are required for the diagnosis and treatment of the psychiatric patient have been obtained, it is necessary to develop a formulation of the case. Unfortunately, case formulation tends to be taught in a casual, nonsystematic fashion. Relatively few training programs provide the resident with detailed instruction on how to prepare a coherent, comprehensive, written case formulation. In the typical trainee's eagerness to complete the written workup of the patient and to initiate treatment, insufficient time is allowed for thinking about the treatment plan in the context of the complex mix of psychological, social, and biological data obtained. Preparation of a case formulation is an exceptional learning and therapeutic device through which the clinician becomes more disciplined, precise, and thorough in his* evaluation and treatment of the patient.

Our book has been designed to be used in conjunction with clinical teaching. For the student to develop increased skill and proficiency in evaluating psychiatric patients, we recommend that thoughts be organized in the form of a written report to be reviewed by an experienced clinician. Several "model" mental status reports and case formulations have been included for the student to use as examples. The reader is encouraged to prepare these repeatedly, because the process of preparing several case formulations provides the clinician with the opportunity to discover specific areas of deficiency in his evaluation and understanding of the patient.

Initially, this text was prepared for psychiatric residents, interns, medical students, psychology students and interns, social work students, nursing students, and other health professionals interested in developing clinical skills. As the book evolved, we realized a secondary audience of experienced clinicians who would appreciate the latest material on the biological evaluation of the patient and a review of neuropsychological testing and rating scales, which are increasingly important in the modern evaluation and necessary to understand certain aspects of current psychiatric literature. Our aim is to provide to the novice and seasoned clinician alike a balanced and comprehensive approach to the evaluation of a patient, which takes into consideration the social, psychodynamic, and biological perspectives.

In developing our outline for the psychiatric history and the mental status examination, we, together with Robert A. Glick, M.D., conducted a survey

---

* We have used the masculine pronoun throughout the book to refer to both male and female health professionals and patients.

of the outlines for psychiatric history and mental status examination used by the Departments of Psychiatry in all American medical schools and the 50 state departments of mental health. We thank all of our respondents (approximately 70%) for filling out our questionnaires. We are particularly grateful to the large percentage who enclosed samples of history and mental status examination outlines currently recommended. We had planned to use those data for a research project; however, the project soon became unmanageable because there were so many different approaches to the task of collecting and organizing clinical data. We had hoped to evolve two or, perhaps, three ideal psychiatric examinations that could be standardized, but this proved naive. For example, many researchers utilize structured questionnaires or rating scales such as the SADS to ensure precise, quantifiable, and valid data. Yet for most clinical purposes, the 78-page SADS would be excessive and unwarranted. Those centers offering broadly based clinical training programs favored outlines such as the one used in this book. Even among these outlines there was substantial variability and inconsistency regarding what was included, what was omitted, and where various data were placed in the psychiatric history and mental status examination. Although we have tried to use *what appeared to us* to be the best features of each system, we often found ourselves making arbitrary judgments. Where appropriate, we have explained the conceptual basis of our hierarchical organization. Additionally, throughout the book, we have adhered as much as possible to widely accepted terminology and to systems of classification that are compatible with DSM III-revised.

To the best of our knowledge, the chapter on the psychodynamic case formulation, with three sample formulations, is the only published work of its kind. Although they are deficient in many ways, the case formulations will provide a useful guide for students of dynamic psychiatry. We wish that there existed a psychodynamics textbook that was written in plain language and provided the necessary theoretical foundation required to prepare a discussion of the patient's key psychodynamics. In the absence of such a text, we have attempted to review and highlight ego psychological aspects of psychodynamic theory and generally to discuss their application in the assessment of psychiatric patients. Therefore, Chapter 6 provides an introductory discussion of mental conflict and ego functions and includes developmental perspectives of both psychological conflict and psychological deficit. We hope that this discussion will stimulate the reader to pursue a number of other sources to acquire additional background knowledge of psychodynamics.

Some information in the section on the biological evaluation will be out of date by the time the book is in print. Knowledge in this area increases by leaps and bounds. Two years ago, when the book was taking shape, our reviewers cautioned us to advise our readers that such imaging technologies as MRI (then called NMR) were still experimental and that it would be some time before they would have clinical usefulness in the evaluation of patients. MRI is already available in most parts of the country, and it is considered an essential tool to confirm elusive diagnoses, such as multiple sclerosis with atypical features.

Finally, we wish to reemphasize that all clinical material has been carefully altered to disguise the identity of patients, while at the same time preserving the important psychopathological and psychodynamic features of the patient. The examples used were chosen because they are representative of the clinical problems typically found in psychiatric practice.

Roger A. MacKinnon, M.D.

Stuart C. Yudofsky, M.D.

Acknowledgments

The inspiration for this book is a classic work on the same subject entitled *Outlines for Psychiatric Examinations* by Nolan D.C. Lewis, M.D., New York State Press, 1943. In its day, this volume was affectionately known as the "Lewis Red Book." For about 30 years, psychiatric residents relied heavily on the Red Book as a guide for eliciting and organizing clinical data.

Patterns of psychiatric education have changed substantially in the past three decades. In our role as teachers of psychiatric residents, we have often wished there were an updated version of the Lewis classic to assist us in our educational task. Thus, we have undertaken the preparation of this modern day derivative.

It is impossible to thank individually each teacher who has contributed to our knowledge of basic clinical psychiatry. Nevertheless, special appreciation is expressed to Hilde Bruch, M.D., Paul Hoch, M.D., Lawrence C. Kolb, M.D., Nolan D.C. Lewis, M.D., Irville H. MacKinnon, M.D., and Sandor Rado, M.D.

We are indebted to the many classes of residents who have helped us to organize and to refine our clinical knowledge, thereby enabling us to present it in a more logical and coherent format. We are also grateful to our residents and our patients for providing us with the clinical examples that have been used throughout the book. We are particularly indebted to the Class of 1985 from the New York State Psychiatric Institute, because they have listened to much of the material in this book and have responded with helpful suggestions and questions. The clinical examples are sufficiently prototypic that a substantial number of readers may feel certain that a particular case refers to one of their patients, or to someone whom they know. Although great care has been taken to preserve the authenticity of the clinical data, at the same time, all identifying material that could render a patient recognizable has been changed.

Our greatest debt is for the many helpful suggestions and criticisms provided by the readers of the individual chapters. We thank the following reviewers, each of whom has devoted significant time and thought to this task.

Arthur Carr, Ph.D.	Ethel Person, M.D.
Frances Cohen, M.D.	Nancy Petersmeyer, M.D.
Richard Druss, M.D.	Ronald Rieder, M.D.
Jean Endicott, Ph.D.	Steven Roose, M.D.
Michael Fetel, M.D.	Harold Sackheim, Ph.D.
Michael Franzen, Ph.D.	Jonathan Silver, M.D.
Robert Glick, M.D.	Robert Spitzer, M.D.
Jack Gorman, M.D.	James Stevenson, M.D.
Fred Kass, M.D.	Milton Viederman, M.D.
Lisa Mellman, M.D.	Scott Wetzler, Ph.D.
Robert Michels, M.D.	Beth Yudofsky, M.D.

Our book is immeasurably improved by their recommendations, which we have attempted to follow.

We also specifically thank Arnold Cooper, M.D., Otto Kernberg, M.D., Robert Michels, M.D., and Roy Schafer, Ph.D. for their criticisms of the section on ego functions, which was used by one of the authors in an earlier publication on that topic.

For assistance in the preparation of our case material, we thank Joanne Ahola, M.D., Charles Schwartz, M.D., and Diane Stone, M.D.

Special gratitude is extended to Richard Druss, M.D. and to Nancy Petersmeyer, M.D. for their line by line comments on a major portion of the book.

Robert Michels, M.D. not only has written a thoughtful and generous foreword but he also has reviewed the entire manuscript and made detailed comments. He truly has extended himself beyond the customary bounds of friendship.

We thank Kathy Woznicki for her patience in the countless hours of typing and retyping the numerous drafts of the manuscipt. We also thank Lorraine Smith, Marge Zamanski, and Mary Siefring for their assistance in typing the manuscript.

To William Burgower, who was the acquiring medical editor, we express particular appreciation for his encouragement and support in planning the book and negotiating the contract. We owe a debt of gratitude to Delois Patterson, our developmental editor, for her recommendations concerning final organization and design decisions. Her cooperation and assistance have been exemplary. To Virginia Barishek, our manuscript editor, we extend our thanks for her meticulous attention to every detail of the manuscript and the extra effort required on her part to meet an early publication date. Finally, we thank J. Stuart Freeman, Jr., editor-in-chief of J.B. Lippincott Company, for his support, enthusiasm, and special production arrangements to allow early publication.

Finally, we thank our families for their support and patience during the many evenings and weekends devoted to this task.

Contents

1. **The Psychiatric Interview**   **1**
Factors Influencing the Interview   4
Diagnostic Versus Therapeutic Interviews   4
The Role of the Interviewer   5
Practical Issues   8
The Data of the Interview   10
Pre-Interview Considerations   18
The Opening Phase   19
The Middle Phase   22
The Closing Phase   27
Subsequent Interviews   30
Interviews with Relatives and Significant Others   31
Conclusion   33

2. **The Clinical Examination of the Patient**   **35**
The Psychiatric History   40
The Mental Status Examination   58
Appendix: Sample Mental Status Examination Reports   78

3. **Biological Testing in Psychiatry**   **85**
Clinical Laboratory Testing in Psychiatry   87
Electrical Diagnosis and Brain Imaging Techniques in Evaluating
    Psychiatric Disorders   110
The Risk–Benefit Ratio of Laboratory Testing   117

4. *Evaluation of Regional Cortical Functioning*   123
Frontal Lobes   *125*
Temporal Lobes   *129*
Parietal Lobes   *137*
Occipital Lobes   *138*
Diffuse Cortical Impairment   *138*

5. *Psychological Testing and Psychiatric Rating Scales*   145
Overview of Psychological Testing and Rating Scales   *146*
Evaluation of Intelligence   *148*
Personality Tests   *151*
Neuropsychological Tests and Assessment   *157*
Clinical Application of Psychological Testing Batteries   *159*
Psychiatric Rating Scales   *165*
Appendix 5-1:   Beck Depression Inventory (BDI) (Short
   Form)   *190*
Appendix 5-2:   Global Assessment Scale (GAS)   *192*
Appendix 5-3:   Hamilton Anxiety Rating Scale (HAMA)   *195*
Appendix 5-4:   Hamilton Rating Scale for Depression
   (HAMD)   *197*
Appendix 5-5:   The Mini-Mental State Examination   *200*
Appendix 5-6:   Overt Aggression Scale (OAS)   *203*
Appendix 5-7:   Wechsler Memory Scale: Form I (WMS)   *206*

6. *DSM III Diagnosis and the Psychodynamic Case Formulation*   213
Multiaxial Evaluation According to DSM III   *214*
The Written Psychodynamic Case Formulation   *219*
Appendix 6-1.   Case Formulation   *250*
Appendix 6-2.   Case Formulation   *259*
Appendix 6-3.   Case Formulation   *267*

***Index*   279**

The Psychiatric
Evaluation in
Clinical Practice

Although great care has been taken to preserve the authenticity and integrity of the clinical data, all patients' names, physical characteristics, and identifying material have been changed.

1

The Psychiatric Interview

Factors Influencing the Interview 4

Diagnostic Versus Therapeutic Interviews 4

The Role of the Interviewer 5
  Reassurance, Understanding, and Empathy 5
  Suggestion and Limit Setting 6
  Building the Patient's Self-Esteem 7
  Interpretation 7

Practical Issues 8
  Time Factors 8
  Space Considerations 9
  Note Taking 10

The Data of the Interview 10
  Systems of Classification 10
  The Patient 11
    Transference 12
    Resistance 14
  The Interviewer 15
    The Inexperienced Interviewer 16
    Countertransference 17

Pre-Interview Considerations 18
  The Patient's Expectations 18
  The Doctor's Expectations 18

The Opening Phase 19
  Meeting the Patient 19

The Development of Rapport   20
   Understanding the Patient   20
   The Doctor's Interest   20
   Confidentiality   20
   The Patient's Shame   21
   Uncovering Feelings   21

The Middle Phase   22
   The Abrupt Transition   22
   The Patient's Personality   23
   Exploring the Past   24
   Needs for Reassurance   24
   Stimulating Curiosity   24
   Using the Patient's Words   25
   Open-Ended Questions   25
   Sensitive Topics   26
   Stressing the Patient   26
   Managing the Patient's Anxiety   27

The Closing Phase   27
   The Patient's Questions   27
   The Treatment Plan   28
   Prognosis   30

Subsequent Interviews   30

Interviews with Relatives and Significant Others   31
   Basic Ground Rules   31
   Seeing the Relative Alone   32
   Reassurance and Questions   33

Conclusion   33

The psychiatric interview is not a casual or random meeting between doctor and patient. Like other physician and patient interactions, the psychiatric interview is based upon the principle that one person is suffering and desires relief and the other person is expected to provide this relief. The patient's desire to be helped enables him to expose personal and often painful thoughts, feelings, and experiences. An atmosphere of trust and openness is facilitated both by the interviewer's empathy and by the patient's awareness of the confidential nature of the doctor–patient relationship.

In those situations where the patient views the doctor as a potential source of help, the physician can obtain a considerable amount of information about the patient and his suffering solely by listening. Nevertheless, there are many cases where the patient is unable to trust the interviewer from the start. In such situations, the physician's success will be contingent upon his expertise as an interviewer. Interviewing is a skill founded upon extensive knowledge of normal and abnormal human behavior. An understanding of psychodynamics, coupled with a mastery of the technical principles of interviewing, are essential for the psychiatrist to function as the expert that the patient expects and deserves.

Actual ingredients of the psychiatrist's efficacy as an interviewer are his sensitivity and his empathic capacity. This is not the same as the offering of a sympathetic ear. Empathy is the ability to place oneself in the plight of another person and then feel what that person would feel in that situation. Empathy, therefore, encompasses more than what the interviewer would have felt in the situation described by the patient. Sympathy, on the other hand, is a more simple concept involving some feeling of compassion for another person's misfortune. The psychiatrist further demonstrates his expertise both by the questions he asks and does not ask and by other skills that will be discussed later in this chapter.

The psychiatrist, like his colleagues in other branches of medicine, is interested in the patient's symptoms, their dates of onset, and significant factors in the patient's life that may explain them. More so than other medical illnesses, diagnosis and treatment of psychiatric illness is based on the total life history of the patient. In addition to specific events, the life history includes the patient's life-style, self-appraisal, and individual coping mechanisms. Those psychiatric symptoms that involve the defensive functions of the ego represent unconscious psychological conflicts. To the extent that the patient defends himself from awareness of these conflicts, he will also conceal them from the interviewer. Therefore, although the psychiatric patient is motivated to reveal himself to gain relief from his suffering, he also is motivated to conceal his innermost feelings and the fundamental causes of his psychological disturbance.

Another factor contributing to the patient's concealing data during the interview is his concern with the impression he makes on others. The doctor, as a figure of authority, may symbolically represent the patient's parents; consequently, his reactions are particularly important to the patient. If the patient suspects that some of the less admirable aspects of his personality are involved in his illness, he may be unwilling to disclose such material until he feels certain that he will not lose the doctor's respect. The psychiatrist's reactions to the patient are significant because they can facilitate or impede the development of trust, which is essential for self-revelation. The patient's perception of the psychiatrist strongly influences what the patient tells or does not tell the physician.

In other specialties of medicine, the physician finds there is less chance of omitting important details of the patient's illness if his interview follows a routine. The experienced psychiatrist avoids over-structured or stereotyped approaches, because he cannot expect to learn things in the same order or always cover the same material in every initial interview.

FACTORS INFLUENCING THE INTERVIEW

Many factors influence both the content and the process of the interview. For example, the nature of the patient's symptoms or his character style significantly influences the transference and the way in which the interview unfolds.

Special clinical situations (such as the patient who is evaluated on a general hospital ward, the patient with psychosomatic symptoms, the psychologically unsophisticated patient, or the emergency room patient) all introduce specific dimensions that shape the interview.

Technical factors also affect the interview, such as telephone interruptions, the use of an interpreter, note taking, and the physical space and comfort of the room.

The first professional who meets with the patient will have a different experience from subsequent interviewers because each encounter changes the patient somewhat. The interviewer's appearance, his rhetorical style, and his theoretical orientation also influence the content and process of the interview. Even the timing of interjections such as "uh-huh" influences the patient's productions as he unconsciously follows the subtle leads provided by the interviewer. In general, the interviewer is nonjudgmental, interested, concerned, and kind. These complex and subtle factors are discussed in detail in MacKinnon and Michels, *The Psychiatric Interview in Clinical Practice*, W.B. Saunders, 1971.

DIAGNOSTIC VERSUS THERAPEUTIC INTERVIEWS

Psychiatric interviewers often draw distinctions between a diagnostic and a therapeutic interview. The interview that is oriented largely toward establishing a diagnosis gives the patient the feeling that he is a specimen of pathology being examined, and therefore actually inhibits him from revealing certain problems. The hallmark of a successful interview is the degree to which the patient and doctor develop a shared feeling of understanding. The psychiatrist who establishes a therapeutic relationship with the patient in the initial interview will thereby elicit more accurate and extensive diagnostic material. In addition, he achieves the advantage of being better able to assess the patient's attitude toward treatment. This will be reflected by the patient's responses to the psychiatrist's therapeutic interventions.

Patients experience some measure of relief by articulating and sharing their symptoms and other problems with a professional person.

THE ROLE OF THE INTERVIEWER

The most important role of the interviewer is to listen to the patient and understand him, and to establish rapport. Through rapport and understanding a mutually acceptable treatment plan will be developed.

Reassurance, Understanding, and Empathy

The novice interviewer frequently feels an undue pressure to provide reassurance or approval. He may use statements that begin "Don't worry," or "That's perfectly normal," that are reassuring but that do not indicate understanding. The reason that such remarks are only briefly helpful stems from the fact that the patient's fears are usually based on some deeper psychodynamic conflict. Frequently, the patient has already been told by his family doctor "not to worry." Nevertheless, the patient continues to worry, and he will keep worrying until someone understands his underlying fears and conflicts. For example, an agoraphobic female patient expressed a fear of going to restaurants. In probing this symptom the psychiatrist learned that the patient was afraid of fainting. Responding with reassurance rather than empathy, the psychiatrist said, "What would be so bad about that? It is unlikely that you would injure yourself in this fashion." Angrily, the patient stated, "How would you like to faint in a restaurant?" The doctor replied, "You're right, I was not understanding your concerns. It would be very upsetting to faint in a restaurant." Later, the patient revealed that she was afraid that if she were to be carried out of the restaurant on a stretcher, her dress might be pushed up, revealing that she had psoriasis on both knees. She subsequently realized through her therapy that the psoriasis symbolized feelings of defectiveness that she felt as a woman. It was only when she and the doctor reached that level of shared understanding that the fear subsided. At that point, the psychiatrist's responses, such as "I can see how badly you felt when . . .," were accepted by the patient and provided her with a feeling of being understood.

In different clinical circumstances from the example described, the interviewer may offer the patient reassurance concerning specific fears without detailed knowledge of the patient's life history and dynamics. An example is the patient who asks, "Do you think I am crazy?" In this case, no experienced psychiatrist would frustrate the patient with the response, "What do you think?" Instead, the patient may be told, "No, you are not crazy, but your concern that you might be crazy is a reflection, in part, that you don't have much confidence in the validity of your feelings, or perhaps in your ability to control them." On other occasions, the patient requires more general reassurance when he asks, "Am I talking about the right things, doctor?" In this situation it is appropriate to nod affirmatively or to reply, "You're doing fine; please continue."

The interviewer utilizes his own empathic responses to facilitate the development of rapport. For example, it is more effective when the patient describes a terrible experience to reply "How awful," rather than "You must have felt awful." When the interviewer replies, "How awful," he is putting himself in the patient's position and responding as he would expect any normal human being to react. The statement "You must have felt awful" seems similar at first glance, but it sounds more detached, objective, and less empathic (Schafer, 1974).

Expressions of emotion by the patient during the interview take priority over other matters. Not only do emotional expressions provide the interviewer with an opportunity to respond empathically, but they also reveal important information about the patient. It is often useful for the physician to name the emotion the patient is displaying. If the patient denies the emotion named by the interviewer but suggests a synonym, the psychiatrist accepts the correction and asks what evoked that feeling, rather than arguing with the patient. Some psychiatrists are reluctant to name a patient's feelings because of concerns about being condescending, controlling, or "telling a patient what to feel." If it is done correctly, the patient feels better understood when the doctor recognizes his (the patient's) emotion. This constitutes an empathic experience, rather than the doctor telling the patient what he should feel.

Suggestion and Limit Setting

The interviewer frequently asks questions, which may serve to obtain information or to clarify his own or the patient's understanding. Questions also can be a subtle form of suggestion, or, by the tone of voice in which they are asked, may give the patient permission to do something. When the interviewer asks, "Did you ever tell your husband how you feel about that?", he is also indirectly providing a suggestion. Thus, the interviewer may suggest that the patient discuss major decisions with him before acting on them, or that it would or would not be a good idea to discuss certain feelings with a specific person at a particular time. The psychiatrist may, at times, give the patient some advice or practical suggestions about his life. Many of the interviewer's activities serve to gratify the patient's emotional need to feel protected or loved. Nevertheless, on occasion, the interviewer may frustrate the patient's need for immediate solutions or reassurance. The therapist cannot make the patient's complex problems disappear by magic, find him a better job, a better spouse, or the like. For example, when a patient asks the therapist, "Do you think I'm attractive?" or "Promise me everything will turn out all right," the clinician must explore with the patient the meaning and implications of these questions rather than complying with a simple and direct "Yes."

In some situations, the interviewer may have to set limits with a patient who has trouble controlling his impulses. In one instance, a patient picked up a chart on the doctor's desk and the interviewer stated, "That chart is private and you may not look at it."

Building the Patient's Self-Esteem

Finally, the interviewer helps to build or maintain the patient's self-esteem when he focuses on the patient's successful achievement and talents. He also can reduce the patient's guilt through interventions that serve to modify the patient's harsh superego.

Interpretation

The interviewer offers interpretations aimed at undoing the process of repression, allowing unconscious thoughts and feelings to become conscious, thereby enabling the patient to develop new methods of coping with these conflicts without the formation of symptoms. The preliminary steps of an interpretation are confrontation (pointing out that the patient is avoiding something) and clarification (formulating the area to be explored). An example occurred with a compulsive man who arrived home for dinner to find his wife clad in a revealing negligee. Insensitive to her sexual mood, he asked, "Aren't you feeling well?" and was surprised and confused by her angry response. The interviewer replied, "I guess you didn't realize that she wanted you to make love with her." The patient responded, "As a matter of fact, the thought crossed my mind briefly, and then I thought that she might not be feeling well." The psychiatrist then asked, "Were you annoyed with her?" "No," the patient replied, "but she could at least have given me time to look at the mail. Maybe I thought she was making a demand on me. I like to be the one who initiates sex. Now I think I understand why she got angry. It was a rejection by me." In this example, the psychiatrist has helped the patient increase his awareness of his repressed anger and his need to be in control of the sexual relationship with his wife.

A complete interpretation delineates a pattern of behavior in the patient's current life, exposes the basic conflict between wish and fear, isolates the defenses that are involved, and helps the patient connect those data with the resulting symptoms. The neurotic pattern is traced to its origin in his early life, its manifestations in the transference are pointed out, and the secondary gain is formulated. It is never possible to accomplish all of these ends in a single interpretation offered in a single session. The earliest interpretations are directed towards the area in which conscious anxiety is greatest, which is usually the patient's presenting symptoms, his resistance, or negative transference. A premature interpretation involves exposing unconscious material before a patient is prepared to deal consciously with the data. A patient perceives a premature interpretation as threatening because it increases his anxiety and thereby intensifies his resistance. Interpretations are first directed at manifestations of the patient's resistance in an empathic and understanding tone that will not make the patient defensive. Students often misinterpret this advice to mean that is is acceptable to tell the patient, "You are being resistant" or "You do not have the right attitude." Actually, it is the therapist who does not have the right attitude in those examples. Consider the case of a person who blames his problems on other people or upon unavoidable circumstances. Here, the interviewer might comment, "If I understand you correctly, you feel that it is really your wife who should be seeing a psychiatrist rather than yourself," or "You seem to be saying that if you no longer had back pain all of your problems in life would be solved."

PRACTICAL ISSUES

Time Factors

Psychiatric interviews last for varying lengths of time. The average consultation or therapeutic interview is 45 or 50 minutes. Interviews with psychotic or medically ill patients are more often brief, because the patient may find the interview stressful or fatiguing after 20 or 30 minutes. Nevertheless, in emergency room interviews or intake evaluations, time periods longer than 50 minutes may be required. In most situations the patient should know in advance approximately how long the interview will last.

The patient's management of time reveals important facets of his personality. Many patients arrive a few minutes early for their appointments. The anxious patient may arrive as much as half an hour early. When a patient arrives unusually early and does not appear anxious, this fact often deserves exploration during the early part of the interview. The patient who arrives significantly late creates a problem for the interviewer. The first time it occurs, the interviewer should listen to the explanation if one is offered. Sympathetic responses are indicated if the patient's lateness were clearly due to circumstances beyond his control. A response such as "I understand how frustrating it is to get a cab on such a rainy day" is preferable to a comment such as "That's quite all right." If the patient indicates a blatant resistance, such as "I forgot all about the appointment," the interviewer could ask, "Did you feel some reluctance about coming?" If the answer is "Yes" the psychiatrist might explore the matter further. However, if the reply is "No," then it is usually better to drop the matter for the time being. It is sometimes appropriate to comment, "Well, we'll accomplish as much as we can in the time remaining." Occasionally a patient is so late for an initial interview that only 5 or 10 minutes remain. This situation calls for sympathy and tact. The time is best used to arrange for another meeting and to get acquainted with the patient. Beginning a discussion of the present illness with so little time can only leave the patient feeling frustrated when he is cut off right in the middle of his story. Interpreting the patient's first lateness will be an exercise in futility and may discourage the patient from returning. If the clinician has the next hour unscheduled, it is appropriate to offer it to the patient.

The physician's handling of time is also an important factor in the interview. Chronic carelessness regarding time indicates a lack of concern for the patient. If the physician is unavoidably detained for a first interview, it is quite appropriate for him to express his regret that the patient was kept waiting.

Space Considerations

Most patients do not speak freely without privacy and assurance that their conversation cannot be overheard. Quiet surroundings offer fewer distractions for both parties. Interruptions are undesirable, and even a brief telephone call may be disrupting. Proper seating arrangements also facilitate the interview. Both chairs should be approximately equal in height so that neither person looks down on the other, and it is desirable that the chairs be placed so there is no furniture between the doctor and the patient. If the room contains several chairs, the doctor indicates his own chair and allows the patient to choose the chair in which he will feel most comfortable. For example, an overly dependent patient prefers the chair closest to the doctor, whereas the oppositional or competitive patient will choose a more distant chair, often the one directly across from the doctor.

Note Taking

Many opinions exist among experienced psychiatrists concerning the quantity and method of note taking. The psychiatrist in training often takes written notes during the session to present the material to a supervisor. That process may disturb either the patient or the interviewer, particularly if the supervisor has requested "verbatim" notes.

Because there is a legal and moral responsibility to maintain an adequate record of each patient's diagnosis and treatment, the need for keeping written records about patients is clear. The patient's record also serves to aid the psychiatrist's memory concerning his patient. Each interviewer must determine what type of information he has the most difficulty remembering, and use this knowledge as a guideline for his own system of recordkeeping.

A common practice is to take fairly complete notes during the first few sessions. After that, most psychiatrists record only pertinent new historical information, important events in the patient's life, medications prescribed and their effects, transference or countertransference trends, dreams, and general comments about the patient's progress. An alternate method is to record these notes directly after the patient's session has ended. Some patients express resentment if the psychiatrist records no notes during the interview. They feel that what they said must not be sufficiently important to record or that the doctor was uninterested. Other patients cannot tolerate note taking because they feel it distracts the psychiatrist's attention from them. Once the patient has expressed his resentment that he does not have the doctor's undivided attention and the physician is empathic, it may be possible to work out a compromise whereby some brief notes can be made during the session. There are times during the interview when the doctor may want to establish a heightened sense of intimacy by putting his pen and paper aside. That practice is customary when the patient discusses such matters as his sex life, his negative feelings about a previous doctor, or when he makes comments about the interviewer.

THE DATA OF THE INTERVIEW

Systems of Classification

There are a number of different ways to classify or organize the data of the interview. One system is content and process. The content of the interview refers both to the factual information provided by the patient and to the specific verbal interventions of the interviewer.

The process of the interview refers to the developing relationship between doctor and patient. Process particularly involves the implicit meanings of the communications. The patient's awareness of the process varies but is usually limited to his trust or confidence in the doctor, or his lack thereof, and, perhaps, his fantasies about him. The interviewer strives for a continuing awareness of the process, which reveals the unfolding of the early transference and countertransference.

Process involves both the manner in which the patient relates to the interviewer and many of the issues in the patient's mental status, such as impulse control. With increasing experience, the interviewer learns to become aware of his own emotional responses to the patient. If he examines those responses in the light of what the patient has just said or done, he may broaden his understanding of the patient and himself. For example, if he feels bored, he may realize that the patient is avoiding emotional contact by a preoccupation with his symptoms. If the psychiatrist feels titillated by the sexual details provided by a patient, he may learn that the patient uses sex as a distraction from other issues.

The data of the interview may also be classified as introspective or inspective. Introspective data refer to the patient's subjective report of his feelings and experiences; such data focus on his inner life. Inspective data refers to the nonverbal behavior of the patient and the interviewer. The interviewer is particularly interested in the symbolic meanings of the nonverbal content. For example, the patient who nervously takes his wedding ring on and off is communicating more than general anxiety.

Still another classification of data concerns the affect and thought content of the interview. As in any other meeting between strangers, both the patient and doctor experience anxiety in the initial interview. Most people find the idea of having to consult a psychiatrist rather upsetting. The patient is anxious about his illness, the doctor's reaction to him, whether or not the physician will be able to help him, and the logistical problems of psychiatric treatment.

The Patient

The interview reveals data about the patient, including his psychopathology, psychodynamics, personality strength, motivation, transference, and resistance.

Frequently a patient comes to a psychiatrist with the expectation that the doctor is only interested in his symptoms and possible deficiencies of character. It is reassuring to such a patient when the psychiatrist shows interest in his assets, talents, and other personality strengths. Some patients will volunteer such information, but others must be asked, "Would you tell me some things you like and find positive about yourself?" Sensitivity and proper timing are required in asking such questions. There is little likelihood that the patient will demonstrate his capacity for joy and pride if, just after revealing embarrassing or painful material, he is asked, "Tell me, what do you do for fun?" It is preferable to lead the patient gently away from upsetting topics, and then allow him the opportunity of a transition period before exploring his capacities for warmth and tenderness.

The interviewer should *always* look at anything the patient has brought to show him. Through those exchanges, some positive aspect of the patient's life is invariably revealed. When the patient spontaneously asks, "Would you like to see a picture of my children?", an interviewer's reluctance to look would be experienced by the patient as indifference or a frank rebuff. Likewise, if the interviewer looks at the picture and returns it without comment, there is little likelihood that the patient will reveal his own capacity for warmth. Rapport is facilitated by the interviewer's interest in and appropriate questions or observations about whatever the patient shows him. Beginning clinicians frequently misunderstand advice they receive about dealing with patients in a neutral manner. They confuse neutrality with being unresponsive. The term *technical neutrality* refers to the psychiatrist not siding with one agency of the patient's mind against another. In other words, the psychiatrist attempts to maintain a position of equal distance between the patient's id, ego, and superego. (This concept is discussed in greater detail in Chap. 6.) Neutrality also refers to the clinician's noninterference with the patient's right to his own values and life choices. The psychiatrist attempts to help the patient better understand his own feelings and thoughts, and thereby make more informed decisions.

Transference

Transference is a process whereby the patient unconsciously and inappropriately displaces on to persons in his current life those patterns of behavior and emotional reactions that originated with significant figures from his childhood. The relative anonymity of the psychiatrist and his role as a parent-surrogate facilitates this displacement on to him. We believe that the patient's realistic and appropriate reactions to his doctor are not transference. Furthermore, we distinguish the positive transference from the therapeutic alliance, which is the relationship between the doctor's analyzing ego and the healthy, observing, rational component of the patient's ego. The therapeutic alliance also has its origin during infancy and is based on the bond of real trust between the child and his mother. Therefore, positive transference is limited to those responses that are truly displaced from childhood figures and are inappropriate. The omnipotent power that the patient delegates to the physician is an example. The same principles apply in defining negative transference, which stems from the child's fear, anger, or mistrust of his parents. Some theoreticians believe that the separation of the positive transference from the therapeutic alliance is artificial and that all of the patient's responses to the physician are transferential in nature. A discussion of that theoretical point is beyond the scope of this book.

Realistic factors concerning the doctor can be starting points for initial transference. Age, sex, personal manner, and social and ethnic background all influence the rapidity and direction of the patient's responses. The patient's desire for affection, respect, and gratification of dependent needs is a prominent form of transference. Requests for special time, financial considerations, pills, matches, cigarettes, tissues, or a glass of water can be concrete examples of such needs or feelings. Because the inexperienced interviewer has great difficulty in differentiating legitimate demands from irrational demands, many errors are made in the management of such matters. This problem can be simplified if it is assumed that all requests have an unconscious transference component. The question is to determine when it is in the best interest of the patient to gratify his request and when it is best to interpret. The decision is based upon the time of the request, its content, the type of patient, and the reality of the situation. For example, at the first meeting a new patient might greet the interviewer by saying, "Do you have a tissue, Doctor?" Such a patient begins the relationship by making a demand. Because immediate refusals or interpretations would be premature and quickly alienate the patient, the psychiatrist simply gratifies the request. Nevertheless, the clinician should make a mental note about this interaction, and seek to learn more about its implications as the treatment evolves.

Omnipotent transference feelings are revealed by remarks such as, "I know you can help me," and "Why do I keep getting into these situations?" and "You must know the answers," and "What does my dream mean?" Try to avoid the cliché, "What do you think?" A more effective comment would be, "Do you feel I'm not being helpful enough?" It is even better to tell the patient, "I need to know more about you, and then, perhaps, I can better answer your question." This response is preferable because it takes the patient's question more seriously in the literal way that a patient expects. Patients become frustrated and angry with psychiatrists who never answer their questions and who instead turn every question back to them. Patients are also annoyed by therapists who invariably interpret what the patient really means as something different from what the question implies. We are not suggesting that an interviewer should never interpret a patient's question or never turn it back to the patient. However, inexperienced clinicians should be cautious not to overuse either technique.

Questions about the interviewer's personal life may involve several different types of transference. However, they most often reveal concern about his status or his ability to understand or help the patient. Such questions are usually about the psychiatrist's age, marital status, ethnic background, place of residence, or training. The experienced interviewer usually recognizes the true nature of the patient's interest and intuitively senses when it is or is not preferable to give the patient a direct answer. With or without a direct reply the doctor can inquire, "What lead you to ask that question?" or after answering the patient's question, he can ask, "Now, tell me what you learned from that information that was important to you." It then may be appropriate to interpret the meaning of the patient's question by stating, "Your question about whether or not I have children sounds as though you want to know if I am able to understand what it feels like to be a parent." On other occasions such questions signify the patient's desire to become a social friend of the psychiatrist. Often this reveals a feeling that he cannot be helped as a patient, or that he considers the role of patient to be degrading. The latter situation is most common in patients who develop competitive transferences and experience the interview as putting them in the "one down" position.

Resistance

Resistance is any conscious or unconscious attitude on the part of the patient that opposes the objectives of the treatment. Any psychological exploration of the patient's symptoms and behavior patterns threatens to expose the underlying conflicts that the patient has partially resolved in the formation of his symptoms and character structure. The same defense mechanisms that removed the basic conflict from the patient's awareness seek to maintain that repression or denial. Toward this end, the patient resists all insight. Even the most highly motivated patient cannot tell the doctor what he does not know about himself.

Resistance may be classified in many ways. Resistance may be expressed by the patterns of communication during the interview. Silence, garrulousness, censoring or editing thoughts, intellectualization, generalization, or preoccupation with one phase of his life (such as symptoms, current events, or the past) are common examples of resistance.

The patient who resists by talking excessively to control the interview can be interrupted by the psychiatrist with a comment such as "I find it difficult to say anything without interrupting you." That intervention may expose the patient's fear of what the physician might want to tell him.

At times, affective display can serve as a resistance to meaningful communication. The hysterical patient often uses one emotion to ward off other deeper and more painful affects: for example, constant anger may be used as defense against injured pride. Arriving late, forgetting the appointment, using a minor physical illness to avoid the session, seductive behavior, and competitive behavior are other examples of resistance.

Silence is also a common form of resistance. Prolonged or uncomfortable silences are rarely useful in an initial interview. The interviewer can address himself to the silence, if it develops, with comments such as "You seem to feel at a loss for words" or "What are you thinking about right now?" or "Perhaps there is something that is difficult for you to discuss." Sometimes interviewers unwittingly provoke silences by assuming a disproportionate responsibility for keeping the interview going. Asking questions that can be answered "Yes" or "No," or providing the patient with multiple choice answers to a question discourages the patient's sense of responsibility for the interview. Such interviewer activity limits the patient's spontaneity and constricts his flow of ideas. The patient retreats to passivity while the interviewer struggles for the right question that will "open the patient up."

Not all silences are a function of resistance. Some patients tolerate silences rather well, and, in fact, often use them to gather their thoughts before speaking. If the patient is engrossed in his story, he may not even notice the silence. When the patient uses silence to edit thoughts, he becomes uncomfortable and thereby provides a clue to the interviewer about the meaning of the silence.

The Interviewer

The principal instrument of the psychiatric interview is the psychiatrist himself. Each psychiatrist brings a different personal and professional background to the interview. His character structure, values, and sensitivity to the feelings of others influence his attitude and behavior toward fellow human beings—patients and nonpatients alike. Differences in the social, educational, and intellectual backgrounds between the patient and interviewer may interfere with the development of rapport. It is an obvious advantage for the physician to acquire as much understanding and familiarity as possible with the patient's subculture. The psychiatrist must know what effects his own personality has on a wide variety of people to recognize and better understand the responses he has elicited in the patient.

The Inexperienced Interviewer

In observing inexperienced interviewers, it is easily recognized that they have certain problems in common as contrasted with their more experienced colleagues. The inexperienced interviewer is more ill at ease with the patient. Consequently, the beginner is more apt to follow his recollections of the outline for psychiatric examination, rather than to follow the cues provided by the patient. The inexperienced interviewer may also feel guilty about practicing on the patient, and may fear that his status as a beginner will be discovered.

In some respects, the inexperienced interviewer is similar to the histology student who first peers into the microscope and sees only myriad pretty colors. As his experience increases, he becomes aware of structures and relationships that had previously escaped his attention. Later, he recognizes an ever increasing number of subtleties. The novice tends to interrupt the patient with a new question before the patient has finished reacting to the last question. With more experience, the interviewer learns whether a patient has completed his answer to a question or whether he merely requires some encouragement to continue his response.

Inexperienced interviewers suffer from two excesses. If the neophyte begins the session by talking too much, he later will tend to talk too little, and will lapse into a state of exaggerated passivity. This occurs more frequently when the interviewer is unable to understand the deeper meaning of the patient's disclosures, or when the interviewer feels anxious, bored, or helpless. The typical pattern is that the novice interviewer starts out with excessive enthusiasm for the challenge of his new task. This is manifested by excessive questioning and inadequate listening. When the patient resists the barrage in whatever manner is consistent with his particular character style, the clinician becomes discouraged and begins to withdraw from the patient. At this point, the physician realizes that the interview is not going well and he then begins a second period of questioning based upon his recollections of the outline. Because these interactions are not related to cues provided by the patient, the interview takes on a disjointed or jerky quality. The basic professional identity of the interviewer starts to assume excessive prominence at this point. The young psychiatrist becomes preoccupied with diagnosis and ruling out organic factors; the young clinical psychologist focuses on psychodynamic and personality factors; the social worker becomes preoccupied with family and social aspects of the patient's life. These comments are overly general; nevertheless, the patterns described are common.

Countertransference

Psychiatrists have two classes of emotional responses to their patients. First, there are reactions to the patient as he actually is. The doctor may like or dislike the patient or even be antagonized by him without countertransference implications, provided these are reactions that the patient would elicit in most people. Second, there are countertransference responses that are specific for an individual psychiatrist. Although inappropriate, those responses can become a useful source of information if the interviewer can allow himself to be aware of them, and uses them to improve his understanding of the patient.

Countertransference may be defined as the psychiatrist responding to aspects of the patient as if he were an important figure from the psychiatrist's past. The more the patient actually resembles figures from the doctor's past, the greater the likelihood of such reactions. A narrower definition of countertransference is the interviewer's unconscious response to the patient's transference. Countertransference reactions include the following: becoming dependent on the patient's praise or approval; intolerance and frustration when the patient is angry; exhibitionistic behavior to court the patient's favor; inability to see inconsistencies in certain interpretations; insisting on his own infallibility; being critical of a prior psychiatrist the patient saw; overidentification with the patient; experiencing vicarious pleasure in the sexual or aggressive behavior of the patient; power struggles; arguing with the patient; and wishing to be the patient's child. Boredom or inability to concentrate on what the patient is saying often reflects unconscious anger or anxiety on the part of the interviewer.

Another common countertransference problem stems from the therapist's failing to see occasions when the patient's observing ego is actually a transference masquerade. The result is an overly intellectualized interview that is devoid of emotion. The direct expression of emotion in the transference frequently will elicit countertransference responses. An example is the doctor who tells the patient, "It isn't really me you are angry at; it is your father." Telling a patient that his feelings are displaced implies that they are not real, and is disrespectful and belittling. Similarly, responding to the patient's anger with a comment such as "It is good that you are able to get angry with me" is contemptuous and is aimed to keep the psychiatrist one up on the patient. The patient's emotions must be taken seriously and dealt with in a forthright and open manner. The mistakes that the novice clinician makes as a result of inexperience or ignorance are not countertransference.

PRE-INTERVIEW CONSIDERATIONS

The Patient's Expectations

The patient's prior knowledge and expectations of the doctor play a vital role as the interview unfolds. In a hospital or clinic setting where the patient does not select the doctor personally, the institutional transference is of considerable importance. In this case the doctor must explore the patient's reasons for selecting a particular hospital or clinic. A pre-interview transference may be disclosed if the patient seems surprised by the psychiatrist's appearance, or remarks "You don't look like a psychiatrist." The doctor may ask, "What did you expect a psychiatrist to be like?" If the patient replies, "Well, someone much older," the interviewer might answer, "Perhaps you feel an older psychiatrist would be more experienced and could help you more quickly." Another patient may express relief by indicating that he had expected the psychiatrist to be a more frightening figure. These statements reveal important early transferential attitudes to the clinician. They provide clues to uncovering wishes or fears that must be understood to help the patient become aware of his unconscious resistance to the treatment.

In private practice, patients are usually referred to a specific doctor. The interviewer is interested to learn what the patient was told about the doctor at the time of the referral. Was he given one name or a list of names? In the latter case, how did he decide which doctor to call first, and was the interviewer the first one he contacted? One patient may indicate that he was influenced by the location of the doctor's office; another may have selected the doctor whose name suggested a particular ethnic background.

The Doctor's Expectations

The interviewer usually has some knowledge of the patient prior to the start of the first meeting. The knowledge may have been provided by the referring physician, or by a nurse or social worker if the patient is seen in a hospital. Some clues about the patient may have been obtained directly by the psychiatrist during the initial telephone call that led to the appointment. Experienced psychiatrists have personal preferences concerning the amount of information they want from the referring source. Some prefer to learn as much as possible; others desire only the bare minimum, on the ground it allows them to interview with a fully open mind.

Any time the interviewer experiences a feeling of surprise when he meets his new patient, he must question himself. Was he misled about the patient by the person who referred the patient, or was his surprise due to some unrealistic anticipation of his own? The positive attraction that the psychiatrist and patient often experience initially is derived chiefly from their unconscious fantasied expectations of each other. As their relationship evolves, the initial somewhat formal behavior is replaced by more intimate behavior that reveals more about the real person of the patient and of the doctor. It is at the point when their magical expectations are threatened by reality that the expertise of the psychiatrist is crucial.

THE OPENING PHASE

Meeting the Patient

The doctor obtains much information when he first meets a new patient. He can observe who, if anyone, has accompanied the patient, and how the patient was passing the time while waiting for the interview to begin. The psychiatrist can greet the patient by name and then introduce himself. Such social pleasantries as "It's nice to meet you" are inappropriate. If the patient is unduly anxious, the doctor might introduce a brief social comment, perhaps by inquiring if the patient experienced any difficulty finding the office. A natural and pleasant manner on the part of the psychiatrist makes the patient feel more at ease.

The experienced interviewer learns much about the patient during the initial greeting, so that he may appropriately vary the opening minutes of the interview according to the patient's needs. A suitable beginning might be to ask the patient to be seated and then to inquire, "What problem brings you here?" or "Would you tell me about your difficulty?" A less directive approach would be to ask the patient, "Where shall we start?" or "Where would you prefer to begin?"

Sullivan (1954) discussed the value of a summary statement about the referring person's communications concerning the patient, or a restatement of what the psychiatrist learned during the initial telephone conversation. It is comforting for the patient who is not self-referred to feel that the psychiatrist already knows something about his problem. An overly extensive presentation of the details is likely to be harmful, because they will rarely seem completely accurate to the patient. In this case, the interview gets underway with the patient defending himself from misunderstanding. General statements are preferable. For example, the interviewer might say, "Dr. Jones has told me that you and your wife have had difficulties," or "I understand that you have been quite depressed." Usually, the patient continues the story, but occasionally the patient asks, "Didn't he give you all the details?" The interviewer could reply, "He did say more than that, but I would like to hear the details directly from you."

The Development of Rapport

Understanding the Patient

To establish rapport, the interviewer must communicate that he has begun to understand the patient. That objective is accomplished both by the doctor's attitude and by the nature of his remarks. He does not wish to create the impression that he can read the patient's mind, but he does want the patient to realize that he has treated other people with similar problems and that he understands those problems—not only neurotic and psychotic symptoms, but ordinary problems in living. For example, if a young housewife reveals that she has four young children and no household help, the interviewer may ask, "How do you manage?" A question such as "Do they ever get on your nerves?" shows a lack of understanding.

The Doctor's Interest

The doctor's interest helps the patient to talk. On one hand, the more the doctor speaks, the more the patient is concerned with what the doctor wants to hear, rather than what is on his own mind. On the other hand, if the doctor is unresponsive the patient feels abandoned and is inhibited from revealing his feelings. Guiding the patient gently with comments such as "Then what happened?" or "Please continue" may suffice except when a more empathic response is required. For example, the interviewer might remark, "A child is bound to be upset by his parents' divorce," or "It sounds as though your mother was able to control you by making you feel guilty." Such comments really do not constitute premature interpretations because they do not deal with unconscious wish and defense. However, they do encourage the patient to reveal more by creating an atmosphere of safety with the psychiatrist.

Confidentiality

Sometimes the patient is reluctant to speak freely because he fears the doctor will betray his confidence. The patient may say, "I don't want you to tell this to my husband," or "I hope you don't tell everything to my internist." The interviewer should assure the patient that his privacy will be maintained. Any lapse in confidentiality will destroy the possibility of effective treatment.

Recent court decisions regarding the psychiatrist's responsibility to the public pose a threat to the confidentiality of the doctor–patient relationship. One problematic situation is that of the patient whom the psychiatrist believes to be a danger to some third party. In this instance the psychiatrist is obligated by law to warn the third party. When a psychiatrist encounters a situation in which the patient could be dangerous to others, it is important that he advise the patient of his obligation to third parties.

Another circumstance that is an increasing threat to confidentiality is third-party payment for treatment. We strongly recommend that the physician not only obtain the patient's written release to provide information to third-party payors, but also show the patient any report to be sent to the insurance company or government agency before mailing it. The patient always has the right to retain his privacy and relinquish the opportunity for financial reimbursement.

The Patient's Shame

At times the patient may seem to bog down or behave evasively. The impasse usually stems from feelings of shame or the patient's concern that the interviewer will judge him. Shame causes the patient to attempt to hide, whereas guilt feelings make him want to confess. The sensitive physician will perceive the distinction and respond with an empathic comment, such as "It's hard to discuss embarrassing topics with a stranger," or "Is there something that makes you feel too ashamed to continue?" It is a mistake to coerce the patient to go further with the use of implied threats, such as "If you don't tell me everything, I won't be able to help you." It is preferable at the start of the evaluation either to let the matter drop or to tell the patient, "Perhaps you can tell me later when you feel more at ease with me." A patient who persists in keeping conscious secrets from the doctor is unable to cooperate in his own best interest, and the doctor may eventually have to tell such a patient that his ability to help is dependent upon and is limited by the patient's capacity to confide in him.

Uncovering Feelings

An effective technique to help the patient become more in touch with his emotions is to ask for specific examples. The patient may make general statements about his life, such as "My husband doesn't understand me," or

"My mother was too protective," or "I wasn't as popular as my brother." When the psychiatrist replies, "Would you give me an example?" or "What do you remember about that?" he is obliging the patient to focus on those events and, in part, to relive them. Further questions should emphasize the patient's role in the experience under discussion, such as "What did you do then?" or "How did you react to that?" That sort of guidance gives the patient an idea of the material that is significant to the interviewer, and the patient will respond accordingly. Furthermore, he may experience some relief from an emotional catharsis, which also encourages him to continue.

In a different situation the patient does not express the feelings that one might expect. For example, if the patient describes an experience where he was able to assert himself and the psychiatrist offers the supportive comment, "That must have made you feel better," and the patient replies, "No," it is necessary to develop the subject further to regain the shared feeling of understanding. It is a mistake for the interviewer to feel merely that he had made an error and to let the issue slide past. When the patient discusses an experience without any apparent feeling, the psychiatrist should ask what the patient felt rather than conclude that the patient experienced no emotion. A patient may be able to discuss the subject without revealing his feelings, which is different from having experienced no emotion.

Frequently, patients struggle to maintain control over their emotions because reliving upsetting experiences awakens their accompanying painful affects. If the interviewer observes that the patient stops speaking and has a tear in his eye, he may comment, "It makes you sad to speak of that," or "You are trying not to cry." Anger is another emotion that may be difficult to acknowledge. When the patient manifests no response, the doctor may indicate that a certain experience would make most people angry. For example, the depressed patient is particularly unable to tolerate his angry feelings and might reply, "No, I only felt hurt." The interviewer accepts that formulation for the time being rather than argue with the patient.

THE MIDDLE PHASE

The Abrupt Transition

An abrupt transition is sometimes required after the patient has discussed his present illness. For example, the psychiatrist might say, "I have a picture of the problems that brought you here, and now I would like to learn more about you as a person," or "Can you tell me something about yourself in addition to the problems that brought you here?" At this point, it is appropriate for the interviewer to devote his attention to the patient's history. Just where to start depends on what aspects of the patient's life have been revealed while discussing the present illness. In most cases the patient talks about his current life before revealing his past. If the patient has not already mentioned his age, his marital status, the length of his marriage, the age and the name of his spouse, the ages and names of his children and parents, his occupational history, a description of current living circumstances, and so forth, the interviewer should ask for those details. It is preferable to obtain as much of that information as possible during the description of the present illness. A question such as "How have your symptoms interfered with your life?" may allow the patient the opportunity to provide data concerning any or all of the topics mentioned previously.

If the patient seems preoccupied with his symptoms, past illnesses, or any other subject, it may be necessary for the interviewer to deflect him, gently but firmly. Deflection can be done with a comment such as "You seem to have trouble getting away from that topic. Is there something about it that you feel I don't understand?", or "We have a lot of things that we haven't discussed yet, and if we don't move on, we may not get to them," or "Our time is limited today, and we haven't yet talked about your marriage."

The number of possible avenues to pursue in the middle portion of the interview is infinite; consequently, it is impossible to provide precise instructions about which choices to make. Most leads provided by the patient should be followed up at the time of presentation. Doing so gives smooth continuity to the interview, even though there may be numerous topical digressions.

The Patient's Personality

When the interviewer has some ideas about the present illness and the patient's current life situation, he may turn his attention to what sort of person the patient is. A question such as "What sort of person are you?" will come as a surprise to most people, because they are not accustomed to thinking of themselves in that fashion. Some patients respond easily, whereas others become uncomfortable and reply with concrete details that reiterate the facts of their current life situation, such as "Well, I'm a lawyer," or "I'm just a housewife." Nevertheless, such answers provide both phenomenological and dynamic information. The first reply was made by an obsessive-compulsive man who was preoccupied with rules and regulations, not merely in his job, but in his human relationships as well. What he was telling the interviewer was, "I am first and foremost a lawyer, and, in fact, I can never cease being a lawyer." The second reply was offered by a phobic woman who had secret ambitions for a career. She was letting the psychiatrist know that she had a deprecatory view of women, particularly women who are housewives. Like the first patient, she was never able to forget about herself.

Some of the questions that pertain to the patient's view of himself were suggested earlier in this section in the discussion of exploring the patient's assets. Questions such as "What things bring you the most pleasure?" and "What things about yourself give you the most pride?" are additional examples. The interviewer may ask the patient to describe himself both as he appears to others and as he appears to himself in major life roles, including family, work, social situations, sex, and situations of stress. It is often revealing to ask a patient to describe a typical 24-hour day. The insightful patient often will experience an increase in his self-awareness while reflecting on this question.

Exploring the Past

Depending on the amount of time available and whether there will be more than one interview, the psychiatrist plans his inquiry into the patient's past. Which past issues are most significant varies with the problems of the patient and the nature of the consultation. This is discussed in greater detail in the next chapter.

Needs for Reassurance

At various times during the interview, the patient may be uncomfortable with the material he is discussing. That feeling of discomfort is due to his wish to be accepted by the interviewer and, what is often more important, because of his fear concerning partial insight into himself. For example, he may pause and remark, "I know lots of people who do the same thing," or "Isn't that normal, Doctor"? or "Do you think I'm a bad mother?" Certain patients may require a reassuring reply to become engaged in the interview; others profit by the doctor's asking, "What did you have in mind?" or "Just what is it that you are concerned about?"

Stimulating Curiosity

Stimulating the patient's curiosity about himself is a fundamental technique in all interviews aimed at uncovering deep feelings. Basically, the psychiatrist uses his own curiosity about the patient to awaken the patient's interest in himself. The psychiatrist's curiosity is best not directed toward the most deeply repressed or the most highly defended issues, but at the more superficial layer of the patient's conflict. The doctor's expressed curiosity about motives of the patient and his loved ones is seldom therapeutic in the first few interviews, because it threatens the patient's defenses and may sound critical. For example, if the psychiatrist were to say, "I wonder why your husband spends more time at the office than is necessary?" the patient might construe this to be a hostile accusation or an innuendo. Similarly, confronting the patient with inconsistencies in his story must be done tactfully, so that the patient does not feel accused of lying or being confused. In that situation, the psychiatrist's tone of voice is all important. He might say in a gentle, nonconfronting tone, "I'm a bit confused. I thought I understood you to say the situation was thus and so," or "Earlier in the session you described your husband as generous, but now you tell me that he keeps you on a very tight budget; do you have conflicted feelings about him?" These interventions focus on the inconsistency without embarrassing the patient, and thus serve to protect his dignity and self-respect.

Using the Patient's Words

Using the patient's own words not only facilitates the development of rapport, but actually helps to avoid the resistance of the patient who argues over terms and different shades of meanings. The technique is particularly important when the psychiatrist wishes to return to a statement the patient has made earlier in the interview. Such occasions occur when the interviewer wants to allow the patient to continue with a point he was developing rather than to deflect him by pursuing another issue that the patient raised while telling his story. An example is a patient who was describing how his impulsiveness had gotten him into trouble with his supervisors at work, when he mentioned, as an aside, "My wife gets pretty upset about it too." After the patient had completed the story of his problems at work, the psychiatrist commented, "You said your wife gets pretty upset too?" thereby introducing another manifestation of the problem while maintaining the continuity in the interview. By developing the patient's own references, it is sometimes possible for the psychiatrist to conduct an entire and thorough interview without having to introduce a new topic.

Open-Ended Questions

In most situations, questions that can be answered "Yes" or "No" place an undue burden on the interviewer and allow the patient to assume too little responsibility for maintaining the progress of the interview. This does not exclude the possibility that it may be necessary to ask an evasive patient for a yes or no answer on certain occasions. Even when the interviewer wants to explore a particular topic, he can phrase his question in such a way as to give the patient the greatest possible leeway in answering. For example, a patient may indicate that her husband seems distant and overly involved with his work. The interviewer can ask, "What things do you do together for fun?" or "Has he always been that way?" or "What things do you argue about?" Those questions may uncover important information, but the interviewer might have learned even more by asking the patient, "Please go on!" or "Tell me more about your marriage."

Sensitive Topics

Tact is required at all times during the interview but particularly when exploring sensitive topics. What makes a given topic sensitive is determined by a complex set of factors, including the patient's predominant character type and the timing of certain events in the patient's life. For example, an obsessive patient may find questions about his financial affairs more difficult to discuss than questions about his sex life. The more recently a traumatic event has taken place, the more difficult it will be for the patient to discuss.

The interviewer can lead into the sensitive areas more gently by reserving such questions until the patient has led the discussion to a related topic. The obsessive patient in the previous example commented that he had received a significant raise when he moved to his new job. The interviewer was then able to ask, "What is your salary now?"

The same principle can be followed when exploring the topic of sex. A young man was describing his awakening interest in girls during his early adolescence. In that context it was easy for the psychiatrist to ask, "What were your first sexual experiences?", a question that led naturally to the discussion of the patient's current sex life.

Stressing the Patient

It is occasionally necessary for the psychiatrist to utilize stress during an interview to help clarify the patient's diagnosis. For example, an elderly patient with a suspected memory deficit was skillful at covering up her problem. Earlier in the interview, the patient indicated that she had been in the hospital for a week. Later in the interview, she referred to having dinner at her sister's home the previous day. The psychiatrist replied, "Are you sure that was yesterday?" The patient hesitated, and the interviewer continued, "You told me earlier that you have been in the hospital for a week; are you having trouble with your memory?" Another example involves determining whether or not a borderline patient may have been psychotic. The psychiatrist's firm but kindly confrontation of the patient's idiosyncratic ideas revealed the presence of a thought disorder, which helped to establish a diagnosis.

When the interviewer has made a stressful confrontation, he should offer the patient some reassurance that is specifically designed to neutralize the effects of the confrontation. The use of stress in an interview does not imply that the patient is to be treated in a callous or insensitive manner. Asking an elderly patient who seems to be confused about the date, "Are you sure?" is stressful to the patient.

Providing too little structure during an interview is a stress for the disorganized patient. Once this technique has demonstrated the patient's disorganization, there is no point in stressing the patient further. The psychiatrist should then provide the requisite structure to help the patient reorganize his thinking.

Managing the Patient's Anxiety

There is an optimum level of anxiety that drives the patient to seek help but does not incapacitate him to the extent that he is unable to tell his story or answer the interviewer's questions. Clinical experience is required to assess accurately the amount of anxiety that is optimum for each patient. If the interviewer has the feeling that the patient may abruptly leave the office or that the patient may not return for a second interview, he has allowed the patient to become too anxious. On the other hand, if the patient seems composed and manages the interview as though it were a social meeting, the interviewer could become more confronting of the patient's evasion of problem areas.

THE CLOSING PHASE

The Patient's Questions

Near the end of the initial interview, 5 or 10 minutes should always be set aside to deal with certain issues. The patient who has been crying needs some time to regain his composure before he leaves the office. A patient who has come with a written or mental list of questions he wanted to ask requires the time to ask them.

The patient has consulted an expert, and he is entitled to a professional opinion concerning his situation. This includes an appropriate formulation of his problem, recommendations concerning treatment, or some other helpful advice. Frequently, such consultations require two or even more appointments.

As the end of the session nears, the psychiatrist can say, "We have about 10 minutes remaining, and perhaps there are some questions you would like to ask." The patient may then reveal crucial material that has been of concern to him throughout the interview. Obsessive patients are noted for that behavior. Most often the patient raises questions pertaining to his illness or to his need for treatment.

In today's world of an informed public, a patient will often ask questions concerning specific modalities of treatment such as psychotherapy, psychoanalysis, behavior modification, hypnosis, pharmacotherapy, group therapy, and marital therapy. Although the patient is entitled to direct answers to his questions at the completion of his evaluation, the psychiatrist can correctly assume that such questions reveal a great deal concerning the patient's motivation for treatment in general and for intensive psychotherapy in particular. They also reveal the role the patient expects to play in the treatment process and the speed with which he expects relief from his symptoms. Significant resistances uncovered at that time may require the psychiatrist to alter his treatment plan. Patients do not always accept their physician's advice, and many passively accept prescriptions that they never fill, both literally and metaphorically.

The Treatment Plan

When the psychiatrist's usual procedure is to recommend a second or even a third interview to complete a thorough evaluation of a complex case, the patient should be so advised before the first appointment. Otherwise, the patient may have come unprepared for a second meeting; and if his questions are not adequately dealt with in the final 10 minutes of the first interview, he may not return for the second appointment. When the patient accepts the need for additional sessions, the interviewer can advise him that adequate time will be reserved at the completion of the consultation to discuss all of the various issues of concern to the patient. Although the more thorough presentation of the psychiatrist's ideas has been deferred, it is still necessary to give the patient some brief summary of the doctor's findings thus far. By presenting the treatment plan step by step, the interviewer can better discover the areas in which the patient has questions, confusion, or disagreement. This cannot occur when the doctor hands down his opinion like a royal decree.

Formal diagnostic labels are of little value to the patient and may even be harmful, because the psychiatrist is unaware of the conscious or unconscious significance they hold for the patient or his family.

The best clues for the proper terminology are often provided by the patient. The patient may say, "I realize it's all in my mind," or "I know it's some psychological hangup," or "I know I have to do something about my relationship with my mother."

Although the patient's statement may have been made earlier in the session, the doctor can utilize it as a foundation for his own formulation, provided the patient really believed what he said. An example of the latter problem is a patient with psychosomatic headaches who said, "I know it's all in my mind, Doctor." The patient does not really accept the psychological cause of his headaches and was merely appeasing the psychiatrist.

The interviewer might start his formulation by repeating the patient's own remark: "As you said before, you do have a psychological problem." The doctor then may refer to what he considers the patient's predominant symptoms, and indicate that they are all interrelated and part of the same condition. It is a good plan to separate the patient's acute problems from those that are chronic. The problems of recent duration are generally the ones that respond most quickly to treatment. By confining the formulation to the major area of disturbance, the psychiatrist avoids the danger of overwhelming the patient with a comprehensive statement covering all of his psychopathology.

When the psychiatrist and patient have mutually identified the major problem areas, the doctor can then move on to the subject of treatment. If several forms of therapy are available, the doctor can acknowledge the fact. Nevertheless, the patient still expects the psychiatrist to advise him concerning the treatment that would be best suited for him. "Best suited" is a complex notion that includes not only the subtleties of diagnosis, but also the patient's emotional, financial, and life situation. On occasion, the patient may reveal his alarm over the treatment plan by a comment such as "You don't really think it's that serious, do you?" or "Well, is there any hope for me?" or "How long do you think the treatment will take?" It is difficult at the onset to predict exactly how long treatment will take, and it is rarely useful to tell a patient that he will require many years of therapy. Instead, the psychiatrist can point out that the acute symptoms will respond first, and that the patient can then reassess his desire for help with the lifelong problems, which would require a longer period of treatment. In that way, the doctor provides the patient and himself with time to explore the interrelationship of acute and chronic symptoms, as well as more time to assess the patient's motivation and capacity to work with deep personality problems. The patient's concern with the duration of treatment is not merely a desire for a magical cure or some other resistance. Therapy is costly both in terms of expense and time involved, and it interferes with other aspects of the patient's life. If there is a time limit on the duration of therapy or if the psychiatrist will not be available as long as the patient expects treatment to last, the patient should be so informed from the onset. Also, the patient deserves to know when the first appointment is arranged if the consultant will not be the treating psychiatrist. If the patient's financial resources play a limiting role in determining the treatment plan, it is the consultant's responsibility to advise the patient where and how to get the most for his money.

Prognosis

The patient may reveal a great deal of concern over his prognosis with comments such as "Well, I'm a real basket case, aren't I?" or "Have you ever seen someone like me get better?" The patient will be helped by the doctor's empathic recognition of his feeling of hopelessness. Nevertheless, prognosis is often difficult to predict early on, and the doctor may harm the patient and his own professional reputation by being overly reassuring and by guaranteeing cures. In the case of the depressed patient, some positive statement concerning the doctor's belief that the patient will recover is part of the therapy.

SUBSEQUENT INTERVIEWS

A single meeting with a patient permits only a cross-sectional study. Therefore, it is a good plan routinely to schedule two appointments, allowing a few days to intervene between the first and second interviews. That time provides both the patient and the psychiatrist an opportunity to reflect on and to react to the first interview. The added perspective provides supplementary information concerning how the patient may react to further treatment. The subsequent interview also provides an opportunity for the patient to correct any misinformation that he provided in the first meeting. It is often helpful to begin the second interview by asking the patient if he has thought about the first interview, and by asking for his reactions to the experience. Another variation of that technique is for the doctor to say, "Frequently, people think of additional things they wanted to discuss after they have left. What thoughts did you have?" The patient may begin to speak at that point, or he may indicate that he had no afterthoughts. In that case, the doctor may pause to allow the patient time to gather his thoughts. If the patient is floundering, the doctor can go back to a topic that the patient had previously discussed productively.

The psychiatrist often learns valuable information when he asks the patient if he discussed the interview with anyone else. If the patient has done so, it is enlightening to learn the details of that conversation and with whom the patient spoke.

There is no set of rules concerning which topics are best put off for the second interview, but in general, as the patient's comfort and familarity with the psychiatrist increases, he will be able to reveal more intimate details of his life.

INTERVIEWS WITH RELATIVES AND SIGNIFICANT OTHERS

In recent years, psychiatrists have developed more flexible attitudes concerning speaking with people who are closest to the patient. Few psychoanalysts now flatly refuse to speak with a patient's spouse or parents, for example. At the other extreme, few psychiatrists obtain history only from other informants on the grounds that the patient is not capable of giving an accurate history. Virtually every modern residency training program provides some experience in family and couples therapy and in crisis intervention involving multiple family members. Those experiences have made it easier for psychiatrists to understand and treat the patient in his life context.

Basic Ground Rules

There are three important guidelines for speaking with the relatives of adult patients. One is to see the patient first. The second is to obtain his permission before speaking with a family member. Comatose, psychotic, or severely disoriented patients are the only exceptions to that rule. The third cardinal rule is not to violate the patient's confidence directly or indirectly. If any information provided by the patient needs to be discussed with a family member, the psychiatrist must obtain the patient's permission first. Where possible, have the patient present during discussions with the family.

The only exceptions to these rules arise when the life of the patient or someone else is in danger. If the psychiatrist cannot obtain the patient's permission to reveal a plan for suicide or homicide and if the patient refuses hospitalization, the psychiatrist has an obligation to advise the family and to recommend commitment. If the psychiatrist cannot obtain the patient's permission to disclose such data, he must at least give the patient the courtesy of telling him that he plans to disclose that information and why. Some part of the patient may be relieved, even though he consciously and overtly objects. The patient's relatives may provide valuable information concerning the patient that helps the psychiatrist arrive more quickly at a treatment plan.

In the case of elderly patients, the opportunity to observe the patient's spouse, parents, or children provides the psychiatrist with an objective view of those people who are vitally important in the patient's life. With the aid of such information, the psychiatrist may be more alert to conflicting data in the views provided by his patient, and may be able help the patient more quickly expand his awareness of certain distortions and conflicting feelings concerning his loved ones.

Seeing the Relative Alone

Some psychiatrists flatly refuse to speak with a relative except in the presence of the patient; others are willing to meet with relatives alone. The second group is further subdivided into those who do and those who do not feel it is essential to report to the patient everything that was said by the relative. There are more risks in *not* reporting all details of a conversation with a relative, and that approach requires training, sensitivity, and judgment regarding what to disclose and what not to disclose of the information provided by the relative. One current school of thought holds that families have no secrets, but only conspiracies not to discuss certain topics. Although the viewpoint applies in many situations, there are still secrets that are best left alone. For example, a relative revealed to the psychiatrist that there was some uncertainty in her mind concerning the paternity of the patient, her 35-year-old son. She had had a brief affair with another man 36 years earlier and had not seen him since. She had worked out the conflict with her husband that precipitated the affair, and had maintained a monogamous relation thereafter. The mother's concern involved unresolved guilt feelings, and there was nothing to be gained by disclosing that information to the patient, who had no suspicion. If it turned out later on that the patient did unconsciously know about this event and was ready to face it, he could always broach the subject with his mother if he felt there were something to be gained.

Interviewing relatives alone is not an innocuous procedure, and it requires much skill.

Reassurance and Questions

It is normal for relatives to feel concern about the illness of their loved one and to have questions concerning the diagnosis and treatment plan, including duration and prognosis of the illness. The same general principles apply as when the psychiatrist discusses such matters with the patient. By first exploring the extent of the relative's knowledge and understanding of the patient's problems, the psychiatrist can often indicate that they have grasped the essentials of the patient's illness without disclosing any confidential information. The psychiatrist may follow the same guidelines in discussing treatment recommendations and prognosis. The relative may express some overt or covert feeling of guilt or responsibility for the patient's illness. It is important that the psychiatrist not collaborate with the patient against his relatives. Doing so would support only one side of the patient's ambivalent feelings, and it alienates the relatives, who may become more distrustful of and antagonistic to the patient, his psychiatrist, and psychiatric treatment in general. The doctor is not a judge, but occasionally he may have some constructive recommendation for the relative who asks, "Is there anything I can do to help?" Suggestions should be practical, and should be something that the patient will respond to favorably and that the relative will be able to follow.

CONCLUSION

The psychiatric interview encompasses all of the basic psychological sciences and requires the integration and clinical application of all of the psychiatrists's training. Although each psychiatrist develops his own stylistic variations, studies show that as interviewers become more experienced, it is more and more difficult for an observing third party to identify correctly his theoretical persuasion.

No professional ever conducts an interview that is totally free of mistakes. The human reality of imperfection provides the psychiatrist with continuing opportunity for professional growth.

SUGGESTED READING

Bird B: Talking with Patients. Philadelphia, JB Lippincott, 1973

Garrett AM: Interviewing: Its Principles and Methods. New York, Family Welfare Association of America, 1942

Gill MM: The Analysis of Transference, Vol 1. New York, International Universities Press, 1982

Gill M, Newman R, Redlich FC: The Initial Interview in Psychiatric Practice. New York, International Universities Press, 1954

Hoyle L, Reiser MF: The Patient: Biological, Psychological, and Social Dimensions of Medical Practice. New York, Plenum, 1980

Kohut H: The Restoration of the Self. New York, International Universities Press, 1977

MacKinnon RA, Michels R: The Psychiatric Interview in Clinical Practice. Philadelphia, WB Saunders, 1971

Menninger K: A Manual for Psychiatric Case Study. New York, Grune & Stratton, 1952

Powdermaker F: The techniques of the initial interview and methods of teaching them. Am J Psychiatry 104:642, 1948

Schafer R: Talking to patients in psychotherapy. Bull Menninger Clin 12:503, 1974

Sullivan HS: The Psychiatric Interview. New York, WW Norton, 1954

Weed LL: Medical records that guide and teach. N Engl J Med 278:593, 1968

Whitehorn JC: Guide to interviewing and clinical personality study. Arch Neurol Psychiatry 52:197, 1944

2

The Clinical Examination of the Patient

The Psychiatric History 40
  Purpose 40
  Techniques 41
  The Psychotic Patient 43
  Organization of Data 43
    Preliminary Identification 43
      Chief Complaint 43
      Personal Description 45
    History of Present Illness 45
      Onset 45
      Precipitating Factors 46
      Impact of the Patient's Illness 46
    The Psychiatric Review of Systems 47
    Previous Psychiatric Illnesses 48
    Personal History 48
      Prenatal History 50
      Early Childhood 50
      Middle Childhood (Ages 3 Years to 11 Years) 52
      Later Childhood (Prepuberty Through Adolescence) 53
      Psychosexual History 53
      Religious, Cultural, and Moral Background 54
      Adulthood 54
        Occupational and Educational History 54
        Social Relationships 55
        Adult Sexuality 55
        Marital History 56
        Current Social Situations 56
        Military History 57
    Family History 57
  Conclusion 57

The Mental Status Examination   58
  Organization of Data   61
    Appearance, Attitude, and Behavior   61
      General Description   61
      Behavior and Psychomotor Activity (Conation)   62
      Attitude Toward Examiner   62
      Speech   63
    Thought Process and Content   64
      Production of Thought   64
      Continuity of Thought   64
      Content of Thought   65
        Preoccupations   65
        Delusions and Referentiality   65
      Abstract Thinking   66
      Concentration and Cognition   66
    Perception   67
      Hallucinations   67
      Illusions   68
      Feelings of Depersonalization and Unreality   68
    Mood, Affect, and Emotional Regulation   69
      Subjective Evaluation   69
      The Interviewer's Observations   70
      Appropriateness   70
    Consciousness (Alertness and Wakefulness)   71
    Orientation   72
    Memory   73
    Impulse Control and Frustration Tolerance   74
    Information and Intelligence   75
    Judgment   76
    Insight   76
  Conclusion   76
Appendix: Sample Mental Status Examination Reports   78

The clinical evaluation of the patient consists of the psychiatric history and the mental status examination. The psychiatric history covers the patient's entire lifetime (Table 2-1), whereas the mental status examination (Table 2-2) describes the patient's mental state at one point in time.

Many psychiatric patients have difficulty in cooperating fully with the physician because they are embarrassed about their problems or because they have difficulty trusting others as a part of their psychological disturbance. Therefore, the better the quality of rapport between patient and clinician, the more honest and forthright the patient will be in telling his story

---

TABLE 2-1. The Psychiatric History (*Anamnesis*)

1. Preliminary identification
   (a) Chief complaint
   (b) Personal description
2. History of present illness
   (a) Onset
   (b) Precipitating factors
   (c) Secondary gain
3. Psychiatric review of systems
4. Previous psychiatric illnesses
5. Personal history
   (a) Prenatal history
   (b) Early childhood
   (c) Middle childhood
   (d) Later childhood (prepuberty through adolescence)
   (e) Psychosocial history
   (f) Religious, cultural, and moral background
   (g) Adulthood
       (1) Occupational and educational history
       (2) Social relationships
       (3) Adult sexuality
       (4) Marital history
       (5) Current social situation
       (6) Military history
6. Family history

---

and answering the physician's questions. Special problems occur in the case of the uncooperative patient. Unless other sources of information are available, the clinician's attention will focus more on the mental status portion of the examination.

In the classical medical model, the history is recognized as subjective, whereas the physical examination is considered a major source of objective information. The mental status examination in psychiatry is comparable to the physical examination in medicine; therefore, it is expected to provide objective data about the patient. Although this is true to some extent, the examiner cannot directly palpate the patient's mind and auscultate his thought processes in the way that he can examine the patient's abdomen or chest. The more the patient trusts the clinician, the more closely the mental status examination approaches the objectivity of the physical examination, which, it must be remembered, still has subjective elements.

Because the psychiatric history and the mental status examination are

---

TABLE 2-2.   The Mental Status Examination

A. Appearance, attitude, and behavior
  1. General description
  2. Behavior and psychomotor activity (conation)
  3. Attitude toward examiner
  4. Speech
B. Thought process and content
  1. Production of thought
  2. Continuity of thought
  3. Content of thought
     (a) Preoccupations
     (b) Delusions and referentiality
  4. Abstract thinking
  5. Concentration and cognition
C. Perception
  1. Hallucinations
  2. Illusions
  3. Feelings of depersonalization and unreality
D. Mood, affect, and emotional regulation
  1. Subjective evaluation
  2. The interviewer's observations
  3. Appropriateness
E. Consciousness (alertness and wakefulness)
F. Orientation
G. Memory
H. Impulse control and frustration tolerance
I. Information and intelligence
J. Judgment
K. Insight

---

presented separately in the written record, the inexperienced physician is inclined to follow the medical model, wherein the history taking is performed separately from the physical examination. This separation is useful during the formative years of the clinician, when it is probably necessary in order to remember significant areas to be explored. Nevertheless, the experienced psychiatrist will be able to describe most of the required aspects of the mental status examination by the time he has completed taking the history, so that the patient never experiences a separate evaluation of his mental processes, even in instances where the patient suffers from serious symptoms, such as hallucinations, delusions, or memory disturbances. The discussion of those symptoms flows naturally from the discussion of the present illness, so that the examiner merely has to ask if the symptoms are noticeable to the patient at the time of the interview.

There are areas of overlap in the psychiatric history and mental status examination. For example, the patient's appearance, manner, dress, level of tension, personal hygiene, and ability to concentrate are described in both sections. The patient's symptoms, which are discussed in the history, are only repeated in the written mental status if the patient actually experiences those symptoms during the examination. However, there are exceptions, such as the patient who has intermittent hallucinations or intermittent alterations of consciousness, which would be described in the mental status despite the fact that the patient did not manifest them during the interview. Another exception would be the patient with phobic symptoms. These symptoms would be described in the present illness section of the history only if they are part of the reasons for the patient's seeking treatment. If this is not the case, the psychiatrist can place the discussion of phobic symptoms under the mental status and cross-reference the symptoms in the history section of the written record, even though the patient is not actually experiencing phobic anxiety or demonstrating phobic behavior during the interview.

A comprehensive psychiatric evaluation should also include a medical history and physical examination. If the interviewer is not medically trained, the patient should be referred for a competent medical evaluation. When the interviewer is medically trained, it is recommended that he take his own medical history and emphasize the review of systems. Many significant clues will be uncovered because the psychiatrist will place a different emphasis than the internist on the review of systems. Many psychiatric disorders are accompanied by physical complaints. A few examples include panic disorder with respiratory and cardiovascular symptoms; depression with vegetative disturbances in appetite, bowel function, and sleep; and a host of psychosomatic disorders involving every organ system. In addition, there is an extensive list of physical conditions, ranging from disorders of thyroid function to brain tumor, which can cause psychiatric symptoms. Refer to one of the standard medical psychiatric textbooks for a more comprehensive discussion of this important topic.

Although the written record must include specific data and adhere to a traditional organized format, the clinician must be ever aware that he is engaging in a therapeutic process with his patient while eliciting information. As in every therapeutic situation, the patient's recollections and responses are accompanied by specific feelings, of which the interviewer must be aware and to which he must be sensitive. The patient's feelings, associations, movements, and reactions to the interviewer provide crucial data that enable the psychiatrist to evaluate both content and process while gaining insight into the continuity between the patient's past and present problems. Although such material as the patient's behavior, slips of the tongue, jokes, or other data concerning his unconscious mental processes emerge as the history is being taken, these data are to be recorded under the mental status examination.

The most common error that the psychiatrist makes while obtaining a psychiatric history is his interference with the patient's natural unfolding of the history by overstructuring the interview with excessive questions or by following a particular interview schedule. It cannot be emphasized too strongly that the organization of the history and the mental status examination outlined in this chapter is for the psychiatric written record; it is not a script to follow during the interview.

THE PSYCHIATRIC HISTORY

Purpose

Psychiatrists, like other specialists in medicine, rely upon a careful history as the foundation for the diagnosis and treatment of every illness. Each branch of medicine has its own method for gathering and organizing an accurate, comprehensive story of the patient's illness. In the general practice of medicine, the usual technique is to secure, in the patient's own words, the onset, duration, and severity of his present complaints; to review his past medical problems; and to question the patient regarding the present function of his organs and anatomical systems. This focus is designed essentially to investigate the function of the tissues and organ systems as they maintain the internal economy of the body, and emphasis is placed on how malfunctions affect the patient's physical state or social patterns. In psychiatry, the history must also convey the more elusive picture of the patient's individual personality characteristics, including his strengths and his weaknesses. The psychiatric history should include insight into the nature of the patient's relationships as well as information about important people in his past and present life. A complete story of the patient's life is impossible to obtain, because it would require another lifetime to tell. Nevertheless, a useful portrayal of the patient's development from his earliest years through the present usually can be developed.

Like other professionals, the novice psychiatrist must progress through certain stages in the mastery of his profession. Whether it be school figures for the skater, finger exercises for the pianist, or the classic third-year medical student history for the future physician, these techniques are time-proven steps to be mastered in the pursuit of professionalism. The relevant historical data that the third-year medical student requires 3 hours to elicit usually can be obtained by the resident in 20 minutes. Similarly, time and experience are required before the novice psychiatrist can respond quickly and directly to the initial cues provided by the patient that tell the clinician how and where to proceed with the history. Many clinical situations or diagnostic categories require particular modification with regard to history taking (MacKinnon and Michels, 1971). For example, in a situation of crisis, whether the patient is neurotic or psychotic, it is usually not appropriate to elicit an extensive story of the patient's past life (unless the patient is a child).

Techniques

The most important technique in obtaining the psychiatric history is to allow the patient to tell his story in his own words and in the order he chooses. Both the content and the order in which the patient presents his history reveal valuable information concerning his deeper feelings. As the patient relates his story, the skillful interviewer recognizes points at which he can introduce relevant questions concerning the various important areas described in the outline of the psychiatric history and the mental status examination.

Although the doctor's questions or comments are relevant, it is not uncommon for the patient to become confused or perplexed. The physician realizes this when the patient knits his eyebrows or says, "I don't understand why you need to know that." The interview will proceed more smoothly if the doctor takes the time to explain what he had in mind and show the patient the relevance of his question. On occasion, as the result of inexperience or an error in judgment, the clinician has pursued an issue that in fact was irrelevant. In that case the doctor can say, "It just occurred to me, but perhaps you are right and it is unimportant." The patient will accept such occurrences without losing confidence in his physician, provided irrelevant questioning does not occur to excess. Every physician will, on occasion, ask the patient a question that elicits information the patient had provided earlier. Often the doctor continues, hoping the patient will not notice or will not care. It is always preferable to remark, "Oh yes, I asked you that earlier," or "Oh yes, you already told me—" and then repeat what the patient had said. Successful physicians often keep a summary sheet of the patient's identifying life data, personal habits, and the names and ages of the spouse and children, if any. Prior to the appointments, they review this material for patients they follow irregularly. In this way they not only keep up with the patient's medical condition, but they avoid asking questions time and time again, such as "Is your child a boy or a girl?" or "Do you smoke?" Although this advice seems simple and obvious, many experienced and competent physicians neglect to follow it.

Some psychiatrists obtain the history by providing the patient with a questionnaire to complete prior to their first meeting. Although that technique saves the psychiatrist time and may be useful in clinics or other places where professional resources are severely limited, that efficiency is obtained at a significant price: it deprives the psychiatrist and the patient of the opportunity to explore the patient's feelings that are elicited while answering the questions. Questionnaires may also inject an artificial quality to the interview when the patient finally meets the psychiatrist, whom he may experience as yet another bureaucratic functionary, more interested in pieces of paper than in him. A good psychiatrist can overcome this undesirable mental set, but it is an unnecessary bit of pseudo efficiency to create it in the first place.

Psychiatric histories are vital in delineating and diagnosing major neurotic or psychotic illnesses. Nevertheless, in the realm of personality diagnosis, many psychiatric histories are of minimal value. This is particularly true when they are limited to superficial reports such as historical questionnaires filled out by the patient.

Another major deficiency in the average psychiatric history is its representation as a collection of facts and events that are organized according to date, with relatively little understanding of the impact of those experiences on the patient or the role that the patient may have played in bringing about those events. The history is often filled with data indicating that the patient went to a certain school, held a certain number of jobs, married at a certain age, and had a certain number of children. Often, none of that material provides distinctive characteristics about the person that would help to distinguish him from another human being with similar vital statistics.

In most training programs, there is relatively little formal psychiatric training in the techniques involved in eliciting historical data. The novice psychiatrist is given an outline and is somehow expected to learn magically how to acquire the information requested. It is unusual for each of his written records to be corrected by his teachers, and is still more unusual for him to be required to rewrite the report to incorporate any suggested corrections. In his supervised psychotherapy training, the resident usually begins with a presentation of the history as it has been organized for the written record, rather than as it flowed from the patient. The supervisor is often unaware of the trainee's skill in the process of eliciting historical information. Supervisors are usually more interested in the manifestations of early transference and resistance than in teaching the technique of eliciting a smooth, flowing history. As a result, this deficit in the supervisor's own training is unintentionally passed on to another generation of young clinicians.

The Psychotic Patient

Major modifications in techniques may be necessary in interviewing a disorganized patient. In the case of the patient who suffers from a psychotic process or from a severe personality disorder, the psychiatrist should provide more structure to elicit a coherent, chronological, organized story of the patient's present illness. The patient's lack of an organizing ego requires the interviewer to provide that support. The purpose is not merely to enable the interviewer to construct a more coherent story; the technique also has a therapeutic value: the patient is able to use the physician's ego to compensate for his own deficit and experience relief from a frightening state of confusion. In that fashion the therapeutic alliance is formed at the same time that the requisite historical data are secured.

Organization of Data

We wish to reemphasize that the organization used in this chapter is solely for the purpose of preparing the written record, and is not to be used as a guideline for conducting the interview, as stated earlier.

Preliminary Identification

The psychiatrist should begin the written history by stating the patient's name, age, marital status, sex, occupation, language (if other than English), race, nationality, religion, and a brief statement about the patient's place of residence and circumstances of living. Comments such as "The patient lives alone in a furnished room," or "The patient lives with her husband and three children in a three-bedroom apartment," provide adequate detail for this part. If the patient is hospitalized, a statement can be included as to the number of previous admissions for similar conditions. In most written psychiatric records, one or more of the above-mentioned items has been omitted. In some instances an omission is the result of a lack of thoroughness by the interviewer, but it frequently reflects a countertransference problem of the interviewer.

CHIEF COMPLAINT

The chief complaint is the presenting problem for which the patient seeks professional help. The chief complaint should be stated in the patient's own words. If the information is not supplied by the patient, the record should contain a description of the person who supplied it and his relationship to the patient. At first glance, this part appears to be the briefest and simplest of the various subdivisions of the psychiatric history; however, in actuality it is often one of the most complex. In many cases the patient does not begin his story with a chief complaint. One or more sessions may be required for the physician to learn what it is that the patient finds most disturbing or why he seeks treatment at this particular time. In other situations, the chief complaint is provided by someone other than the patient. For example, an acutely confused and disoriented patient may be brought in by someone who provides the chief complaint concerning the patient's confusion. Occasionally, a patient with multiple symptoms of long duration has great difficulty explaining precisely why he seeks treatment at a particular time. Ideally, the chief complaint should provide the explanation of why the patient seeks help now. That concept must not be confused with the precipitating stress (often unconscious in nature) that results in the collapse of the patient's defenses at a particular time. The precipitating stress may be equally difficult to determine. Usually, the ease of determining the chief complaint correlates directly with the ease of determining the precipitating stress. At times the physician uncovers the chief complaint in the course of looking for a precipitating stress, or in considering what the patient unconsciously hoped to accomplish in pursuing the consultation.

An example illustrating the usefulness of determining the patient's expectation of the psychiatrist is the woman who arrived at the psychiatrist's office feeling distraught after her husband confronted her with the fact that he had been unhappy with their relationship for the past 10 years. She felt depressed and upset about his request for a separation, and she was convinced that her husband was going through a midlife crisis. She was certain that he did not know what he was feeling, and that in actuality, they had been happily married during all their years together. Although she consulted the psychiatrist voluntarily, she did not believe that she suffered from a psychiatric illness. She believed that her reaction to the confrontation with her husband was quite normal. She wanted the psychiatrist to interview her husband, convince him that he was going through a phase for which he might require treatment, and advise him that he should remain with her. Although she did not see herself as a patient, she had some striking personality pathology that, at the time, was egosyntonic and not directly involved in her reason for seeking psychiatric help. She was unaware of her inability to look critically at her own behavior, its effects on others, or her tendency to project her own tension state onto her husband. These traits were central aspects of her neurotic character and accounted for the fact that she was never able to accept treatment for herself.

PERSONAL DESCRIPTION

Although a detailed description of the patient appears at the beginning of the mental status portion of the record, it is useful to have a brief, nontechnical description of the patient's appearance and behavior as it might be written by a novelist. What is required is not a stereotyped medical description of a "well-developed, well-nourished, white male," but rather, a description that brings the person to life in the eyes of the reader. The following description is a good illustration of what is desired:

> Mr. A is a 5 feet, 5 inch-tall, powerfully built, heavyset man with coarse features and a swarthy complexion, who appeared quite unfriendly. His short, curly, dark brown hair is parted on the side, and one is immediately aware that his gaze follows the interviewer's every move. He creates an intimidating image as he nervously paces the floor, and repeatedly looks at his watch. He spontaneously says, "I gotta get outta here, Doc. They're comin' to get me, Doc!" His perspiration-drenched tee shirt is dirty and is tucked into his paint-stained, faded jeans. He appears younger than his stated age of 30, and he obviously has not shaved for several days.

Significant omissions in the description of the patient may result from a lack of careful observation, or they may reflect countertransference on the part of the examiner. In the example above, the most common countertransference problem would be the omission of the frightening aspect of the patient.

History of Present Illness

ONSET

The psychiatrist must provide an adequate amount of time during the initial interview to explore those details of the patient's presenting symptoms that are most relevant to the patient's decision to consult a psychiatrist at this time. Inexperienced psychiatrists, particularly those with an interest in psychodynamic psychiatry, often have difficulty determining precisely when an illness begins. They frequently feel that the present illness must have begun sometime in the patient's early life, perhaps even during the first 2 years. Although such developmental concepts are useful in understanding the patient's psychodynamics, they are of relatively little value in determining when the patient's current failure in adaptation began. For that reason, it is essential to evaluate the patient's highest level of functioning, even though this may not be considered healthy by normative standards. The patient's best level of adaptation must be considered the baseline from which his current loss of functioning is measured and when maladaptive patterns first appeared. Most often, a relatively unstructured question such as "How did it all begin?" leads to an unfolding of the present illness. A well-organized patient is able to present a chronological account of his difficulties.

PRECIPITATING FACTORS

As the patient recounts the development of the symptoms and behavioral changes that culminated in his seeking assistance, the psychiatrist should attempt to learn the details of the patient's life circumstances at the time these changes began. When asked to describe these relationships directly, the patient is often unable to give correlations between the beginning of his illness and the stresses that occurred in his life. A technique referred to as the "parallel history" is particularly useful with the patient who cannot accept the relationship between psychological determinants and psychophysiological symptoms. In eliciting a parallel history, the interviewer returns to the same time period covered by the present illness, but later in the interview. he specifically avoids making his inquiry in phrases that suggest that he is searching for connections between what was happening in the patient's life and the development of the patient's symptoms. The psychiatrist, without the patient's awareness, makes connections (*i.e.*, the parallel history) between stresses that the patient experienced and the development of his disorder. The patient may notice some temporal connection between a particular stress and the appearance of his symptoms that impresses him and arouses his curiosity about the role of emotional factors in his illness. Nevertheless, by premature psychological interpretations concerning the interrelationship of the stress and the symptom, the psychiatrist may undermine that process and intensify the patient's resistance. Unless the patient makes a spontaneous connection between his emotional reaction to a life event and the appearance of his symptoms, the physician should proceed slowly. (See Chap. 6 for a discussion of defense mechanisms and symptom formation.)

IMPACT OF THE PATIENT'S ILLNESS

The patient's psychiatric symptoms or behavioral changes have a significant impact on the patient and his family. The patient should describe activities or emotional experiences in which he cannot participate, and how he and his family adapt to these limitations. This is the secondary loss of the symptom.

The secondary gain of a symptom may be defined as the indirect benefits of illness, such as obtaining extra affection from loved ones, being excused from unpleasant responsibilities, or obtaining extra gratification of one's dependency needs, as opposed to the primary gain that results from the unconscious meaning of the symptom.

The ways in which the patient's illness has affected his life activities and personal relationships highlight both the secondary loss and the secondary gain of the patient's illness. In attempting to understand the secondary gain, the interviewer must explore, in a sympathetic and empathic fashion, the impact of the patient's illness on his own life and the lives of his loved ones. The physician must be careful to communicate to the patient this understanding of the pain of the patient's illness and the many losses that result from his symptoms. An implication that the patient may unconsciously benefit from being ill would immediately destroy the rapport the physician has established. For example, a married woman with three children complained of severe backaches with no apparent physical abnormalities. After listening to the description of her pain, the psychiatrist asked, in a sympathetic voice, "How do you manage to take care of the housework?" "Oh," replied the patient, "My husband has been very kind; ever since I have been sick he helps after he comes home from work." The psychiatrist did not interpret the obvious secondary gain, but mentally stored, for later use, the clue that the husband may not have been very helpful or understanding of his wife's feelings concerning her housekeeping role before the onset of her backaches. In subsequent meetings, the psychiatrist explored that area with the patient, who, after her resentment unfolded, became aware of the secondary gain of her backaches.

The Psychiatric Review of Systems

After the psychiatrist has completed his initial study of the patient's present illness, he can inquire about the patient's general medical health and carefully review the functioning of the patient's organ systems. Emotional disturbances are often accompanied by physical symptoms. The systems review is the same one as performed by an internist, but through the particular perspective of a psychiatrist. No psychiatric evaluation is complete without statements concerning the patient's sleep patterns, weight regulation, appetite, bowel functioning, and sexual functioning. If the patient has experienced a sleep disturbance, it would be described here unless it is part of the present illness. Inquire whether the insomnia is initial, middle, terminal, or a combination, and what remedies the patient has attempted. Other organ systems commonly involved in psychiatric complaints are the gastrointestinal, cardiovascular, respiratory, urogenital, musculoskeletal, and neurological systems.

It is a logical time to inquire about dreams while asking the patient about sleep patterns. Freud stated that the dream is the royal road to the unconscious. Dreams provide valuable insight into the patient's unconscious fears, wishes, and conflicts. Repetitive dreams and nightmares are of particular value. Some of the most common themes are of food (either the patient is being gratified or the patient is being denied while others eat), aggression (the patient is involved in adventures, battles, or chases, most often in the defensive position), examinations (the patient feels unprepared, is late for the examination, or cannot find the proper room), helplessness or impotence (the patient is shooting at someone with a gun that is ineffective; the patient is fighting and his blows seem to have no effect on the opponent; or the patient is being chased and is unable to run or to cry for help), and sexual dreams of all varieties, both with and without orgasm. Also record the residual feelings of the patient regarding anxiety, and revealing associations or feelings while recounting the dream.

It is useful to ask the patient for a recent dream. If the patient cannot recall one, the interviewer might say, "Perhaps you will have one between now and our next appointment; if you do, try to make a note of it." The patient frequently produces a dream in the second interview that reveals his unconscious fantasies about the physician, treatment, his illness, or all three.

Fantasies or daydreams are another valuable source of unconscious material. As with dreams, the psychiatrist can explore and record all manifest details and attendant feelings.

Previous Psychiatric Illnesses

The section on previous psychiatric illnesses is a transition between the story of the present illness and the personal history. Here, prior episodes of emotional or mental disturbances are described. The extent of incapacity, the type of treatment received, the names of hospitals, the length of each illness, and the effects of prior treatments should all be explored and recorded chronologically.

Personal History

In addition to studying the patient's present illness and current life situation, the psychiatrist needs an equally thorough understanding of the patient's past life and its relationship to his presenting emotional problem.

In the usual medical history, the present illness gives the physician important information that enables him to focus his questions in his "review of systems." Similarly, because it is impossible to obtain a complete history of a person's life, the psychiatrist uses the patient's present illness to provide significant clues to guide him in further exploration of the personal history. When the interviewer has acquired a general impression of the most likely diagnosis, he can then direct his attention to the areas that are pertinent to the patient's major complaints and to defining the patient's underlying personality structure. Each interview is modified according to the patient's underlying character type as well as according to important situational factors relating to the setting and circumstances of the interview. (For a more detailed discussion of these factors, refer to MacKinnon and Michels, *The Psychiatric Interview in Clinical Practice*, 1971.) To modify the form of the interview, the psychiatrist must be familiar with the psychodynamic theory of psychological development and with the phases and conflicts that are most important for each condition. In that way, he may concentrate the questions in the areas that will be most significant in explaining the patient's psychological development and the evolution of the patient's problems.

With a patient with obsessive-compulsive symptoms, for example, the psychiatrist should study obedience–defiance conflicts, early relationships to authority figures, and how power struggles were dealt with in the patient's home. The psychiatrist should also inquire about the patient's development of rigidity and tyranny of conscience and history of early-life rituals. He can expect to find conflicts over the patient's control of aggressive and sexual impulses.

Another example is that of a patient with an antisocial personality, which should lead the interviewer to focus his exploration on different aspects of the patient's history of relationships with figures of authority as well as peers and subordinates. He may begin with the patient's interaction with parents and teachers, and then continue into the area of conflicts with the law. With such a patient, one should also determine whether the patient's problem stems from a failure in the development of conscience (superego), poor impulse control (ego deficits), or whether biological factors such as learning disabilities, attention deficit disorder, or low frustration tolerance played a role. The history may reveal the patient's success in getting away with things and failure to develop appropriate conscience mechanisms. In this situation, questions designed to discover the unconscious collaboration on the part of one or both parents are appropriate, as are questions about overt sociopathic behavior on the part of the parents. Questions about lying, cheating, and stealing may be gently worked into the interview by the clinician, who should indicate an understanding of the patient's lifelong struggle against impulses that other people have learned must be controlled. A clinician who asks questions of this type to a patient with obsessive personality disorder would be experienced by the patient as inappropriate and offensive.

A thorough psychodynamic explanation of the patient's illness and personality structure requires an understanding of the intricate ways in which the patient reacts to the stresses of his environment and the recognition that the patient has been in some way responsible for his current situation and choice of environment. Through an understanding of the interrelationship between external stress and the patient's tendency to seek out situations that frustrate him, the psychiatrist develops a concept of the patient's core intrapsychic conflict.

The personal history is perhaps the most deficient section of the typical psychiatric record. It is usually divided into the major developmental periods of prenatal, infancy, early childhood, middle childhood or latency, puberty, adolescence, and adulthood. The personal history usually begins with some statement about whether the patient was breast fed or bottle fed, followed by statements of questionable accuracy concerning the patient's toilet training and early developmental landmarks such as sitting, walking, and talking. That entire area may be condensed in a statement such as "Developmental landmarks were normal." Just what of value one learns from the fact that the patient was breast fed or bottle fed and weaned at the age of 6 months has always mystified us. The psychiatrist might replace those routine and often meaningless inquiries by an attempt to understand and utilize new areas of knowledge germane to child development, as explained below.

PRENATAL HISTORY

In the prenatal history, the psychiatrist considers the nature of the home situation into which the patient was born and whether the patient was planned and wanted. Were there any problems with the mother's pregnancy and delivery? Was there any evidence of defect or injury at birth? What were the parents' reactions to the gender of the patient? How was the patient's name selected?

EARLY CHILDHOOD

The early childhood period considers the first 3 years of the patient's life. The quality of mother–child interaction during feeding is certainly more important than whether the child was breast or bottle fed. Although an accurate account of this experience is difficult to obtain, it is frequently possible to learn whether, as an infant, the patient presented problems in feeding, was colicky, or required special formulas. Early disturbances in sleep patterns or signs of unmet needs, such as head banging or body rocking, provide clues about possible maternal deprivation. In addition, it is important to obtain a history of caretakers during the first 3 years. Were there auxiliary maternal objects? The psychiatrist should discover who was living in the patient's home during early childhood and should try to determine the role that each person played in the patient's upbringing. Did the patient exhibit problems at any early period with stranger anxiety or separation anxiety?

It is helpful to know if the loving mother and the disciplining mother were one and the same person. In one case, a child received most of her love from a grandmother, but was trained and disciplined by a maid. In her adult life, she rejected housework, which was associated with the cold punitive authority of the maid, but pursued a career in music, which had served in her childhood as a connection to her loving grandmother. The fact that her actual mother had not enjoyed child rearing and had been emotionally distant caused further problems in maternal identification. It was not surprising that the patient did not have a cohesive sense of herself as a woman and had great difficulty integrating her career with being a wife and mother.

The patient's toilet training is another traditional area of limited value in the initial history. Although an age may be quoted, the problem is that useful and accurate information concerning the more important interaction between parent and child usually is not remembered. Toilet training is one of the areas in which the will of the mother and the will of the child are pitted against each other. Whether the child experienced toilet training chiefly as a defeat in the power struggle or whether he experienced it more as enhancing his own mastery is of critical importance for characterological development. However, this information usually is not possible to ascertain during the evaluation.

Unmet emotional needs, as well as exaggerated power struggles, give rise to various problems in childhood including thumb sucking, temper tantrums, tics, nightmares, fears, eating disorders, excessive masturbation, bed wetting, and nail biting.

The patient's siblings and the details of his relationship to them are other important areas that often are underemphasized in the psychiatric history. The same deficiency is often reflected in the psychodynamic formulation as well. Psychodynamics are too often conceptualized only in terms of oedipal or pre-oedipal conflicts. Other psychological factors such as sibling rivalries and positive sibling relationships may significantly influence the patient's social adaptation. The death of a sibling before the patient's birth or during his formative years has profound impact on developmental experience. The parents, particularly the mother, may have responded to the sibling's death with depression, fear, or anger, which may have resulted in their being incapable of providing adequate emotional nourishment to their other children. Siblings may also have played a critical role in supporting one another emotionally, and may have provided an opportunity to develop multiple alliances and to have significant support at times when the patient experienced feelings of rejection or isolation from the parents.

The emerging personality is a topic of crucial importance. Was the child shy, restless, overactive, withdrawn, studious, outgoing, timid, athletic, friendly? Play is a useful area to explore in studying the development of the child's personality. The story begins with the earliest activities of the infant who plays with bodily parts, and gradually evolves into the complex sports and games of adolescents. This portion of the history not only reveals the child's growing capacity for social relationships, but it also provides information concerning his developing ego structures. The clinician should seek data concerning the child's increasing ability to concentrate, to tolerate frustration, to postpone gratification, and, as he became older, to cooperate with peers, to be fair, to understand and comply with rules, and to develop mature conscience mechanisms. The child's preference for active or passive roles in physical play also should be noted. The development of intellectual play becomes crucial as the child becomes older. His capacity to entertain himself—playing alone, in contrast to his need for companionship—reveals important information concerning his developing personality. It is useful to learn which fairy tales and stories were the patient's favorites. Such childhood stories contain all of the conflicts, wishes, and fears of the various developmental phases, and their themes provide clues concerning the patient's most significant problem areas during those particular years.

The psychiatrist should ask the patient for his earliest memory and for any recurrent dreams or fantasies that occurred during childhood. The patient's earliest memory is significant if it reveals, even in a gross sense, some affective quality. Memories that involve being held, loved, fed, or playing carry a positive connotation for the overall quality of the patient's earliest years. On the other hand, memories that contain themes of abandonment, fear, loneliness, injury, etc. have the negative implication of a traumatic childhood.

MIDDLE CHILDHOOD
(AGES 3 YEARS TO 11 YEARS)

In the middle childhood section, the psychiatrist can address such important subjects as gender identification, punishments used in the home, who provided the discipline, and who influenced early conscience formation. The psychiatrist can inquire about early school experiences, especially about how the patient first tolerated being separated from his mother. Data about the patient's earliest friendships and peer relations are valuable. The psychiatrist should ask about the number and the closeness of the patient's friends, whether the patient took the role of leader or follower, his social popularity, and his participation in group or gang activities. Early patterns of assertion, impulsiveness, aggression, passivity, anxiety, or antisocial behavior often emerge in the context of school relationships. A history of the patient's learning to read and the development of other intellectual and motor skills is important. A history of minimal brain dysfunction or of learning disabilities, their management, and their impact on the child is of particular significance. A history of nightmares, phobias, bed wetting, fire setting, cruelty to animals, and compulsive masturbation is also important in recognizing early signs of psychological disturbance.

LATER CHILDHOOD
(PREPUBERTY THROUGH ADOLESCENCE)

The unfolding and consolidation of the adult personality occurs during later childhood, an important period of development. The psychiatrist should continue to trace the evolution of social relationships as they achieve increasing importance. During this time, through relationships with peers and in group activities, a person begins to develop independence from his parents. The psychiatrist should attempt to define the values of the patient's social groups and determine whom the patient idealized. That information provides useful clues concerning the patient's emerging idealized self-image.

The clinician should explore the patient's academic history, his relationships with teachers, and his favorite curricular and extracurricular interests. The psychiatrist should ask about his hobbies and participation in sports and inquire about any emotional or physical problems that may make their first appearance during this phase. Common examples include feelings of inferiority, weight problems, running away from home, smoking, and drug or alcohol use or abuse. Questions about childhood illness, accidents, or injuries are always included in thorough history taking.

PSYCHOSEXUAL HISTORY

Inasmuch as the sexual history is often the most personal and embarrassing area for the patient, it can be useful to elicit this material all at one time. It will be easier for the patient to answer the physician's questions if they are asked in a matter-of-fact, professional manner. Such a concentration of attention on the patient's sexual history provides a therapeutic structure that is supportive of the patient and that makes sure the therapist will not fail, as a result of countertransference, to obtain relevant sexual data. Much of the history of infantile sexuality is not recoverable, although many patients are able to recollect sexual curiosities and sexual games played during the ages of 3 years to 6 years. The interviewer should ask how the patient learned about sex and what attitudes he felt his parents had about his sexual development and sex in general. The interviewer can inquire about sexual transgressions against the patient during childhood. Those important incidents are conflict laden and are seldom voluntarily reported by the patient. The patient often experiences relief when a sensitively phrased question allows him to reveal some particularly difficult material that he otherwise might not have recounted to the psychiatrist for months or even years.

No history is complete without a discussion of the onset of puberty and the patient's feelings about this important milestone. Female patients should be questioned about preparation for the onset of their menses, as well as about their feelings concerning the development of the secondary sexual changes. Children who develop unusually early or unusually late typically suffer embarrassment and often take elaborate measures to conceal their differences from their peer group. Any exception to that general principle is well worth understanding. The adolescent masturbatory history, including the content of fantasies and the patient's feelings about them, is significant. The interviewer should routinely inquire about dating, petting, crushes, parties, and sexual games. Attitudes toward the opposite sex should be examined in detail. Was the patient shy and timid, or was he aggressive and boastful with the need to impress others by his sexual conquests? Did the patient experience anxiety in sexual settings? Was there promiscuity? Did the patient participate in homosexual, group masturbatory, incestuous, aggressive, or perverse sexual behavior?

RELIGIOUS, CULTURAL, AND MORAL BACKGROUND

The psychiatrist should describe the religious and cultural background of both parents as well as the details of the patient's religious instruction. Was the family attitude towards religion strict or permissive, and were there any conflicts between the two parents over the religious education of the child? The psychiatrist should trace the evolution of the patient's adolescent religious practices to his present beliefs and activities. Even though the patient may have been raised without formal religious affiliation, most families have some sense of ethnic and social class identity. Furthermore, each family has a sense of social and moral values. These typically involve attitudes towards work, play, community, country, the role of parents, children, friends, and cultural concerns or interests.

ADULTHOOD

Occupational and Educational History.   The psychiatrist should explore the patient's choice of occupation, the requisite training and preparation, his ambitions and long-range goals. What is the patient's current job and what are his feelings about it? The interviewer should also review the patient's relationships at work with authorities, peers, and, if applicable, subordinates. He should then describe in his writeup the number of jobs the patient has had, their duration, and the reasons for changes in jobs or job status.

Social Relationships. The psychiatrist should describe the patient's human relationships, with emphasis on their depth, duration, and quality. What is the nature of his social life and his friendships? What types of social, intellectual, and physical interests does he share with his friends? By depth of relationships, we refer to the degree of mutual openness and sharing of one's inner mental life as measured by norms of the patient's cultural background. By quality of relationships, we refer to the patient's capacity to give to others and his capacity to receive from them. How much are his relationships colored by idealization or devaluation? Are people used narcissistically to enhance the patient's sense of status and power, or does he truly care about the inner well-being of others?

A question often arises concerning the patient who has few, if any, friends. First, the clinician explores the nature of the few relationships that the patient has maintained, even if they are limited to one or two family members. Next, the interviewer attempts to understand why the patient has so few friendships. Does a fear of rejection cause him to remain aloof from others? Does he passively wait for others to take the initiative in friendships? Does he feel unlikable and reject overtures from others? Does he lack the requisite social skills to negotiate a friendship? Does he overwhelm people with excessive needs for intimacy, and thereby alienate himself from friends? The major character disorders all show some disturbance in this crucial area of functioning. For example, the compulsive personality typically is excessively controlling in his relationships with others, whereas the hysteric is seductive and manipulative.

For a detailed discussion of how personality types can be recognized and the ways in which the interview should be modified accordingly, refer to MacKinnon and Michels, *The Psychiatric Interview in Clinical Practice*, 1971.

Adult Sexuality. Although the written record has organized adult sexuality and marriage into separate categories, in the conduct of the clinical interview it is usually easiest to elicit that material together. The premarital sexual history should include sexual symptoms such as frigidity, vaginismus, impotence, premature or retarded ejaculation, and sexual perversion.

The positive aspects of both premarital and postmarital sexual experiences should be described. Menopause is described here when it has occurred.

Marital History.   In this section, the psychiatrist describes each marriage or other sustained sexual relationship that the patient has had. The story of the marriage should include a description of the courtship and the role played by each partner. The evolution of the relationship should be described, including areas of agreement and disagreement, the management of money, the roles of the in-laws, attitudes toward raising children, and a description of the couple's sexual adjustment. The last description should include who usually initiates sexual activity and in what manner, the frequency of sexual relations, sexual preferences, variations, techniques, and areas of satisfaction and dissatisfaction for each partner. It usually is appropriate to inquire if either party has engaged in extramarital relationships, and, if so, under what circumstances and whether the spouse learned of the affair. If the spouse did learn of the affair, describe what happened. The reasons underlying an extramarital affair are just as important as its subsequent effect on the marriage. Of course, these questions should be applied to the spouse's behavior as well as the patient's.

Homosexual "marriages," or sustained sexual relationships in which a residence is shared with a person of the same sex, are becoming increasingly common. In such cases, it is appropriate to explore most of the same areas suggested for heterosexual marriages.

No marital history is complete without describing the patient's children or stepchildren. Include the names and ages of all children, living or dead, a brief description of each, and a detailed discussion of his or her relationship to the patient. Make an assessment of the patient's capacity to function adequately in the parental role. Attitudes toward contraception and family planning are important.

Current Social Situations.   The psychiatrist should inquire about where the patient lives and include details about the neighborhood and the patient's particular residence. Include the number and types of rooms, the number of family members living in the home, the sleeping arrangements, and how issues of privacy are handled. Particular emphasis should be placed on nudity of family members and bathroom arrangements. Ask about family income, its sources, and any financial hardships. If there has been outside support, inquire whether it was public assistance or from other family members, and the patient's feelings about it. If the patient has been hospitalized, have provisions been made so that he will not lose his job or home? Will financial problems emerge because of the illness and associated medical bills? The psychiatrist should inquire about who is caring for the children at home, who visits the patient in the hospital, and how frequently visits occur.

Military History. With the cessation of the draft, it is predictable that younger psychiatrists may overlook the patient's military history. Nevertheless, for those patients who have been in the military, it has usually been a significant experience. The psychiatrist should inquire about the patient's general adjustment to the military, and whether he saw combat or sustained an injury. Was he ever referred for psychiatric consultation, did he suffer any disciplinary action during his period of service, and what was the nature of his discharge?

Family History

Recent contributions from the field of genetics demonstrate the importance of hereditary factors in a variety of emotional disorders. A statement about any psychiatric illness, hospitalizations, and treatments of family members, particularly the patient's parents, grandparents, siblings, and children, or any other important family members, should be placed in this part of the report. In addition, the family history should describe the personalities of the various people living in the patient's home from childhood to the present. The psychiatrist should also define the role each has played in the patient's upbringing and his current relationship with the patient. Informants other than the patient may be available to contribute to the family history, and this source should be cited in the written record. (For a brief discussion of the technique of interviewing family members, refer to Chap. 1.) Frequently, data concerning the background and upbringing of the patient's parents suggest probable behaviors that they exhibited toward the patient, despite their wishes to the contrary. Finally, the psychiatrist should determine the family's attitude toward and insight into the patient's illness. Does the patient feel they are customarily supportive, indifferent, or destructive?

Conclusion

In summary, we would like to emphasize the following points. (1) There is no single method to obtain a history that is appropriate for all patients or all clinical situations. (2) The patient's psychotherapy is not postponed or interrupted for the purpose of data collection. (3) It is necessary to establish rapport and to obtain the patient's trust and confidence before the patient will cooperate with treatment. (4) The history is never complete or fully accurate. (5) The description of the patient, the psychopathology, and the developmental history should all fit together. (6) The patient's mental life should be linked with his symptoms and behaviors. (7) Psychodynamics and developmental psychology explain the important connections between past and present. Without this foundation, psychotherapy is not based on a theory of personality development but on concepts about communication and the therapeutic relationship. Therefore, the psychiatrist is unable to exploit the potentials of reconstructive or psychogenetic approaches. (8) No psychiatrist can answer every question raised in this chapter for any patient he treats.

THE MENTAL STATUS EXAMINATION

Systematic attempts at modern psychiatric diagnosis date back to the 19th century with the system devised by Kraeplin. Because these early attempts to develop a systematic nomenclature began with the most seriously ill patients, early definitions of the symptoms and components of mental functioning focused on major disturbances of mental processes. Thus, the mental status examination was devised initially for the description and understanding of the psychoses.

Modern psychiatrists have broadened the number of categories of psychiatric diagnoses and have objectified the criteria for each diagnosis. Therefore, it is essential that the data base be broadened concomitantly to strengthen the scientific foundation for the recognition and categorization of mental phenomena.

The contemporary mental status examination should describe and classify all areas or components of mental functioning. It must relate to substance use disorders, organic mental disorders, organic brain syndromes, schizophrenic disorders, affective disorders, somatoform disorders, dissociative disorders, psychosexual disorders, and last, but not least, personality disorders. The mental status examination has traditionally only included data pertaining to the patient's conscious mental life. Nevertheless, when the patient makes hostile jokes about mental illness, or makes slips of the tongue referring to his wife as his mother, he is revealing important information to be understood and placed in the written record.

The mental status examination can be defined as a standardized format in which the psychiatrist records his observations of the patient's appearance, attitudes, behavior, affective functioning, thought processes, consciousness, perceptual apparatus, orientation, memory, judgment, intelligence, and impulse control. As stated earlier, several of these areas require subjective information provided by the patient and cannot be assessed with the same objectivity as can be obtained from an examination of the retina. A patient's responses are not constant, and the patient's appearance may depend on the circumstances of and the time when the mental status examination is performed. The same patient examined by a different psychiatrist may be found to have a different mental status, and the same physician may find a different mental status on a different day of the week.

Outlines for the mental status examination have changed relatively little since the 1940s. In consulting the leading textbooks of psychiatry, one readily sees that each book gives a similar but somewhat different organization of the examination. Several years ago, we studied the forms for mental status examination in use at each of the various state departments of mental hygiene and most of the university departments of psychiatry. Although there were basic similarities, many individual variations of the mental status were found (unpublished study, MacKinnon R, Yudofsky S, Glick R).

Personality or character diagnosis can be based largely on the patient's history, or on the nature of the patient's interaction with the psychiatrist, if the clinician has developed the requisite skills to accomplish this complex and subtle task.

Regardless of whether he will use the process data of the examination and his subjective reactions to the patient, the clinician must acquire some understanding of ego function. Otherwise, his descriptions of character type will be superficial and will lack richness of clinical detail.

The areas of ego weakness (mental illness) are only a part of the total picture of any patient. The concept of ego strength (mental health) is as essential in differentiating two patients with schizophrenia as it is in differentiating two patients with histrionic personality disorder. The psychiatrist utilizes his knowledge of ego strength to assess the severity of the patient's disorders. (For a discussion of these important topics, refer to Chap. 6.)

Some areas of ego functioning, although included in many mental status examinations, are not described in a way that is useful for the diagnosis of mental disorders. Other areas of ego functioning have been omitted altogether. For example, disorders of impulse control are nowhere to be found in the typical mental status outline, nor is there any category where one can record the sublimatory capacity of the ego, or the capacity for object relations. (Inferential data could be gathered about the capacity for object relations from the psychiatric history.) The fact that one can use either the data from the history or the data from the interactions with the psychiatrist contributes to the inescapable blurring of the boundaries between the history and the mental status parts of the report.

Many outlines for the mental status examination contain items that, although of questionable value, are nonetheless passed on from one generation of psychiatrists to the next. An example is "The Cowboy Story" in Lewis, *Outlines for Psychiatric Examinations* (1943). The story is listed as a test for memory function, more particularly for immediate retention and recall. The theme of the story is of a cowboy and his dog, which does not recognize him in his new clothes but does recognize him when he returns in his old familiar clothes. The patient is asked to repeat the story and to explain its meaning. However, the instructions regarding the scoring of the patient's response pertain only to memory, although the interviewer is advised to determine whether or not the patient seems to comprehend the meaning of the story. How does one score the response if, after repeating the story, the patient says, "Dogs recognize their masters more by smell than by sight. The writer of that story must never have owned a dog." Or what if the patient has never owned a dog, has a limited fund of information, and, on that basis, fails to recognize the absurdity of the story? A different patient may examine the deeper metaphor of the story, whereas still another patient may merely find the story boring and irrelevant to his concerns, and dismiss the examiner with a comment such as, "I don't know what it means." Another patient might merely remain silent. Nevertheless, the story has been passed on from one generation of psychiatrists to another without a critical evaluation of its usefulness.

In doing a mental status examination, avoid using this outline as a checklist that structures the interview. Once the interviewer is familiar with the material to be covered, he (as stated earlier) should elicit most of this information at the same time he is taking a history. The separation of the history and the mental status in the written report is important for the organized study of the patient, his illness, and his reactions to his illness. In the interview, such a separation is artificial and will be resented by the patient. Use common sense and clinical acumen in deciding what questions to ask. It is poor clinical judgment to ask patients questions that have no relevance to their problems.

The overutilization of psychiatric terms in the mental status report will not present an adequate picture of the patient or his illness. Give examples from the patient's behavior that substantiate your particular conclusions. When another person is reading the mental status, the direct quotations of the patient and your objective description of his behavior create the most vivid impression. One can transmit a better picture of a person by recording the mental status in the form of a biographical paragraph rather than in the form of a long list of items. The material to be covered is included in the following discussions (see Table 2-2). One should, as stated earlier, include not only statements about pathological findings but also about health and personal assets (ego strengths; see Chap. 6) in each of the areas described below. The question always arises with trainees concerning statements in the written report pertaining to significant negatives. The general principal is, if a mental status question were relevant to ask the patient, then the answer belongs in the written report. For example, in the case of a patient with a severe agitated depression, feelings of depersonalization, and hypochondriacal ideas, the subject of delusions should always be raised. If no delusions are present, this is a significant negative. In the case of a patient with an acute onset of delirium, agitation, and tremors, the presence or absence of hallucinations should be described. In the case of a patient with suspiciousness, hostility to the examiner, and referentiality, specific statements should be made concerning delusions, thought insertion, thought withdrawal, etc. Such findings are of vital importance to the person who reads the mental status in the future in the same way that including findings of normal function in a physical examination (*e.g.*, normal sinus rhythm) may later have value in estimating changes in the patient's health. Two sample mental status reports have been included at the end of this chapter.

Organization of Data

Appearance, Attitude, and Behavior

GENERAL DESCRIPTION

The general description of the patient begins with comments about the overall physical and emotional impression he conveys to the interviewer as reflected by his clothing, grooming, physical health, facial expressions, posture, and dominant attitude towards the physician. In describing the patient physically, the examiner obtains information from the patient, or, if necessary, from the relatives concerning changes from his normal appearance, attitudes, and behavior. Behavior is a final common pathway, and therefore, it expresses multiple determinants. The important issue is what drives the behavior and how it has changed from the patient's normal state (character). A patient's character is what differentiates him from others of a similar social-cultural background. For example, depending on the context, the descriptive statement "The patient speaks slowly" may relate to a cultural norm, a character trait, or to a manifestation of depression. Likewise, the observation that a patient had "a one-day growth of beard" has different significance for a depressed man who had shaved every day for 30 years than it did for a college student returning from a camping trip.

The patient's degree of poise, the amount of anxiety he manifests, and the manner in which it is expressed are part of the general description. These aspects, together with his appearance in relationship to his stated age and his attractiveness, should be covered in a narrative paragraph that would allow someone who does not know the patient to recognize him easily in a room full of other people. Avoid vague and editorial words such as "unkempt," "inappropriate," or "pleasant looking." What is attractive to one clinician may be unappealing to another. Instead, describe the patient's appearance precisely, such as "Ms. B. has fine features, shoulder length dark brown hair, and brown eyes. She was dressed in a plaid skirt, a plain white blouse, and penny loafers. Her only jewelry was simple gold earrings, and she wore no makeup or nail polish, but she radiated a feeling of quiet beauty."

BEHAVIOR AND PSYCHOMOTOR ACTIVITY (CONATION)

Behavior and psychomotor activity refer to the examiner's observations both of the quantitative and qualitative aspects of the patient's motor behavior. Certain components of the patient's personality structure may be revealed here, as well as behavioral indications of a probable psychotic disorder. An example of the latter would be, "The patient paced the room nervously, staring at the interviewer, and, on several occasions, started to punch at the wall. He pulled his punch at the last instant."

The psychiatrist should describe the patient's overall psychomotor activity precisely, such as "The patient sat immobile in his chair for 45 minutes, never once changing his position, staring into space." This is more informative than stating, "The patient shows severe psychomotor retardation" with no description.

The psychiatrist must also note any specific abnormalities such as dystonias, restlessness, tics, twitches, gesticulations, stereotyped behavior such as echopraxia or echolalia, or posturing with catatonic rigidity or flexibility. Echolalia, or repeating the words of others in echo fashion, is usually classified as a disorder of speech. Nevertheless, it could be argued that this is merely another variety of echopraxia, or mimicking the behavior of others. Both phenomena are part of normal play in young children, but in adults they are usually a sign of a serious mental illness. Last, but not least, comment on the patient's gait, agility, and coordination.

ATTITUDE TOWARD EXAMINER

It is necessary for the psychiatrist to be aware of his own responses to the various personality types of patients before the attitude of the patient is determined and documented. Overly subjective and countertransferential distortions are common in this section of the mental status examination.

The psychiatrist must be aware of the kinds of responses he elicits from patients of varying types. For example, a patient who is paranoid and anxious while under the influence of hallucinogens will respond and relate differently to a psychiatrist who is warm, supportive, and reassuring than he will to a psychiatrist who is removed, reproachful, and nondirective. *In the process of taking a mental status, the examiner is eliciting, as well as documenting, information.* The attitude of the patient may be assessed in the areas of cooperativeness, friendliness, trust, purposefulness, maturity, seductiveness, ingratiation, hostility, contentiousness, evasiveness, guardedness, and other characteristics. Again, it is important to be descriptive rather than to label the patient. An acceptable description would be "The patient stated that he viewed the psychiatric consultation as an unnecessary intrusion. He offered that he distrusted the motives of all psychiatrists and did not wish the examiner 'to try and poke around in my personal business.'"

SPEECH

Speech is somewhat artificially separated from thought, although it is chiefly through speech that thought is revealed. Traditionally, this part of the report is used to describe the physical characteristics of speech, although a number of textbooks confuse speech and thought. Disordered thought processes are reflected in certain language impairments such as incoherent speech, word salad, clang associations, and neologisms. The patient with incomprehensible verbal productions is unable to communicate with others. Some psychiatrists consider this the only evidence of a true thought disorder. For this reason, these severe language impairments also could be included under disturbances of thought. (See discussion of continuity of thought.) The decision to include them here is quite arbitrary. Errors of classification are often made by describing personality traits as a function of speech, for example, garrulous or taciturn. In the traditional outline, speech may be described in terms of its overall quality, its rate of production, and its quantity. Speech may be rapid, slow, pressured, hesitant, emotional, monotonous, loud, whispered, slurred, mumbled, or mute. Impairments of speech such as stuttering are included in this section. A sample statement would be, "The patient spoke loudly and rapidly with exaggerated emphasis. There were few pauses between words, sentences, or paragraphs. It was necessary for this examiner to raise his voice and to repeat questions in order to interrupt the patient's incessant flood of words. Nonetheless, the patient's articulation remained intact to the degree that his words were readily heard and understood by the staff in the nursing area over 50 feet away from the closed examining room."

Thought Process and Content

The term *thought disorder* is controversial in psychiatry; thus, it is used in various ways by different clinicians. For some psychiatrists, the term *formal thought disorder* has become a euphemism for schizophrenic thought. Many others do not accept that narrow usage of the term, and consider thought disorder to include all disorders of thinking that affect language, communication, or thought content. This is the area of the mental status examination with the greatest amount of variation from one outline to another. The reduction of the thought process into component parts is artificial and is used to facilitate the teaching process. In the clinical setting, such parts overlap considerably. Thought disorders are often accompanied by disturbances of emotion.

PRODUCTION OF THOUGHT

The psychiatrist should comment on the overall amount of thought and its rate of production. The patient may have too many thoughts pressing for expression all at once, or he may have a paucity of ideas. Rapid thinking, carried to an extreme, is called *flight of ideas*. Other patients may exhibit slow or hesitant thinking. Because thought is typically expressed verbally, each of these impairments of rate, quantity, or continuity of thought has a corresponding impact on the patient's speech. This categorization is obviously somewhat arbitrary.

CONTINUITY OF THOUGHT

The second component of the stream of thought involves the continuity of ideas. Do the patient's replies really answer the questions he was asked, and does the patient have the capacity for goal-directed thinking? Is there a clear cause and effect relationship in the patient's thinking? Does he have loose associations? Other disturbances of the continuity of thought involve statements that are tangential, circumstantial, rambling, evasive, or perseverative. Blocking is an interruption of the flow of thought (and consequently speech) before an idea has been completed. The period of silence may last seconds or minutes, and the patient indicates that his "mind went blank" during the blocking. Circumstantiality indicates the loss of goal-directed thinking. In the process of explaining one idea, the patient brings in many irrelevant details and parenthetical comments and the interviewer may need to interrupt the patient to help him reach his point. Distractability is a disturbance of thought process in which the patient loses the thread of the conversation and pursues other thoughts stimulated by various irrelevant external or internal stimuli.

Distractability may also be manifested when the patient attempts to attend to or concentrate on tasks such as reading, writing, playing a game, or watching television. The inability to concentrate is different from the state of boredom. Boredom is an affective experience derived from deficiency of emotional involvement; or on the other hand, it may be a defense against excessive emotional involvement. The bored person usually can concentrate on the right topic. The patient with impaired concentration is not usually bored and is more likely anxious over his inability to focus his mind.

CONTENT OF THOUGHT

Preoccupations. Disturbances in content of thought are subdivided into two major categories. The first is preoccupation, which may involve the patient's illness, environmental problems, obsessions, compulsions, phobias, suicide, homicidal ideas, hypochondriacal symptoms, or specific impulses. Because those abnormal thoughts appear in a wide variety of neurotic and psychotic illnesses, psychiatrists disagree whether or not those symptoms should be considered disorders of thought.

The question often arises of where in the mental status to include material that demonstrates unconscious concerns, such as dreams, slips of the tongue, or jokes. For example, during the psychiatric examination, a depressed patient reported the following dream: "I was standing beside a lake when I noticed a woman's body floating face down near the shore. There were a man and a woman standing by. The man said something about trying to rescue her but the woman said that it was too late—she had overdosed. Then I looked more closely at the body and I realized that it was me." Even if the patient denied suicidal feelings, which she did not, this dream belongs in the mental status. An acceptable alternative would be to place it under disorders of mood, as part of the description of the patient's depression.

Slips of the tongue or jokes may also be included in this section if they seem to be a preoccupation of the patient. Otherwise, include them under appearance and behavior, whichever is more appropriate. Perhaps, as the mental status evolves, a separate section will be devoted to unconscious material. We would favor such a development, but at the present time, it is somewhat of a departure from tradition even to include unconscious material in the mental status examination.

Delusions and Referentiality. The second category of disturbances of thought content involves delusions, ideas of reference, thought insertion, etc. The content of any delusional system should be described, and the physician should attempt to evaluate its organization and the patient's conviction as to its validity. The manner in which a delusion affects the patient's life is appropriately described in the history of the present illness. Somatic delusions should be included here. Are the delusions isolated or are they associated with a pervasive attitude in relationship to the environment, such as suspiciousness with paranoid delusions? Ideas of reference and ideas of influence should also be described, as well as how such ideas began, their content, and the meaning that the patient attributes to them.

ABSTRACT THINKING

Abstract thought is the last and most advanced level of thought to evolve in a person's development. The way in which the patient conceptualizes or handles his ideas reveals his capacity for concept formation. The ability to abstract can be tested through similarities, differences, absurdities, the capacity to use and understand metaphor, and the ability to understand the meaning of simple proverbs. A skilled clinician does not need to ask the patient to interpret proverbs in order to make an accurate evaluation of his capacity to think abstractly. It is difficult to assess the reply of a patient who finds the proverbs boring and irrelevant to his problems. His concrete answer may be only a reflection of his attitude to the interviewer's question, or it is also possible that the patient's thinking may be overly concrete or overly abstract. Proverbs have limited value in modern psychiatric diagnosis because concrete responses can occur in organic and functional psychoses, or in people with a low IQ and little education. Concrete thinking means the patient is unable to comprehend metaphor or analogy and only understands the literal meaning of words and sentences.

Some schizophrenic or manic patients may show overly abstract thinking. Here, the patient makes complex philosophical statements in a language that is comprehensible, but the listener cannot grasp the meaning of the patient's sentences. The patient who uses metaphor or analogy appropriately in his conversation with the psychiatrist has demonstrated a capacity for abstract thinking. More formal testing of this patient's capacity for abstraction is unnecessary.

CONCENTRATION AND COGNITION

The patient who has disorientation or memory impairment will reveal these problems during the history taking. The psychiatrist then attempts to explore the patient's difficulty concentrating and thinking clearly in situations of daily living. For example, if the psychiatrist has detected a possible organic mental impairment, he can inquire if the patient has trouble with mental tasks such as counting the change from $10.00 after a purchase of $6.37. If that task is too difficult, easier problems may be substituted.

Subtracting serial 7s from 100 is a traditional part of every formal mental status examination. That simple task requires both concentration and cognitive capacities to be intact. It may not always be clear to the examiner whether the patient's difficulty in performing this task is due to anxiety, a disturbance of mood, some alteration of attention, or at times a combination of all three. In any event, the psychiatrist should attempt to estimate which of these functions seems to be responsible for the patient's difficulty. If the patient cannot perform serial 7s he may be asked to attempt simpler arithmetic tasks. The test may be omitted when comparable ability is demonstrated during the interview. The skilled and sensitive clinician does not humiliate the patient by asking questions that are too difficult or too easy.

Perception

Perception is the process of organizing and interpreting sensory data by utilizing previous experience. This complex process combines the integration of external stimulus with internal response. Strictly speaking, perception is the awareness of objects or qualities that follow the stimulation of sense organs, such as visual, auditory, gustatory, olfactory, tactile, and kinesthetic. Perception is distinct from awareness that results from memory. In the mental status examination, hallucinations, illusions, hypochondriacal complaints, and hysterical symptoms such as hysterical anesthesia are commonly listed under disorders of perception. Delusions are occasionally incorrectly categorized under disorders of perception, and are properly placed under thought process and content in the mental status examination. In other outlines of the mental status, hallucinations and illusions have been categorized under the heading of disorders of thought content. We believe that until someone can demonstrate that hallucinations and delusions result from the same basic disturbance in the brain, they are better listed in separate categories.

HALLUCINATIONS

When discussing disorders of perception, the sensory system involved should be described. A hallucination is the apparent perception of an external object without a basis in the person's sensory field. What occurs in a hallucination is that an internal mental event is mistakenly attributed to an external source. In functional psychosis the most common type of hallucination is auditory, but visual hallucinations and tactile hallucinations are more common in organic psychoses. When describing the occurrence of a hallucination in the mental status report, it is not adequate to state simply, "The patient complained of auditory hallucinations." Rather, the circumstances in which the hallucinations occur, the content of the hallucinations, and the effect of the hallucination on the feelings and behavior of the patient must also be detailed. A hallucination does not imply that the patient believes in the reality of his perception, but only that it is a realistic perceptual experience. In effect, the patient who says "Yes" to the question, "Are you hearing voices?" is indicating that he does not believe they are real people.

Hallucinosis is a psychotic state in which the patient is hallucinating despite the fact he is alert, well oriented, and has a clear sensorium. Hallucinosis commonly occurs in the presence of alcohol or hallucinogenic drugs.

ILLUSIONS

An illusion is a perceptual misinterpretation of a real external sensory experience. An example would be the anxious person alone in his home who mistakes the movement of curtains at the open window for the intrusion of burglars. In certain patients with hypochondriasis and with hysterical symptoms, there are marked distortions and misperceptions related to body feelings.

A description of auditory hallucinations for the mental status is reported as follows: "The patient complained of being tormented by a high-pitched female voice. This voice most commonly would be experienced when the patient was in the presence of other people, and would comment disparagingly upon the patient's appearance and behavior. During the course of her psychiatric evaluation, the patient disclosed that the voice said, 'Don't answer the doctor's questions. He thinks you're ugly and stupid. He hates you and wants to get you into trouble.' The patient's responses to hearing the voice were to become frightened and guarded in the interview situation."

FEELINGS OF DEPERSONALIZATION AND UNREALITY

Many psychiatrists believe that feelings of depersonalization and derealization are examples of perceptual disturbances. Unlike hallucinations, they may be found in a wide variety of neurotic and personality disturbances. Most clinical descriptions of these states indicate a disturbance of the patient's sense of reality. On some occasions there is a perceptual component to the description, but on other occasions the patient states, "Things don't seem real" or "I feel disconnected from people." These disturbances usually have an affective component in that the patient feels numb or sometimes frightened by the experience. When such feelings are induced by hallucinogenic drugs, the patient may enjoy them.

Of particular significance are the more bizarre feelings of deadness or being out of one's own body. The patient may describe a feeling as if there were an invisible glass partition between himself and others. Another patient reports that "My hands no longer seem familiar and feel like those of a stranger," or that "My hands have changed and are just like my father's." Feelings of derealization are expressed in statements such as "The world seems different and strange; nothing looks familiar" or "The world looks unreal."

Mood, Affect, and Emotional Regulation

Mood may be defined as a pervasive and sustained emotion that colors the patient's perception of the world. The term *affect* refers to briefer responses. One might liken mood to seasonal climate whereas affect is likened to the weather of the day. Although many authors use affect and emotion interchangeably, others define emotion as a complex feeling state with psychic, somatic, and behavioral components. According to this definition, affect is the external manifestation of emotion. Another author reverses this position and considers affect as the subjectively experienced feeling. In this book, the terms will be used interchangeably.

SUBJECTIVE EVALUATION

The psychiatrist should evaluate the patient's emotional reactions and the way that he experiences and describes them. Ask the patient for information about his feelings at the time of the interview as well as what range of emotions he experiences in general. One should ascertain the intensity of his emotions. Describe disturbances of emotional regulation such as rapid mood swings, or difficulty initiating, sustaining, or terminating an emotional response. Inquire about depression, sadness, or the wish to die, which is discussed in this section. Thoughts of committing suicide, including plans, are enumerated under thought preoccupations. Sudden or unplanned actions the patient has taken to end his life are considered a disorder of impulse control.

The psychiatrist should note whether the patient remarks voluntarily about his feeling state or whether it is necessary to ask the patient how he feels. Statements about the patient's mood should include a discussion of its depth, intensity, duration, and fluctuations. Some of the common moods include depressed, somber, irritable, cheerful, expansive, euphoric, apathetic, fearful, guilty, and angry.

THE INTERVIEWER'S OBSERVATIONS

To portray accurately the patient's full affective capacity or range of emotionality, the interviewer must cover a diversity of topics flexibly. The patient's dominant mood will limit the range of emotions expressed in the interview. Therefore, the psychiatrist must vary the subject matter to assure a true test of whether or not the patient shows a constriction or limitation of affect. If the interviewer fails to tap the patient's full affective range, the patient's affect cannot be fairly labeled as constricted. In assessing range of affect, the psychiatrist must also be aware of the marked cultural differences in affective expression. One can use the same criteria in assessing the affective capacity of an Englishman and an Italian, but it is necessary to utilize the patient's subjective awareness of his own emotions. The two persons in question may both experience their emotions to an equal degree, but the outward manifestations are, for cultural reasons, quite different in the two patients. Other patients have learned to simulate emotions but do not really experience their feelings deeply. The examiner should comment on the patient's affect as broad or restricted, on its depth and range, and on its quantity.

In the normal expression of affect, there is a variation in facial expression, tone of voice, use of hands, and general body movements. When affect is restricted, both expressive range and intensity are clearly reduced. In blunted affect, the intensity of affective expression is severely reduced. With flat affect, one should perceive virtually no signs of affective expressions. The patient's voice would be monotonous and his face immobile. It may be difficult to differentiate flat affect from severely retarded depression. The interviewer should note any lability of affect and then attempt to characterize the dominant affect of the interview, if there is one. Blunted, flat, and shallow refer to the depth of affect; depressed, proud, angry, fearful, anxious, guilty, euphoric, and expansive refer to particular affects.

APPROPRIATENESS

The *appropriateness* of the patient's emotional responses is considered in the context of the subject matter the patient is discussing. For example, it is appropriate for the paranoid patient who is describing a delusion of persecution to be frightened or angry about what he is experiencing. A lack of anger or fear in this context would be inappropriate affect. Some psychiatrists reserve the term *inappropriate affect* for the schizophrenic patient. An example would be a schizophrenic patient who smiled while discussing the death of a beloved child because of the entry into the patient's mind of a simultaneous thought that amused her, but which was apparently unrelated to her feelings about her child's death. This is an example of dissociation between affect and ideation that originally was described by Bleuler. In another patient, the smile over the death of a brother might relate to a hatred for the brother, with whom she had a lifelong rivalry. Therefore, she did not feel grieved nor saddened by the loss, but rather relieved. In this case, the patient's affect would be appropriate if she were able to smile while discussing his death. The psychiatrist who states in the mental status report that "the patient has inappropriate affect," is providing only partial data. A descriptive statement, such as "While describing the tragic death of her brother, the patient continuously giggled and smiled," is preferable.

The psychiatrist wishes to understand what elicited any emotion that the patient displays during the interview. When the cause and effect are apparent, the psychiatrist need not inquire what elicited the feeling. But the interviewer's failure to inquire about emotional responses he does not understand deprives him of opportunities to facilitate rapport. For example, if a patient begins to cry during the interview for no obvious reason, it is appropriate for the interviewer to state, "I am not certain of the reasons for your tears." In some situations, the patient may not understand his own emotional response. That circumstance provides an important opportunity for the physician and patient to collaborate to enable the patient to increase his understanding of his own feelings.

Consciousness (Alertness and Wakefulness)

Disturbances of consciousness usually indicate organic brain impairment, including the effects of drugs. An exception is seen in the altered level of consciousness found in fugue or dream states. The term *clouding of consciousness* describes a dual impairment of the mind. One impairment is reduced wakefulness, the other is an impairment of the capacity to sustain attention to environmental stimuli or to sustain goal-directed thinking or behavior. Clouding or obtunding of consciousness is frequently not a fixed mental state. The typical patient manifests fluctuations in his level of awareness of the surrounding environment. Drowsiness or somnolence is often found in acute delirium. Minor impairments of consciousness may be expressed by decreasing ability to perform mental tasks, heightened effort, perseveration, frequent hesitation, startling, or irritability. The patient who has an altered state of consciousness often shows some impairment of orientation as well, although the reverse is not true. The patient with a stuporous depression and the catatonic patient may be totally unresponsive, but there is no alteration in those patients' states of consciousness.

Orientation

True disturbances in orientation are usually found only in organic mental disorders. It is common for a patient who has been hospitalized for several months to miss the date by a day or two. That mistake is not a sign of disorientation but is the result of sensory deprivation and a loss of interest or contact with the environment. A normal person may mistake the date by as much as 2 days in the middle of a month-long vacation and may temporarily mistake the day of the week by 1 day without showing signs of organic impairment. A good history usually reveals whether or not the patient is fully oriented, and the psychiatrist should not insult the patient or make himself appear foolish by asking unnecessary questions about orientation. Where the history has provided clues that the patient has some organic problem, the manner in which he answers the interviewer's questions about the orientation may provide useful clues. For example, if, when asked to name the season, the patient looks out the window, the interviewer has found a deficit. The sensitive physician corrects the patient's errors in a respectful manner and makes a therapeutic effort to improve the patient's contact with his environment.

Disorders of orientation are traditionally listed according to time, place, and person. Organically caused impairment in orientation usually appears in that order, and as the patient improves, the impairment will clear in the reverse order. It is necessary to determine whether the patient can give the correct date. In addition, if he is in a hospital, does he know how long he has been there? Does the patient behave as though he is oriented to the present? In questions about the patient's orientation for place, it is not sufficient that the patient be able to correctly state the name and the location of the hospital; he should also behave as though he knows where he is. If more subtle signs of disorientation to place are suspected, the interviewer may ask the patient the routes and the means by which he would travel from the hospital to his home. In assessing orientation for person, the interviewer asks the patient whether he knows the names of the persons who are around him and whether he understands their roles in relationship to him. It is only in the most severe instances that the patient does not know who he is; in those cases the psychiatrist must be careful to differentiate a disorientation for the person from a delusion in which, for example, the patient believes that he is Jesus Christ. When impairments for orientation are suspected, it is useful for the examiner to consult the patient's chart or the nurses' notes, or to speak with the patient's relatives or ward personnel. Disorders of orientation are often inconstant; for example, the patient may show no impairment at the time of the examination, although he may be up wandering about the ward in a state of confusion at night.

Memory

An intact memory requires that the perceptual apparatus registers impressions in the brain (registration) to be stored (retention), and which must be retrieved or recognized when needed (recall). Memory changes have been traditionally divided into four areas: remote memory, recent past memory, recent memory, and immediate retention and recall. Disturbances of immediate retention and recall may be due to difficulty in concentration (faulty registration), or may be the result of impaired retention or recall. Disorders of consciousness (alertness) are frequently involved in such difficulties.

Although the traditional view is that remote memory is better preserved in dementia than is recent memory, there is differing opinion concerning the matter. Some psychiatrists and psychologists think that the patient's apparent capacity to recall remote events is actually due to constant repetition and reinforcement of the same material, and that detailed testing of remote memory shows that it is just as impaired as recent memory.

Many patients with dementia confabulate to cover up their memory impairment. This is usually an unconscious defense mechanism designed to spare the patient either anxiety or humiliation about his incapacity.

The experienced clinician does not find it necessary to ask the patient structured questions about his memory, because he has learned much about that function during the interview. If the history does reveal memory problems, he then asks the patient questions that seem appropriate and are relevant to the patient's life or the difficulties from which he is suffering.

Recent memory may be checked by asking the patient about his recollection of things he discussed with the physician earlier in the interview. He also can be asked about current events in the news, or he may be asked at that point if he recalls the interviewer's name. Asking the patient to repeat seven digits forward and then backward is a traditional test for concentration and immediate retention. Nevertheless, the results are often difficult to evaluate. Adults with residual minimal brain dysfunction may show particular difficulty in repeating the digits backward or may even reverse numbers in repeating them forward. Patients who routinely respond to test questions with anxiety may have difficulty with the digit span. Impaired concentration may also interfere with the patient's ability to repeat digits.

If the examiner has any questions concerning functions that may be impaired, detailed psychological testing should be performed. Finally, no assessment of memory function is complete without determining the effects of the deficit on the patient and making note of what compensatory mechanisms the patient has developed to cope with his loss of capacity.

Impulse Control and Frustration Tolerance

Impulse control refers to a person's ability to control the expression of his aggressive, hostile, fearful, guilty, affectionate, or sexual impulses in situations where their expression would be maladaptive. Loss of impulse control means a failure of the ego to control such impulses, which are then acted upon in spite of the patient's conscious wish for self-control. There are situations in which the patient's behavior would be considered impulsive in spite of the patient's claim that he could have controlled his actions if he so desired. An example is the man under the influence of alcohol who pinches the buttocks of a woman at a cocktail party. The next day he feels embarrassed and apologizes.

The mode of impulse discharge can be verbal or behavioral. Manifestly, to tell the boss to "go to hell" is a loss of impulse control, but to punch him is an even more serious loss of control.

Certain behaviors are misdiagnosed as a loss of impulse control. An example is the ego-syntonic expression of impulses that is maladaptive only because of the negative responses elicited from others. Here, the psychopathology is usually in the superego. The patient could control the impulse, but he believes that control is unnecessary.

An example occurred when the doctor was called out of his office for a moment. When he returned, the patient handed him his pen and said, "I borrowed your pen for a moment; I hope you don't mind." The doctor replied, "Oh no, it's quite all right." Only later did he realize that this particular pen had been inside his closed briefcase, which was on his desk. The patient could have controlled this impulse but he saw no reason to do so because he did not realize that he, in fact, had crossed a social boundary. This example could be described in the opening section of the mental status report as part of the description of the patient's behavior.

Impulse control is a function that has not traditionally been a part of the mental status examination. It may be disturbed in a variety of emotional disorders, including neurotic disorders, dementias, schizophrenias, affective disorders, and character disorders. Also included in this category should be certain instances of impulsive, suicidal, or assaultive acts, sexual exhibitionism, and the like, where sustained planning has not been associated with the act. A patient may show subtle evidence of this problem in the doctor's office by trying to read his own chart or something else on the interviewer's desk. In another instance, the patient may seem contained throughout the interview, but reveal a lack of control on the way out. An example of that problem occurred in the case of a woman who showed appropriate behavior throughout the interview but who, at the end of the interview, walked over to the resident psychiatrist, pinched his cheek, and said "You're so cute; are you married?"

The patient who paces the floor during the interview is designated as agitated or restless. If he picks something up from the desk that does not belong to him or pounds his fist on the wall, he also has a loss of impulse control.

A related but different area of disturbance is the effectiveness of a person's delay mechanisms, or in other words, his ability to tolerate frustration. Frequently, the patient's loss of impulse control is a direct result of his low frustration tolerance. His impulses have an urgent quality. The patient experiences a state of inner tension that demands immediate relief. Because the patient can rationalize his actions, it requires careful questioning to classify the behavior accurately. For example, a female patient received a telephone call at home from another woman who claimed to be having an affair with her husband. A short time later, the patient ran to her husband's closet and cut the legs off all his pants. Without information pertaining to the patient's inner state of mind, it would be impossible to be certain that this was not a carefully planned vindictive act. In other words, premeditation rules out loss of impulse control.

In clinical practice, the patient with impaired impulse control and a low frustration tolerance usually has superego deficits as well.

Information and Intelligence

While taking the patient's history, the psychiatrist has learned about the patient's formal and self-education. Therefore, it is *unnecessary* for the experienced psychiatrist to say to the patient, "Now I am going to ask you some simple, silly questions about your general knowledge." The psychiatrist who apologizes to the patient for asking "silly questions" conveys that it is he who is silly. It is insulting to the patient to be asked questions that are too easy for him. If the psychiatrist is uncertain about the patient's ability to function at his level of basic intellectual endowment, he should ask questions that are relevant to the patient's educational and cultural background. If the patient shows some organic mental impairment, that will be revealed during the history taking as the psychiatrist attempts to explore the ways in which the patient experiences his deficit in the problems of daily living. If the examiner has any question about the patient's intellectual functioning, specific psychometric tests should be performed by a trained psychologist. (See Chap. 5.)

Judgment

During the course of the history taking, the examiner should have been able to assess many aspects of the patient's capacity for social judgment. Judgment is required in the countless daily decisions one makes in setting priorities and anticipating the consequences, both short term and long range, for each choice one makes. The ability to conceptualize the likely outcome of one's behavior is not the only prerequisite for good judgment. A person must translate the analytical component of judgment into action in order to have good judgment. If the patient shows some impairment of judgment, the psychiatrist should describe examples. The psychiatrist often assesses judgment by hypothetical questions such as "What would you do if you found a stamped, addressed letter in the street?" Such questions are harmless, but they are often unsatisfactory for testing an ego function as complex as judgment.

Insight

Insight refers to the depth or extent of the patient's awareness and understanding of himself. Insight begins with the recognition of the problem and his relationship to it. In some cases the patient may exhibit a complete denial of his illness. In other instances he may show some awareness that he is ill, but may blame the fact on someone else or on other external factors. He may acknowledge that he has an illness, but ascribe it to something unknown or mysterious in himself.

Intellectual insight is present when the patient can recognize that he is ill and can acknowledge his role in his symptoms or failures in adaptation. Nevertheless, a major limitation to intellectual insight is that the patient is unable to apply this knowledge to alter his future experience. True emotional insight is present when the patient's awareness of his own motives and deep feelings leads to a change in his personality or behavior patterns. He becomes open to new ideas about himself and the important people in his life.

The preceding discussion of insight applies to patients who are neurotic or have character disorders. In the schizophrenic patient or the organic patient, insight is present if the patient realizes that he is ill and that the problem is in his own mind. If the patient with dementia states, "I can't remember things anymore and I get confused," insight is present.

Conclusion

In summary, we offer the following conclusions: (1) The formal mental status examination has changed relatively little since the 1940s. This, in part, has led to a proliferation of rating scales. (2) The contemporary mental status examination should describe and classify all areas or components of mental functioning. (3) Data pertaining to the patient's unconscious mental life may be included. (4) The patient's mental illness is only a part of the total picture of any patient. The psychiatrist utilizes his knowledge of ego strength to assess the severity of the patient's disorder. (5) The patient's mental status is not constant and can be influenced by the manner of the examination. (6) A contemporary model of the mental status examination has been presented with a discussion of areas of current controversy. (7) The purpose of the outline is for the organization of the written record only. It is not a schedule to follow in the interview.

SUGGESTED READING

Garland L, II: The problem of observer error. Bull NY Acad Med 36:570, 1960

Kramer M, Ornstein PH, Whitman RM, et al: The contribution of early memories and dreams to the diagnostic process. Compr Psychiatry 8:344, 1967

Langs RJ: Earliest memories and personality. Arch Gen Psychiatry 12:379, 1965

Lewis NDC: Outlines for Psychiatric Examinations, 3rd ed. Albany, New York State Department of Mental Hygiene, 1943

Lieberman MG: Childhood memories as a projective technique. J Proj Tech 21:32, 1957

Lyerly SB, Abbott PS: Handbook of Psychiatric Rating Scales (1950–1964). Bethesda, National Institute of Mental Health, 1966

MacKinnon RA, Michels R: The Psychiatric Interview in Clinical Practice. Philadelphia, WB Saunders, 1971

Mayman M: Early memories and character structure. J Proj Tech Pers Assess 32:303, 1968

Menninger KA, Mayman M, Pruyser PW (eds): A Manual for Psychiatric Case Study, 2nd ed, p 61. New York, Grune & Stratton, 1962

Ryback R: The Problem-Oriented Record in Psychiatry and Mental Health Care. New York, Grune & Stratton, 1974

Spitzer RL: Immediately available record of mental status exam: The mental status schedule inventory. Arch Gen Psychiatry 13:76, 1965

Spitzer R, Endicott J: DIAGNO: A computer program for psychiatric diagnosis utilizing the differential diagnostic procedures. Arch Gen Psychiatry 18:746, 1968

Spitzer R, Endicott J: DIAGNO II: Further developments in a computer program for psychiatric diagnosis. Am J Psychiatry 125 (Suppl):12, 1969

Spitzer R, Endicott J: Can the computer assist clinicians in psychiatric diagnosis? Am J Psychiatry 131:523, 1974

Spitzer R, Endicott J, Cohen J: Constraints on the validity of computer diagnosis. Arch Gen Psychiatry 31:197, 1974

Spitzer RL, Fleiss JL, Burdock EI, et al: The mental status schedule: Rationale, reliability, and validity. Compr Psychiatry 5:384, 1964

Spitzer RL, Fleiss JL, Endicott J, et al: Mental status schedule: Properties of factor-analytically derived scales. Arch Gen Psychiatry 16:479, 1967

Spitzer RL, Fleiss JL, Kernohan W, et al: Mental status schedule: Comparing Kentucky and New York schizophrenics. Arch Gen Psychiatry 12:448, 1965

Stevenson I: The Psychiatric Examination. Boston, Little, Brown, & Co, 1969

Ulett G: Automation in a state mental health system. Hosp Community Psychiatry 25:77, 1974

APPENDIX. SAMPLE MENTAL STATUS EXAMINATION REPORTS

Mrs. C. is a 56-year-old widowed Jewish female who was brought to the psychiatrist's office by her married daughter, with whom she lives in a three-bedroom house in a middle-class suburb of New York.

The Report

At the time of the interview, Mrs. C.'s clothes were wrinkled, loose-fitting, and clean. Her hair was combed carelessly. She wore no makeup, although her daughter states that she routinely uses makeup when she is well. During the course of the interview, she sat in a hunched over position with her hands in her lap and rarely changed her position in the chair. She appeared sad, and spoke softly and without emphasis. Mrs. C. took long pauses between each sentence, and often sighed loudly and deeply after questions were posed to her. Although she was polite and made efforts to cooperate with the psychiatrist, she was only able to respond to simple questions requiring brief answers. She asked that questions be repeated and responded to many others by saying, "I just don't know what to say." On several occasions in the process of responding to a particular question, the patient would pause and say, "Doctor, I just forgot the question you asked. Would you mind repeating it?"

Mrs. C. was preoccupied with "being a bad mother" and with having "disgraced her entire family." Despite the protestations of her daughter, the patient persistently ruminated about her (the patient's) responsibility for a miscarriage that her daughter had experienced 3 years previously. When asked to explain her responsibilities for the miscarriage, the patient said, "All the world knows that it was my fault. Just ask anybody. When you are corrupt and evil, you are punished." The patient also expressed her belief that she was emitting "foul odors from my brain." She stated that the odors were related to "to evil thoughts that I can't get off my mind." The patient declined to share with the examiner just what these thoughts were. She did state that although she herself could not smell the odors, "everybody else can smell them." Mrs. C. conceded that she felt "hopeless," but she stated that she would "never seriously consider suicide" because of religious convictions and prohibitions. She admitted to feeling incapable of happiness, and she cried openly when discussing her daughter's miscarriage.

She denies hallucinations or feelings of unreality and depersonalization. When asked to subtract 7 from 100 and to keep subtracting 7s serially, the patient responded, "100, 93, 85, 79." There were long pauses between each number and after the fourth number was volunteered, the patient said, "Doctor, I just can't go on anymore. I can't think. I'm very stupid." Mrs. C. correctly identified the year but stated that she thought the date was September 21, when in fact the date was September 25. She was fully oriented to place and to person. Her memory for remote events was intact, but she had some difficulty with the recollection of recent events. For example, she was unable to recall that she had gone to the grocery with her daughter the previous weekend. She was able to recall six figures forward, but only three figures backwards. She was able to repeat three terms—a tree, a tablecloth, and a job—immediately after they were spoken by the examiner. However, after an interval of 5 minutes, Mrs. C. could only recall one term, the tree, and could not recall the other two terms—even after hints from the examiner. Mrs. C. stated that she did not feel that she could benefit from psychiatric care. She stated that she did not feel that she suffered from a medical or psychological problem. "My problem" she said, "is that I have disgraced myself and my entire family. I am an evil person and have the kind of sickness that neither doctors nor anybody else can help. It would be better if I were dead." Nevertheless, she denied any suicidal thoughts.

It was not possible to assess validly her general fund of information or her intelligence because of her depression. She showed very little insight into the fact that she is ill. She realized that she was seeing a psychiatrist, but she believes her daughter brought her for treatment of the foul odor emanating from her brain.

DISCUSSION

Among the principles illustrated in the mental status examination (MSE) report are the following:

   1.   *A mental status examination is meaningful only in the context of other baseline data.* In the case of Mrs. C., her daughter reported that prior to her illness, the patient was meticulous about her hygiene and appearance. She also stated that her mother was normally animated and witty and that her speech formerly had been spontaneous and expressive. The change in Mrs. C.'s appearance and speech constitute important clinical data. For another patient, however, who was perennially unkempt and whose speech was characteristically slow and unmodulated, these descriptions would have different clinical implications.

   2.   *The MSE report should be descriptive as opposed to impressionistic.* In the MSE report, rather than stating that Mrs. C. "was delusional," the examiner included Mrs. C.'s delusions as described in her own words. As opposed to a statement of whether or not her affect was "appropriate," Mrs. C.'s affect was reported in the context of her thinking. In this case, her restricted affect and depressed mood are appropriate in the context of her morbid and self-accusatory thoughts. One should avoid making such statements in the written report as "Mrs. C. exhibited poor insight." Rather, strive to describe, in the patient's own words, his feelings about the source of his symptoms as well as the approach that the patient prefers to take (if any) to achieve relief.

   3.   *Avoid drawing "hard and fast" diagnostic conclusions from specific deficits or disturbances in the mental status.* Mrs. C. showed dysfunction related to concentration (*i.e.,* difficulties of subtracting 7 from 100 serially), with orientation, and with memory. Nevertheless, one cannot judge conclusively from these data that she was suffering from an organic brain syndrome. In Mrs. C.'s case, the diagnostic conclusion of her psychiatrist was that she was suffering from major depression with delusional features. He chose to hospitalize her and to treat her with an antidepressant agent and supportive psychotherapy. Within 5 weeks, Mrs. C.'s appearance, mood, affect, and thought processes had returned to normal. However, the patient continued to demonstrate poor capacity to subtract serially 7s from 100, or to repeat more than six digits forward and three backwards. The patient revealed that since childhood she had difficulty with numbers and with arithmetic, and that letter reversals in her handwriting and typing were common. It was the final conclusion that this difficulty was a residue of a learning disability and not evidence of any early organic impairment.

   4.   *Follow the standardized format in the written MSE report.* The examiner must, of necessity, be selective about which data are to be included and which excluded. To avoid the lengthy and monotonous reports (which discourage careful review by colleagues in clinical settings), emphasis should be placed upon those significant dysfunctions in the mental status that relate to the diagnosis and treatment of the presenting problem. It is necessary to include pertinent negatives. The MSE report states that Mrs. C. *did* *not* exhibit auditory or visual hallucinations, which may have been present in a patient with depressed mood and with delusions. Pertinent negatives also are to be included in the written MSE report for purposes of clarification or emphasis. The examiner included the fact that Mrs. C. *did not* admit to suicidal plans or intentions for medical/legal purposes. To fail to document that a depressed patient was questioned by the psychiatrist about suicide may have legal (*i.e.*, negligence) implications if that patient were later to commit suicide. In addition, the examiner included the data that Mrs. C. was *not* able to smell "the odors" in order to help make the distinction between a disorder of thought and a disorder of perception.

Mr. D. is a 19-year-old single black male college student who was brought to the emergency room of a large general hospital by his parents, with whom he lives in a two-bedroom apartment.

The Report

Mr. D. wore neatly pressed khaki pants, a fresh, blue, buttoned-down oxford shirt, a conservative tie, and appears fashionable and well groomed. His short-cropped hair, close shave, slim physique and youthful manner combined to make him seem younger than his stated age of 19 years. Sitting erectly on the front of his chair, Mr. D. looked directly into the eyes of the examiner as he spoke with enthusiasm. His loud speech and his clear enunciation of each syllable of each word conveyed a slightly unnatural quality, not dissimilar to that of a classical actor delivering lines from a play. The patient gave long, rambling responses to the examiner's questions. Although he did not exhibit loosening of associations, he would frequently stray from the subject of the questions (tangentiality). For example, when asked to name the courses he was presently taking in college, Mr. D. began by discussing his physics class, he next talked about nuclear energy, then he digressed to a lengthy discussion of the threat of nuclear war, and finally offered a detailed plan for nuclear disarmament "which I will take to Russia to help forge a real and lasting peace between us and the Russians." He never returned to the subject of the other courses that he was presently taking in college.

Mr. D. stated his belief that he was endowed with "special powers" to bring about good in the world. He revealed his belief that the central intelligence agency (CIA) communicated to him through "satellites, microwaves, and a receiver that they implanted in my brain when I was just an infant." In addition, he felt that television newscasters gave him coded signals about "special missions of peace, which I am soon to carry out in the national interest." He stated his belief that "Through a secret transmitter in my brain I have the ability to change the thinking of world leaders from hate and greed to love and charity." He also stated that the CIA had the capacity to monitor his thoughts "through the receivers which they implanted." Therefore, he found it necessary to concentrate on thinking "only positive and peaceful thoughts." He added, "I would be in personal danger if I allowed my mind to think base and animalistic thoughts."

The patient admitted to hearing various sounds, "like radio static or rushing noises" that were associated with his "transmitter." He also said that he heard the voices of "agents" who would issue him instructions. On several occasions during the course of his examination, Mr. D. abruptly paused and appeared distracted. When asked about his behavior, he revealed that an "agent" was giving him orders about the way to answer questions. He denied that the voice gave him instructions to harm himself or other people. He denied, as well, visual hallucinations or other perceptual disturbances.

Mr. D. demonstrated difficulty with abstract thought throughout his evaluation. He tended to be both excessively abstract as well as concrete. In addition, he overpersonalized concepts. When asked to interpret the parable "people who live in glass houses shouldn't throw stones", he responded, "Stones last forever, they are a link between the creation of the universe, mankind, and myself. Glass is made from sand which is also particles of stone; and man is made from dust which is even finer particles of stone. The parable means that all things on this earth are touching and that I, as man, am in contact with everything." The patient was intelligent, well-informed, and could use numbers and calculate with great facility.

Although Mr. D. stated that "he was the happiest human being alive," he rarely smiled or varied, in any way, his affective expression. His appearance did not give evidence of dysphoria, irritation, or anger. Rather, the mood and affect of the patient appeared overcontrolled and restricted and gave him a wooden quality. He did not admit to feeling, at the present time, anxiety, sadness, loneliness, guilt or any other feeling or mood other than "happiness."

He was oriented in all spheres and showed no impairment in memory. He was, in fact, able to recall 12 digits forward and 10 digits backwards. The patient showed impaired judgment. For example, when asked what he would do if he were the first to notice that a fire broke out in a movie theatre, he responded, "I would use my brain transmitter to communicate with specialists in the Air Force who are trained to manage fires in military airports. It would be a simple matter for them to rush in the necessary equipment to assist me in extinguishing the fire." Mr. D. did not feel that he suffered, in any way, from a psychological problem. Rather, he viewed his psychiatric examination as a "special consultation for the doctor." He stated that he would agree to treatment "if the doctors believe that medical science can use my assistance."

DISCUSSION

Among the principles illustrated in this MSE report are the following.

1. *The mental status examination is meaningful only in the context of other baseline data.* Mr. D.'s psychiatrist concluded that the patient suffered either from a schizophrenic disorder or from a manic episode as part of a major affective disorder. The psychiatrist attempted to utilize historical data in an effort to arrive at a more definitive diagnosis. He learned that the symptoms described in the mental status examination emerged 8 months prior to the time that the patient presented to the emergency room. The psychiatrist also learned that since adolescence the patient was isolated and withdrawn, with almost no friends. He would spend his vacation periods and weekends away from school alone in his room. The patient's energy and activity levels, his ability to concentrate, and his need for sleep had remained stable over the past several years. Although these data increased the psychiatrist's concern that Mr. D. was suffering from a schizophrenic disorder, the physician did not feel that there were sufficient data to arrive at a conclusive diagnosis. The psychiatrist chose to treat the patient with both lithium and an antipsychotic agent and to follow the patient's course before forming a conclusive diagnostic impression.

2. *The MSE report should be descriptive as opposed to impressionistic.* The MSE report of Mr. D. provides a "written picture" of the way the patient appeared at a given time. The examiner's detailed description of the dress and physical appearance of the patient might have important diagnostic significance years later. In schizophrenic illness, for example, there is usually a progressive deterioration of appearance and personal hygiene. Such a deterioration does not commonly occur in manic-depressive illness. If the patient were to appear in the same emergency room 10 years later and dress and look similarly to the fashion described in the original MSE report, this might be one piece of data to help confirm the diagnosis of an affective illness. Similarly, by describing the content of the patient's delusions in the patient's own words, rather than saying that "the patient suffered from grandiose delusions with ideas of reference, ideas of influence, thought insertion, and thought withdrawal," comparisons may be made with the patient's disordered thinking in the future. If, for example, 5 years later the patient appears in an emergency room with delusions that are more paranoid, more bizarre, and more fragmented, this change in the patient's thinking may have important diagnostic and treatment implications.

3.   *Avoid drawing "hard and fast" diagnostic conclusions from specific deficits or disturbances in the mental status.* Kurt Schneider described a number of first-rank symptoms for schizophrenia. Among these symptoms were the experience of having one's thoughts controlled, the capacity to project one's thoughts to others, and the experience of having one's actions controlled or influenced from the outside. Many other investigators later questioned the specificity of Schneider's first-rank symptoms of schizophrenia. They pointed out that such symptoms can be found in numerous other psychiatric conditions. In the case of Mr. D., his "Schneiderian symptoms" would be consistent with either a diagnosis of schizophrenia or manic illness.

3

Biological Testing in Psychiatry

Clinical Laboratory Testing in Psychiatry 87
  Neuroendocrine Testing 87
    The Dexamethasone Suppression Test 88
      Description of Test Procedures 88
      Range of Normal Results 88
      Clinical Indications 89
      Neurophysiological Basis 89
      Areas of Controversy 90
      Side-Effects and Complications 90
    The Thyrotropin-Releasing Hormone Test 91
      Description of Test Procedures 91
      Range of Normal Results 91
      Clinical Indications 92
      Neurophysiological Basis 92
      Areas of Controversy 92
      Side-Effects and Complications 92
    The Thyroid Function Tests 92
      Description of Test Procedures 92
      Clinical Indications 93
      Areas of Controversy 95
      Side-Effects and Complications 95
  Blood Level Measurements of Psychiatric Medications 96
    Lithium 96
      Description of Test Procedures 96
        Laboratory Testing Before Initiating Lithium Treatment 96
        Monitoring Lithium Levels 98
      Areas of Controversy 99
    Tricyclic Antidepressants 101
      Laboratory Testing before Initiating Tricyclic Antidepressant
      Treatment 101

Description of Test Procedures   102
Clinical Indications   103
Areas of Controversy   104
Antipsychotic and Other Medications Used for Psychiatric Symptoms   104
The Evaluation of Toxicities and Drug Side-Effects   105

Electrical Diagnosis and Brain Imaging Techniques in Evaluating Psychiatric
*   Disorders   110*
Electroencephalogram (EEG)   110
Computed Tomography (CT)   112
Magnetic Resonance Imaging (MRI)   114
Imaging Based on Brain Function: Positron Emission Tomography and
    Regional Cerebral Blood Flow   115
Positron Emission Tomography (PET)   115
Cerebral Blood Flow (CBF)   117

The Risk-Benefit Ratio of Laboratory Testing   117

For nearly a century, psychiatric investigators have searched for biological tests with sufficient sensitivity and specificity to aid in diagnosing the major affective illnesses and the schizophrenias. Thus far, no test, by itself, is pathognomonic of a major "functional" psychiatric illness. Rather, diagnostic procedures and laboratory values, at best, may *supplement* data from the psychiatric history and mental status examination to aid in arriving at a correct diagnosis. Although virtually any laboratory test may be of value in the psychiatric evaluation (*i.e.*, complete blood count, urinalysis, blood urea nitrogen), laboratory tests are particularly valuable when affective, perceptual, or cognitive symptoms are secondary to physical diseases affecting the central nervous system. Prototypic examples are depression associated with hypothyroidism, in which there are decreased protein-bound iodine and decreased thyroxine levels; euphoria associated with multiple sclerosis in which the gamma globulin level in the cerebral spinal fluid is increased; paranoia associated with a left temporal epileptic focus with a high voltage, low-frequency rhythm on electroencephalogram; and episodic discontrol of rage and violent behavior in the presence of a limbic mass revealed on computed tomographic (CT) scan.

This chapter will focus on the role of biological tests that may be useful in either tracing or ruling out the relationship between psychiatric symptoms and organic illness.

It is imperative that the clinician not only be able to assess the potential value of a diagnostic test, but also its limitations. The sensitivity of a laboratory test refers to its ability to detect the abnormality in question. Sensitivity concerns how often false-negative results are encountered. For example, a test with a sensitivity of 95% for a particular disease indicates that it will not be detected in 5% of the patients with that disease. The specificity of a test defines the degree to which the abnormality revealed by a particular test is restricted to those persons who have the disease in question. This may be expressed in how often false-positive results are encountered with that test. For example, a test with a specificity of 80% for a particular disease indicates that 20% of the results suggesting that that particular disease is present, will be inaccurate and in fact will not be due to the disease in question. An example of a test wherein the specificity has been questioned is the dexamethasone suppression test for depression, which will be reviewed later in this chapter. Certain investigators have reported that "positive" dexamethasone suppression test results may be found in patients who do not have depression but, in actuality, have other medical disorders. The psychiatrist should also be intimately familiar with how a laboratory test is actually administered. Some tests may be psychologically threatening for psychiatrically ill patients. This may be a factor in deciding when during the course of the patient's illness the test should be conducted. The clinician should allot sufficient time to explain to the patient (and to the patient's family, if indicated) the rationale of the test, the manner in which it will be administered, and whether or not pain, discomfort, or side-effects are likely. Finally, the patient and family should be made aware of the cost of all laboratory tests to make an informed assessment about whether or not the potential benefits outweigh the expense.

Clinical Laboratory Testing in Psychiatry

Neuroendocrine Testing

Psychiatrists have long attempted to ascertain the underlying pathophysiology of certain specific psychiatric syndromes. For example, the sleep disturbances, appetite changes, and decreased sexual interest inherent in major depressive illness suggest alterations in hypothalamic and pituitary function. It is logical to explore whether such changes may be reflected in abnormalities in neuroendocrine values, which could be measured and thereby aid in establishing the diagnosis. Current research on depression demonstrates the existence of neurohormonal changes involving the hypothalamic–pituitary axis. Most scientists do not believe that these changes constitute the underlying cause of the condition. Nevertheless, patients and their families are prone to overestimate the present state of scientific knowledge. They wish to believe that a specific cause of their illness has been found, that the cause is detectable by a definitive laboratory test, and that when the test reverts to normal (after the physician has administered the appropriate drug), they will be cured. The clinician can explain that neuroendocrine changes may be reactions to complex changes related to psychological stresses, or other biopsychosocial interactions, and that underlying predispositions may persist even after normalization of laboratory results.

The Dexamethasone Suppression Test

DESCRIPTION OF TEST PROCEDURES

In administering the dexamethasone suppression test (DST), the patient receives an oral dose of 1 mg of dexamethasone at midnight. Most methods specify that blood be drawn at 4 PM and again at 11 PM the same day for determination of serum cortisol concentrations. Other methods of administering the DST have been proposed. In a more elaborate system, a patient receives 1 mg of dexamethasone orally at midnight. Blood samples are then taken at 8 AM, noon, 4 PM, and midnight for radioimmunoassay of plasma cortisol concentrations. It is proposed that increased sample points increase the sensitivity of the test. The patient may eat regularly and continue with his or her usual life routines during the test. Table 3-1 summarizes the most commonly utilized method of administering the DST.

RANGE OF NORMAL RESULTS

Plasma cortisol concentrations greater than 5 μg/100 ml are considered "positive DSTs," or nonsuppression. Proponents of the DST propose that a

---

TABLE 3-1. Dexamethasone Suppression Test Protocol

1. The patient receives an oral dose of 1 mg of dexamethasone at midnight.
2. Blood samples are taken the following day at 4 PM and 11 PM for radioimmunoassay of plasma cortisol concentrations.
3. Plasma cortisol concentrations of greater than 5 μg/100 ml are considered "positive," or nonsuppression of cortisol.

positive DST implies the presence of a major depressive episode as well as other psychiatric disorders that may be related to depression.

CLINICAL INDICATIONS

Proponents of the test state that a positive DST has clinical usefulness in the following situations: (1) The diagnosis of a major depressive episode; (2) Monitoring the treatment of depression—advocates state that a return to normal suppression of cortisol during treatment suggests a positive treatment response, whereas a failure to return to normal suppression of cortisol implies an incomplete treatment response; and (3) aid in preventing relapse. An example of the last indication is a patient with recurrent affective illness who becomes moderately lethargic, shows decreased concentration in the work setting, and exhibits diminished capacity for recreational pursuits. In such a case, reduced suppression of cortisol following the administration of dexamethasone may indicate that antidepressant agents should be reinstated before a full-blown, major depressive episode emerges.

NEUROPHYSIOLOGICAL BASIS

Dexamethasone is a synthetic glucocorticoid that affects the hypothalamic and limbic regions of the brain in the regulation of corticotropin, or ACTH release. Figure 3-1 represents suppression of plasma cortisol in a patient

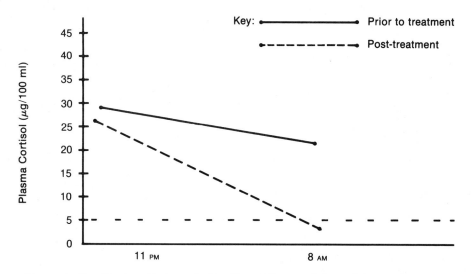

Plasma fasting (8 AM) cortisol result after 11 PM, 1.0 mg oral dose of dexamethasone

FIG. 3-1. Dexamethasone suppression test results for patient with major depression.

with major depression before and 6 weeks after the initiation of treatment with a tricyclic antidepressant medication. The dexamethasone was administered at 11 PM. Studies have shown that many depressed patients, when compared to nondepressed controls, have elevated cortisol levels in serum and urine. Also, in certain depressed patients, high free cortisol levels in cerebral spinal fluid and in plasma, coupled with the absence of normal nocturnal inhibition of cortisol secretion in some depressed patients, indicate that hypothalamic–pituitary functioning is impaired. Sachar hypothesized that cortisol hypersecretion in patients with depression reflects a disinhibition of the hypothalamic–pituitary–adrenocortical axis secondary to a decrease in catecholamine activity in the hypothalamus, which, in normal persons, inhibits ACTH secretion. Carroll and associates suggest a clinical use for these findings by applying a test previously utilized by endocrinologists for evaluating the hypothalamic–anterior pituitary–adrenocortical axis. The DST measures a patient's capacity to suppress cortisol levels after oral administration of dexamethasone. Carroll and associates reported that the test showed a 67% sensitivity and a 96% specificity for the diagnosis of major depressive episodes for inpatients.

AREAS OF CONTROVERSY

Proponents of the DST maintain that the failure to suppress plasma cortisol is extremely rare in other psychiatric disorders, with false-positive rates of 5% to 10%. Critics of the DST report the sensitivity of the test is low (ranges of 50% to 70%), and report that there is a significant percentage of patients with clear major depressive illness who fail to show suppression on the DST. Critics of the DST also maintain that the test is of little practical benefit beyond the data that can be obtained through psychiatric history taking and careful mental status examination. They contend that clinicians may fail to recognize the low sensitivity of the test, and thereby fail to treat depressed patients with psychopharmacologic agents. Opponents of the DST also contend that the test is not so specific as Carroll initially maintained, so that "positive results" may be found in an extensive array of psychiatric and medical illnesses. Also, the test may be less sensitive and less specific in outpatients with depression, in patients with weight loss, and in patients who abuse drugs or who are on certain medications.

SIDE-EFFECTS AND COMPLICATIONS

Proponents of the DST report infrequent adverse physical and psychological side-effects from the oral dose of 1 mg of dexamethasone, and they believe that the several venipunctures involved in the procedure are minor inconveniences when compared to the painful and destructive potentiality of undiagnosed and untreated depression. Critics of the DST contend that certain clinicians overutilize the procedure with the result of unnecessary discomfort and expense for the patients.

The Thyrotropin-Releasing Hormone Test

DESCRIPTION OF TEST PROCEDURE

In administering the thyrotropin-releasing hormone (TRH) test, a 500-μg dose of synthetic thyrotropin-releasing hormone (TRH) is injected intravenously, usually at 8 AM, to a patient who is at bed rest after receiving no food or fluids since midnight. Through an indwelling venous catheter, samples of blood are taken before TRH is injected and then at 15 minutes, 30 minutes, 60 minutes, and 90 minutes after TRH administration. The change in TSH following TRH administration (delta TSH) is derived by subtracting the highest level of TSH secretion from that secured at baseline. It is important to note that lithium may inhibit thyroid function and make the results difficult to interpret for the diagnosis of affective illness. Table 3-2 summarizes the TRH test procedure.

RANGE OF NORMAL RESULTS

Increased TSH is defined as a value above 15 μIU/ml. Decreased TSH is a level below 7 μIU/ml. Normal values for TSH changes following administration of thyrotropin-releasing hormone are in the range of 7 μIU/ml to 15 μIU/ml.

TABLE 3-2. TRH Test Protocol

1. Patient takes nothing by mouth after midnight and is at rest in bed by 8:30 AM
2. Indwelling venous catheter is placed and a normal saline drip is started to keep the line open.
3. At 8:59 AM blood is taken through a three-way stopcock for determination of T_3RU, T_3RIA, T_4, and TSH levels (reverse T_3 is optional).
4. At 9 AM 500 μg of TRH (protirelin) is slowly given IV over a 30-s period. Side-effects from the infusions may include a transient sensation of warmth, desire to urinate, nausea, metallic taste, headache, dry mouth, chest tightness, or a pleasant genital sensation. These effects are generally short-lived and mild.
5. Blood samples are taken through the stopcock before the TRH is administered and at 15, 30, 60 and 90 min after infusion to measure changes in TSH.

CLINICAL INDICATIONS

Advocates of the thyrotropin-releasing hormone test propose it to be useful in providing biological data to support the diagnosis of major depression, particularly in combination with the dexamethasone suppression test. A decrease in TSH (<7 μIU/ml) is said to occur wth major depression. Other investigators have suggested that the test may be useful in separating bipolar patients with major depression from unipolar patients with major depression. Differentiating bipolar from unipolar depression is accomplished based on the observation that bipolar patients show exaggerated response of TSH to TRH injection as opposed to the blunted response of unipolar patients. Proponents suggest uses for the TRH test similar to those of the DST, such as monitoring response to treatment and alerting the clinician to impending relapse.

NEUROPHYSIOLOGICAL BASIS

Thyrotropin-releasing hormone (TRH) is a polypeptide in the hypothalamus. Upon release, it causes the secretion of TSH from the anterior pituitary. Thereafter, TSH stimulates the thyroid to release the thyroid hormones T_3 and T_4.

AREAS OF CONTROVERSY

Some investigators feel that the test lacks specificity, particularly in patients with hyperthyroidism, alcoholism, and other psychiatric disorders. Critics question the usefulness of the TRH test, as well as its costliness. The test is expensive in terms of manpower (at least five samples must be taken over a 2-hour interval), and of the laboratory costs of TSH measurements.

SIDE-EFFECTS AND COMPLICATIONS

Critics of the test believe that patients may exhibit autonomic discomfort upon TRH infusion. In addition, the patient is subjected to the discomfort and risks associated with the presence of an indwelling venous catheter for 2 hours.

The Thyroid Function Tests

DESCRIPTION OF TEST PROCEDURES

There are many points along the hypothalamic–anterior pituitary–thyroid axis where thyroid dysfunction can occur. Previously, the most common screening test was to measure only the levels of circulating thyroid hormones: serum T_3 and T_4 values. More accurate and sensitive measurements of thyroid function can now be obtained by combining several tests of hypothalamic–pituitary–thyroid gland function. Total bound T_3 and T_4 are measured by radioimmunoassay of the patient's serum. The T_4 level is altered by changes in the protein binding of the hormone, which can occur during use of oral contraceptives and other drugs, during pregnancy, and with illness. It is also important to account for the binding of T_3 and T_4 by using resin uptake techniques. This is accomplished by determining the number of available binding sites for T_3 and T_4 on serum proteins such as thyroid-binding globulin (TBG), and thereby determining a free thyroxine index (FTI). Thyroid-stimulating hormone can be measured directly. The TRH test as described previously is also a sensitive provocative test of thyroid function both at the pituitary level and at the level of the thyroid gland itself. Note that the serum protein bound iodine test has been largely replaced by thyroxine (T_4) assay, which is more specific. All tests mentioned are accomplished by serum measurements from small quantities of venous blood. Table 3-3 summarizes the most commonly utilized tests of thyroid function.

CLINICAL INDICATIONS

It has long been recognized that patients with hypothyroidism, or diminished thyroid function, show many clinical features similar to those seen in major depressive illness. It must be recalled that the onset of hypothyroidism is gradual and that the first signs are often revealed in the psychiatric examination. Symptoms such as weakness, tiredness, stiffness, poor appetite, constipation, disturbance in menstrual function, and vague muscular pains are commonly found in patients with hypothyroidism, depression, or both. Speech is often slowed and monotonous in character, and intellectual changes may occur, including poor memory, reduced reaction time, apathy, and drowsiness. In severe cases of hypothyroidism, frank psychosis with hallucinations, perceptual disorders, and delusions may occur. For these reasons the evaluation of any patient suspected of having major depressive episodes must include a systematic evaluation of thyroid function. This is particularly true in patients with previous psychiatric treatment in which their depressive symptoms have failed to respond to standard psychopharmacologic and psychotherapeutic interventions.

Many investigators propose that a careful evaluation of thyroid function is essential in all patients with symptoms of depression and that the frequency of thyroid disease among patients with depression is much higher than that in a matched control group. The most commonly utilized tests to screen for hypothyroidism are measurements of T_3 and T_4. Investigators

TABLE 3-3. Popular Thyroid Function Tests *

Type of Test	Normal Values	Cost ($)	Interference
IN VITRO (SERUM TESTS)			
T_4	4.5–13 μg/100 ml 58–167 nmol/l	6–20	Changes in TBG, drugs, etc.
Resin T_3 uptake	25%–35%	2–10	Changes in TBG, drugs, etc.
T_7 and ETR	Combinations of values for T_4 and resin T_3 uptake		
TSH	0–10 μlU/ml 2–7 μlU/ml	35	Pituitary disease
T_3RIA	80–200 ng/100 ml 1.2–3.1 nmol/l	36	Changes in TBG, drugs, etc.
Autoantibodies	Absent	25–50	
IN VIVO TESTS			
Radioiodine uptake (^{131}I, ^{123}I)	10%–25%/24 h	50–80	Never use in pregnancy: iodides T_3 and T_4 therapy, antithyroid drugs, thyroiditis
Thyroid scan radioiodine	Both lobes homogeneous	70	Iodides T_3, T_4 Never use in pregnancy
TRH injection	TSH increase to 2× control	100	
TSH stimulation	No effect or increased uptake	100	
T_4 suppression	Uptake reduced to half of original value	100	Heart disease or other contraindication of T_4 therapy
HISTOLOGY (BIOPSY)			
Fine needle aspiration biopsy (FNAB)	Normal cytology	23	Inadequate sample
Cutting needle biopsy (CNB)	Normal cytology	†	Significant danger of hemorrhage

* Tests are listed in order of decreasing frequency of practical application. Adapted from Halsted JA, Halsted CH (eds): The Laboratory in Clinical Medicine: Interpretation and Application, 2nd ed. Philadelphia, WB Saunders, 1981

† Cost data vary from laboratory to laboratory.

such as Sternback, Gold, Pottash, and Extein recommend that in the depressed population far more sensitive testing of thyroid function is necessary. They advise the use of thyroid-releasing hormone to detect modest changes in thyroid function before those changes that can be measured through assessment of T_3 uptake, T_4, and TSH. These investigators have shown that a significant number of patients without abnormalities in T_3, T_4, and baseline TSH show augmented TSH response to TRH. Table 3-4 summarizes changes in thyroid function tests in patients with hypothyroidism. These investigators propose that there is a significant percentage of depressed patients with mild hypothyroidism whose clinical signs or symptoms are not recognizable upon physical examination but whose mental symptoms may respond to thyroid replacement regimen.

AREAS OF CONTROVERSY

Although endocrinologists and psychiatrists agree that patients with hypothyroidism often are depressed, they disagree regarding the prevalence of hypothyroidism among populations with major depression. Gold and associates report a 10% incidence of previously undiagnosed hypothyroidism in studies of approximately 400 depressed or lethargic patients and recommend a systematic thyroid workup—including a TRH test—for all patients with depression. Critics feel that few patients with depression have hypothyroidism, and that the TRH test is expensive and adds little to routine thyroid screening in the detection of hypothroidism in depressed populations.

SIDE-EFFECTS AND COMPLICATIONS

Side-effects and complications of thyroid function tests are few, and are limited to those associated with simple venipuncture. However, TRH infusion may induce nausea, hypotension, and other autonomic symptoms.

TABLE 3-4. *Thyroid Function Test Changes in Patients with Hypothyroidism*

1. Serum T_4 concentration is *decreased.*
2. Serum free thyroxine is *decreased.*
3. Serum T_3 concentration is *decreased.*
4. Serum T_3/T_4 ratio is *increased.*
5. Serum T_3 uptake is *decreased.*
6. Serum PBI is *decreased.*
7. Serum thyroxine-binding globulin is *normal.*
8. Serum thyroid stimulating hormone is *increased.*

There are risks and discomfort associated with the presence of an indwelling venous catheter for 2 hours.

Blood Level Measurements of Psychiatric Medications

Lithium

Introduced by Cade in 1949 for the treatment of patients with manic-depressive illness, lithium was the first psychiatric medication in which broad laboratory monitoring of blood levels became an important component of clinical treatment. Lithium is an alkaline metal similar to sodium, potassium, magnesium, and calcium. It is available in the conventional carbonate form, which is completely absorbed by the gastrointestinal tract and reaches a peak serum level in 1 to 2 hours. Lithium is also available in a slow-release preparation, in which peak serum levels are reached in approximately 4 hours to 5 hours. The drug is not bound by plasma proteins and has an elimination half-life of approximately 24 hours. The vast majority of lithium is excreted through the kidneys, a process that depends upon glomerular filtration rate as well as sodium balance. Reabsorbed primarily in the proximal tubules along with sodium, decreased plasma sodium levels may initiate a compensatory increase in sodium reabsorption, which will be accompanied by lithium reabsorption. *Thus, decreased plasma sodium levels, which may result from excessive sweating, from diuretics, or from reduced sodium intake, may result in dangerously high lithium levels.* Lithium is distributed nonuniformly throughout the body and reaches equilibrium about 5 days to 7 days after administration. Serum lithium is measured accurately by flame emission (flame photometry, flame spectrometry) or by atomic absorption spectrophotometry. Both procedures are highly accurate, widely available, and relatively inexpensive.

DESCRIPTION OF TEST PROCEDURE

Laboratory Testing Before Initiating Lithium Treatment.   Prolonged use of lithium can result in specific irreversible pathological changes. *Before initiating lithium treatment, baseline studies must be done to diagnose any preexisting kidney, thyroid, or cardiac illness. Structural kidney damage is the most common irreversible effect of long-term lithium treatment.* Although there is debate among clinicians whether the well-documented changes in the kidney (including interstitial fibrosis in the tubular regions and focal glomerular atrophy) can cause clinically significant morbidity, the physician nonetheless should carefully monitor the renal function of every patient receiving lithium. Monitoring renal function consists of the following:

1. Taking a careful medical and family history to detect the possible presence of hereditary kidney disease;
2. Conducting a specific review of the genitourinary system that might uncover other types of kidney impairment (secondary to diabetes mellitus, hypertension, toxic substances, etc.);
3. Performing a complete physical examination; and
4. Laboratory assessment of renal functions, which includes urinalysis, blood urea nitrogen and serum electrolyte testing, estimation of 24-hour creatinine clearance, calculation of 24-hour urine volume and 12-hour dehydration testing, followed by measurement of urine osmolality.

The renal function of patients receiving maintenance doses of lithium must be reassessed every 6 months, and more frequent specific assessments may be necessary if the patient has preexisting problems with kidney function.

The second chronic adverse reaction that occurs with long-term use of lithium involves thyroid functioning. Lithium inhibits several steps in the synthesis and metabolism of thyroid hormones. Specifically, lithium may inhibit the iodination of tyrosine, the release of T_3 and T_4, and the iodine uptake by the thyroid gland. Lithium also diminishes peripheral metabolism of thyroid hormones as well as the stimulating effects of TSH. About 30% of the patients receiving maintenance doses of lithium develop consistently increased levels of TSH, approximately 5% develop hypothyroidism, and 3% develop diffuse, nontender goiter. Therefore, the clinician must screen for signs and symptoms of preexisting thyroid disease prior to initiating lithium treatment. Specifically, laboratory tests should include TSH, T_4, T_4I (the free thyroxine index), and measurements of T_3 resin uptake. During the course of treatment, TSH measurements should be done every 6 months, and a complete battery of thyroid tests should be repeated on a yearly basis.

Thirdly, hematologic and cardiovascular changes also occur with extended lithium treatment. Mild to moderate elevations of white blood cell count are common with both acute and chronic treatment with lithium. Although this disorder is reversible with the discontinuation of lithium, a complete blood count with differential should be taken prior to initiating lithium treatment, and on a yearly basis with maintenance treatment. Lithium has multiple effects upon the heart. ECG changes in patients without preexisting heart disease include T-wave flattening, U-waves, and suppression of the sinoatrial node. In patients who are known to have cardiac disease, lithium may induce ventricular premature contractions, and conduction changes, including first-degree atrial ventricular block, and irregular or slowed sinus node rhythms. Rarely, ventricular tachycardia, cardiomyopathy, and congestive heart failure may also develop. Therefore, prior to initiating lithium, secure a cardiac history, perform a complete physical examination of the cardiovascular system, and obtain a baseline ECG. The ECG should be repeated approximately 1 month after initiation of lithium, and also should be repeated on a yearly basis. If any changes in the patient's cardiac status emerge while the patient is receiving lithium, evaluation by a qualified cardiologist is critical. Patients on prolonged lithium treatment may develop mild diabetes insipidus. In most patients, urinary output increases from 2 to 3 liters a day. Frequently, patients replace the extra liter of lost fluid with carbonated beverages or other calorie-containing fluids. In this fashion, they may increase their caloric intake as much as 1000 calories per day, and often incorrectly attribute their weight gain to the lithium. Fasting blood sugars and urine testing for glucose and ketones should be taken prior to initiating lithium treatment, and should be repeated on a yearly basis.

Monitoring Lithium Levels. Although it has long been recognized that the therapeutic benefit of lithium is directly related to serum levels, in our experience, errors in measurement of serum lithium levels are commonplace. The most common error in monitoring lithium levels relates to the standardization and the timing of blood drawing in relation to the last administered dose of lithium. Without such standardization, serum levels have far less clinical meaning. It is well known that blood samples that have been obtained within only a few (1 to 10) hours of the last oral dose of lithium have considerably higher concentration than samples taken 12 or more hours later. However, it is less appreciated that there are also wide variations in serum lithium levels taken more than 12 hours after the last oral dose. It is important to standardize the drawing of the patient's blood sample at exactly the same number of hours following the evening dose so that clinical comparisons can be drawn. A recommended approach is always to draw levels in the morning precisely 12 hours after the last dose. Secondly, ensure that the patient is compliant and consistent. For example, a patient who is prescribed 300 mg of lithium carbonate four times a day but who skips one or two doses daily will have varying blood levels. For such a patient, clinical correlations—whether related to therapeutic or adverse effects of lithium—may not be reliable. In the patient without kidney impairment, blood levels should be obtained 2 days after the initiation of treatment. If levels are increased gradually, weekly lithium levels are adequate until stable steady-state blood levels are achieved. However, if impaired renal function is present, or if treatment is initiated with rapidly increasing doses, more frequent blood level sampling (every 2 days) may be necessary to monitor for toxicity. Serum lithium levels should be taken once or twice a week until the patient's symptoms and blood levels stabilize, and thereafter, once per month for the initial 6 months of treatment. Each change in the oral lithium dose will require approximately 7 days before the serum lithium level equilibrates. After the first 6 months of maintenance treatment in which lithium levels are stable, the clinician may check the serum lithium approximately every 2 months to 3 months to monitor for changes in levels.

The guiding principle for treatment with lithium is to use the lowest possible effective dose to avoid side-effects. In general, for acute mania therapeutic serum levels are from 0.8 meq/l to 1.5 meq/l. In maintenance treatment, 0.5 meq/l to 1.0 meq/l is the most commonly recommended range. Toxicity related to serum levels is generally considered to occur in levels above 2.0 meq/l, although certain sensitive patients may exhibit toxic symptoms at much lower levels. Life-threatening intoxication occurs at levels above 3 meq/l, whereupon hemodialysis should be strongly considered. Tables 3-5 and 3-6 summarize laboratory testing required before lithium treatment and during lithium maintenance treatment.

AREAS OF CONTROVERSY

Among researchers and clinicians there is little dispute about the essential role of lithium monitoring when the drug is used clinically to treat affective illness. However, controversy does exist related to the following areas:

1. Methods of beginning lithium treatment and estimating dosage requirements;
2. The frequency of monitoring lithium levels;
3. The levels that are therapeutic for both the treatment of acute mania and for maintenance treatment.

Cooper and co-investigators recommend an initial 24-hour serum lithium level as a prognosticator of dosage requirements. His group recommends giving an initial single dose of 600 mg of lithium carbonate and taking a serum lithium level at 24 hours. This level can then be used to predict the daily dose necessary to achieve a steady-state therapeutic serum level. Other investigators and clinicians have been unable to confirm the predictive value of this test, and feel that the multiple variables that occur in actual clinical practice result in this procedure having little practical application. We recommend gradually adjusting the lithium dosage based on the patient's previous serum levels and clinical response as the safest and most effective procedure to determine the ultimate oral dose for maintenance treatment. With regard to the frequency of monitoring serum lithium levels, we recommend the procedure described earlier in the chapter for the patient whose clinical state is uncomplicated by medical illness. We emphasize that the psychiatrist should closely follow the patient's clinical condi-

TABLE 3-5.   Laboratory Tests Prior to the Initiation of Lithium

1. Complete blood count
2. Serum electrolyte test
3. Blood urea nitrogen test
4. 24-h creatinine clearance test
5. 24-h urine volume test
6. 12-h dehydration test for urine osmolality
7. TSH
8. T_4
9. T_4I (free throxine index)
10. T_3 resin uptake
11. Fasting blood glucose
12. Urinalysis
13. Urine for glucose and ketones
14. ECG

tion, and that with any suggestion of side-effects or toxicity, a lithium level should be drawn. The greatest amount of controversy related to lithium monitoring centers around the range of therapeutic serum levels and whether or not lowering maintenance levels actually reduces structural kidney and thyroid damage. Because the requisite data are not yet available to settle this important issue, we recommend maintaining the lowest serum lithium level possible, while at the same time preserving the therapeutic effects.

Tricyclic Antidepressants

More than twelve tricyclic antidepressant agents either are currently marketed in the United States or are expected to be introduced by 1990. Of these, only three drugs have been studied to the point that significant correlations have been established between blood level measurements and clinical responses. These medications are imipramine, desmethylimipramine, and nortriptyline. Although no specific correlation has been drawn in the laboratory between blood levels of amitriptyline and clinical response, clinical experience indicates that therapeutic response is, in fact, related to increasing blood levels of amitriptyline. All tricyclic antidepressants are lipid-soluble and completely absorbed by the gastrointestinal system. Their biologic availability is markedly reduced by the effects of "first pass" he-

---

TABLE 3-6. Laboratory Tests for Patients
Receiving Lithium Maintenance Treatment

1. Complete blood count, yearly
2. Serum electrolyte test, yearly
3. Fasting blood glucose, yearly
4. Blood urea nitrogen test, yearly
5. TSH, every 6 mo during the first year, and yearly thereafter
6. T_4, T_4I, and T_3 resin uptake, yearly
7. 24-h creatinine clearance test, yearly
8. 24-h urine volume test, yearly
9. ECG, yearly
10. Serum lithium levels
    (a) Biweekly until stable steady-state blood levels are achieved
    (b) Once per month during the initial 6 mo of treatment
    (c) Every 2 mo–3 mo thereafter*

---

* Any change in the patient's clinical state will necessitate more frequent monitoring of the relevant laboratory value.

patic elimination. Elimination of the drug is accomplished by tissue and plasma protein binding and by efficient elimination through hepatic metabolism. Elimination half-lives vary widely from patient to patient. This variability has served as an impetus for investigators and clinicians to attempt to relate blood level measurements of tricyclic antidepressants to clinical response. Of principal concern is the group of patients who are rapid metabolizers of tricyclics and whose failure to respond clinically to standard oral doses may be secondary to low plasma levels. In addition, it has been established that a small percentage of patients are slow metabolizers of tricyclic antidepressants. Such patients may have inordinately high blood levels of tricyclics despite standard oral doses. Should such high levels of antidepressants go undetected, cardiac toxicity and other serious side-effects are possible.

LABORATORY TESTING BEFORE INITIATING
TRICYCLIC ANTIDEPRESSANT TREATMENT

Before initiating treatment with tricyclic antidepressants, baseline studies must be done to diagnose preexisting cardiac, hematologic, or liver disease. Patients who have had recent myocardial infarctions, who have congestive heart failure, or who have left bundle branch block are at high risk with the use of tricyclic antidepressants. Bone marrow suppression including agranulocytosis, eosinophilia, and thrombocytopenia may occur. Because most tricyclics are metabolized by the liver, any condition affecting the function of the liver is a potential hazard. Finally, concomitant use of tricyclic antidepressants with monoamine oxidase inhibiting compounds may result in hyperpyretic crisis, malignant hypertension, or severe central nervous system dysfunction including grand mal seizures.

We recommend the following laboratory studies before the initiation of tricyclic antidepressants: complete blood count (CBC) with differential, serum electrolyte levels, blood urea nitrogen level, liver function tests, urinalysis, and an electrocardiogram. We suggest that the CBC with differential and the electrocardiogram be repeated 1 month after the initiation of imipramine and every 6 months thereafter as long as the patient remains on antidepressants. In the presence of abnormal findings on any of these tests, appropriate medical consultation is required before initiating pharmacotherapy.

Pretreatment evaluation for electroconvulsive therapy (ECT) includes a standard medical history and physical examination. The laboratory testing includes the standard blood and urine tests previously described prior to treatment with tricyclics. In addition, lumbosacral spine films in patients over 50 years of age or in patients who have an increased risk for compression fractures of the spine must be taken. Electroencephalogram and CT scans are also indicated to rule out a space-occupying brain lesion, which is the major contraindication to ECT. Evidence of untreated or malignant hypertension, congestive heart failure, and evidence of a recent myocardial infarction are also, in most cases, contraindications to the use of ECT.

DESCRIPTION OF TEST PROCEDURES

Once the patient has taken a sufficient quantity of an antidepressant for an adequate period of time (*e.g.*, 250 mg of imipramine daily for 3 weeks), the drug achieves a condition of steady state. Thereafter, the patient's blood should be drawn approximately 10 hours to 14 hours after the last dose of medication. This is usually accomplished by drawing the patient's blood in the morning, prior to the administration of the usual antidepressant dose. Special attention must be paid to collection and preparation of the specimen. It is essential that test tube stoppers not contain the compound tris-butoxyethyl phosphate, because contamination from this substance results in erroneous quantitative analyses of tricyclics. Currently, only Venoject blood collection tubes and specially marked Becton–Dickinson Vacutainer blood collection systems are suitable. Specimens should be centrifuged as soon as possible after collection, and the plasma or serum components re-tained. Once the specimen has been collected and correct patient identification of the specimen has been ensured, care must be taken to preserve the sample. Tricyclic antidepressants are stable up to 1 year in frozen plasma and up to 5 days in plasma at ambient room temperature. Caution must be taken to forward the specimen to laboratories with proper equipment and extensive experience in analyzing tricyclic antidepressant levels. The American Psychiatric Association Task Force on the Use of Laboratory Tests in Psychiatry reported that the analysis of antidepressants is significantly less developed and controlled than the analyses of other drugs that are currently monitored for therapeutic purposes. The Task Force found a coefficient of variation among laboratories in excess of 30%. Therefore, it is important for the clinician to select carefully the laboratory to analyze tricyclic antidepressant levels, and to research their methods of quality assurance.

CLINICAL INDICATIONS

Data from the scientific literature show clear relationships between blood level measurement and clinical outcome with the drugs imipramine, desmethylimipramine, and nortriptyline. At present, the relationship of blood levels of amitriptyline to therapeutic outcome is controversial. Of ten different studies, three show a linear relationship, three reveal a "therapeutic window" effect, and four show no relationship between amitriptyline blood level and outcome. The reason for these discrepancies remains unproved.

When the combined blood level of imipramine and its demethylated metabolite exceeds 200 ng/ml of plasma, the percentage of patients who achieve therapeutic response is higher than at lower levels of the drug. With desmethylimipramine, three large studies have shown a linear relationship between drug concentration and outcome. Unlike imipramine and desmethylimipramine, nortriptyline has been found to have a specific "therapeutic window" wherein favorable antidepressant responses occur. Plasma concentrations of nortriptyline below 50 ng/ml or above 150 ng/ml are associated with poor clinical response. Therefore, it is essential, with the use of nortriptyline, to ensure that the patient's blood levels are within the 50 ng/ml to 150 ng/ml range. Unlike imipramine and desmethylimipramine, increasing nortriptyline beyond 150 ng/ml will result in a loss of the antidepressant effect. There is a curvilinear relationship between blood level measurements and clinical outcome for nortriptyline, as opposed to the linear relationship for both imipramine and desmethylimipramine.

Blood level measurements of antidepressant agents are useful in the following clinical situations:

1. For patients whose depressive illness does not respond to the usual oral doses of the respective antidepressant agent

2. For patients who are at high risk because of age or medical illness and who would best be treated with the lowest effective dose of the drug
3. In cases where rapid treatment is urgent, such as in the acutely suicidal patient. Achieving a therapeutic blood level in the briefest time possible is an advantage in this situation.
4. Where a question exists regarding the patient's compliance in taking the medication
5. Where the patient's depression responds to an antidepressant, and the level is recorded to be utilized in the event of later recurrence. It is important to note that published data are minimal concerning the relationship between blood levels and therapeutic response to tricyclics in patients with panic or anxiety disorders.

AREAS OF CONTROVERSY

Certain clinicians question the overall utility of blood level measurements of antidepressants. They propose that good estimates of tricyclic antidepressant levels can be obtained by observing side-effects such as dry mouth, hypotension, and sedation. They propose increasing the dose of tricyclic antidepressants (other than nortriptyline) until either a therapeutic response is achieved or side-effects become prohibitive. These clinicians maintain that this approach avoids unnecessary expense to patients, the inconvenience of venipuncture, and the possibility of confusing or inaccurate laboratory results.

Antipsychotic and Other Medications Used for Psychiatric Symptoms

Originally, it had been hoped that the ability to measure blood levels of antipsychotic agents would lead to clear definitions of therapeutic ranges, as have been determined for lithium. Although radioimmunoassay and other methods are becoming increasingly precise for measuring chlorpromazine levels, at present there is little agreement as to what constitutes a therapeutic level of this antipsychotic agent. Some investigators report that levels of chlorpromazine above 100 ng/ml are not associated with increasing therapeutic benefit, but often result in toxic symptoms. Nevertheless, it is clear that psychoses of many patients respond at blood levels significantly lower than 100 ng/ml of chlorpromazine. It appears that below 100 ng/ml, therapeutic levels vary widely in populations of patients who are matched for age, sex, weight, and symptoms. When treating acute psychoses, experienced clinicians raise the dose of antipsychotic agents until the patient's symptoms resolve or until disabling side-effects emerge. Thereafter, the dose of antipsychotic agent is gradually reduced to the lowest amount that still maintains the therapeutic response. Although accurate plasma levels of haloperidol, thioridazine, and other commonly utilized antipsychotics are also now available, even less is known regarding therapeutic ranges of these agents than is understood for chlorpromazine. Similarly, accurate plasma levels may be measured for other psychiatric medications, such as anticonvulsive agents, beta blocking agents, benzodiazepines, and stimulants, but at this time there are no definitive data about therapeutic blood levels for their use in treating psychiatric disorders. Although therapeutic plasma ranges have been established, for example, for carbamazepine in the treatment of complex partial seizure disorders, these levels may not correspond to the therapeutic levels in the treatment of manic symptoms. The principal value of measuring blood levels of the agents just discussed is for assessing and monitoring toxic levels.

The Evaluation of Toxicities and Drug Side-Effects

Psychiatrists are frequently consulted to evaluate patients who have (1) attempted suicide by drug overdose; (2) who may have psychiatric side-effects of prescribed medications; (3) who may have psychiatric symptoms secondary to alcohol, hallucinogens, or other substances of abuse; or (4) who may have psychological changes secondary to environmental poisons. In the United States there are approximately 100,000 poisoning fatalities annually, and studies have shown that 26% of suicides involve poisons. It has also been estimated that for every so-called "successful suicide" there are 15 to 20 attempts at suicide. Therefore, the total number of nonfatal poisonings exceeds 1 million per year. In addition, a wide variety of medications comprising virtually every category and classification of drugs has been implicated in the initiation of psychiatric side-effects. These agents may induce changes in mental status due to their inherent central nervous system activities, which do not necessarily involve toxic levels of the drugs.

The clinical laboratory is utilized for the detection and quantification of agents that may be implicated in substance-induced organic mental disorders. This classification deals with the various organic brain syndromes that are caused by the direct effects of substances on the central nervous system. These effects may include intoxication, idiosyncratic reactions, and withdrawal effects, as well as hallucinosis, delusional disorders, and affective disorders that are related to the inherent properties of the substance. The clinical laboratory is also essential in assessing organic brain syndromes that are secondary to substance-use disorders. This diagnostic class refers to affective and behavioral changes associated with regular use of substances that affect the central nervous system, but are not prescribed for specific therapeutic conditions. DSM-III utilizes three criteria to define substance abuse. These criteria are (1) A pattern of pathological use; (2) impairment in social or occupational functioning caused by the pattern of pathological use; and (3) a disturbance in social or occupational functioning of a duration of at least 1 month. Five classes of substances are associated with both abuse and dependence. These include alcohol, barbiturates or similarly acting sedatives or hypnotics, opioids, amphetamines or similarly acting sympathomimetics, and cannabis. Certain of these substances such as amphetamines, barbiturates, and opioids are used medically as well as abused recreationally. Three classes of substances are associated with abuse, but may not cause physiologic dependence. These include cocaine, phencyclidine (PCP) or similarly acting arylcyclohexylamines, and hallucinogens.

Toxicities may also occur secondary to ingestion of heavy metals such as lead, mercury, arsenic, manganese, and calcium as well as from fumes and gases in gasoline, and insecticides. However, toxicities are most commonly associated with alcohol, over-the-counter drugs, prescription drugs, and drugs of abuse.

In the assessment of a potential change in mental status secondary to toxicity, "assessing and treating the patient, not the poison" is a guiding principle. Priorities in the evaluation of a patient for a toxicity include the history provided by the patient and other informants, the patient's physical examination, his mental status, and the continuing monitoring of his vital signs and clinical condition. Relying solely for guidance on specific laboratory values may be misleading. For example, a blood alcohol level of 300 mg% in a patient who rarely drinks may be near the lethal level for that patient, whereas the same blood alcohol level may not even result in intoxication for another person who is a chronic alcoholic. The pharmacokinetics of a particular agent or toxic substance include such properties as its half-life, its distribution in the body, and its route of excretion. Knowledge of pharmacokinetics is crucial in treatment decisions such as whether to utilize diuresis, dialysis, or hemoperfusion. A thorough discussion of toxicokinetics is beyond the scope of this book.

The frequency with which substances are involved in toxicities or psychiatric side-effects reflects both the clinical properties of the respective agent as well as its availability and degree of usage in society at large. For example, at one time the emergency room psychiatrist was frequently called upon to evaluate and treat patients with mental status changes secondary to LSD use. At present, the marked emotional lability, acts of impulsiveness, and belligerence secondary to phencyclidine abuse are commonplace, whereas organic hallucinosis caused by LSD is relatively rare. It is important for the clinician to be aware of patterns and fashions of substance use and abuse in his community and to be apprised of those laboratories that can do fast and accurate analyses of such substances.

The clinical laboratory is utilized to screen a patient's blood, urine, and tissues for the presence of substances that may lead to organic brain disease, and where possible to provide quantitative analyses of toxic substances. Emergency rooms commonly utilize "drug screens" that may quickly assess the presence of a potentially toxic agent. Such screens are assays of serum, urine, vomitus, and body tissues (such as hair for PCP) as indicated. A common battery will include the following: (1) serum tests for presence of salicylates and a urine screen for acetaminophen; (2) a serum test for alcohol (urine is utilized only if serum levels are not available, and quantification of alcohol levels is vital); (3) qualitative and quantitative analyses of methanol and isopropanol from serum; (4) urine tests for the presence of opiates and benzodiazepines. If opiates or benzodiazepines are detected, quantitations are performed from serum. Table 3-7 summarizes the therapeutic, toxic, and

(*Text continues on p. 110.*)

TABLE 3-7. Blood Level Data for Clinical Assessment in Psychiatry

Drug	Blood Levels		
	Therapeutic or Normal	*Toxic*	*Lethal*
Acetaminophen (Tylenol)	1.0–2.0 mg%	15.0 mg%	150.0 mg%
Acetylsalicylic acid (salicylate)	10–30.0 mg%	>39.0 mg%	50.0 mg%
Aminophylline (theophylline)	1.0–2.0 mg%	3.0–4.0 mg%	21.0–25.0 mg%
Amitriptyline (Elavil)	5.0–20.0 μg%	>50.0 g%	1.0–2.0 mg%
Amphetamines	2.0–3.0 μg%	50.0 μg%	200.0 μg%
Arsenic	0.0–2.0 μg%	0.10 mg%	1.5 mg%
Barbiturates			
Short acting	0.1 mg%	0.7 mg%	1.0 mg%
Intermediate acting	0.1–0.5 mg%	1.0–3.0 mg%	>3.0 mg%
Phenobarbital	1.5–3.9 mg%	4.0–6.0 mg%	8.0–>15 mg%
Barbital	1.0 mg%	6.0–8.0 mg%	>10.0 mg%
Bromide	5.0–30 mg%	50–150 mg%	200 mg%
Carbamazepine (Tegretol)	0.8–1.2 mg%	>1.5 mg%	
Chloral hydrate (Noctec)	0.2–1.0 mg%	10.0 mg%	25.0 mg%

TABLE 3-7.   *(Continued)*

Drug	Blood Levels		
	Therapeutic or Normal	*Toxic*	*Lethal*
Chlordiazepoxide (Librium)	0.1–0.3 mg%	0.55 mg%	2.0 mg%
Chlorpromazine (Thorazine)	0.05 mg%	0.1–0.2 mg%	0.3–1.2 mg%
Cocaine	5.0–15.0 μg%	90.0 μg%	0.1–2.0 mg%
Codeine	2.5–12.0 μg%		20.0–60.0 μg%
Desipramine (Norpramin)	15.0–30.0 μg%	>50.0 μg%	1.0–2.0 mg%
Diazepam (Valium)	0.05–0.25 mg%	0.5–2.0 mg%	>2.0 mg%
Digoxin	0.06–0.20 μg%	0.21–0.90 μg%	1.5 μg%
Diphenhydramine (Benadryl)	1.0–10.0 μg%	0.5 mg%	>1.0 mg%
Dolophine (methadone)	30.0–110.0 μg%	0.2 mg%	>0.4 mg%
Doriden (Glutethimide)	0.02–0.08 mg%	1.0–8.0 mg%	3.0–10.0 mg%
Doxepin (Sinequan)	10.0–25.0 μg%	50.0–200.0 μg%	>1.0 mg%
Ethanol		100.0 mg% (legal intoxication)	350.0 mg%
Haloperidol (Haldol)	0.05–0.9 μg%	1.0–4.0 mg%	
Imipramine (Tofranil)	15.0–25.0 μg%	50.0–150.0 μg%	0.2 mg%
Lead	0.0–30.0 μg%	130 μg%	110.0–350.0 μg%
Lithium	0.42–0.83 mg% (0.6–1.2 mEq/l)	1.39 mg% (2.0 mEq/l)	>3.47 mg% (>4.0 mEq/l)
LSD		0.1–0.4 μg%	
Meperidine (Demerol)	0.03–0.10 mg%	0.5 mg%	3.0 mg%
Meprobamate	0.8–2.4 mg%	6.0–10.0 mg%	14.0–35.0 mg%
Mercury	0.0–8 μg%	100 μg%	600.0 μg%
Methamphetamine	0.02–0.06 mg%	0.06–0.5 mg%	1.0–4.0 mg%

TABLE 3-7. *(Continued)*

Drug	Blood Levels		
	Therapeutic or Normal	*Toxic*	*Lethal*
Methanol		20.0 mg%	>89.0 mg%
Methaqualone (Quaalude)	0.3–0.6 mg%	1.0–3.0 mg%	>3.0 mg%
Methylphenidate (Ritalin)	1.0–6.0 μg%	80.0 μg%	230.0 μg%
Morphine	10.0 μg%		5.0–400 μg% (free morphine from heroin)
Nortriptyline (Aventyl)	12.0–16.0 μg%	0.05 mg%	1.3 mg%
Oxycodone (Percodan)	1.7–3.6 μg%	20.0–500.0 μg%	
Paraldehyde	2.0–11.0 mg%	20.0–40.0 mg%	>50.0 mg%
Pentazocine (Talwin)	0.01–0.06 mg%	0.2–0.5 mg%	1.0–2.0 mg%
Perphenazine (Trilafon)	0.5 μg%	100.0 μg%	
Phencyclidine (PCP)		0.7–24.0 μg%	100.0–500.0 μg%
Phenytoin (Dilantin)	1.0–2.0 mg%	2.0–5.0 mg%	>10 mg%
Primidone (Mysoline)	0.5–1.2 mg%	5.0–8.0 mg%	10.0 mg%
Propoxyphene (Darvon)	5.0–20.0 μg%	30.0–60.0 μg%	80.0–200.0 μg%
Propanolol (Inderal)	2.5–20.0 μg%		0.8–1.2 mg%
Quindine	0.03–0.6 mg%	1.0 mg%	3.0–5.0 mg%
Quinine	0.18 mg%		1.2 mg%
Thioridazine (Mellaril)	0.10–0.15 mg%	1.0 mg%	2.0–8.0 mg%
Trifluoperazine (Stelazine)	0.08 mg%	0.12–0.3 mg%	0.3–0.8 mg%

(Reprinted with permission: Winek L: Drug and Chemical Blood-Level Data. Pittsburgh, PA, Fisher Scientific, 1985) lethal levels of medications that are most commonly involved in the initiation of psychological symptoms.

ELECTRICAL DIAGNOSIS AND BRAIN IMAGING TECHNIQUES IN EVALUATING PSYCHIATRIC DISORDERS

Electroencephalogram (EEG)

Technical methods of amplifying and measuring electrical activity in the brain through electrodes placed on the scalp were introduced in 1929. In obtaining an electroencephalogram (EEG) recording, 16 electrodes are placed in standardized positions over the scalp. In addition, reference electrodes are positioned on the ears and at the vertex. Utilizing great amplification, a 7-mm deflection is calibrated to correspond with a 50-μV discharge in the brain. These deflections are recorded on a tracing that consists of 8 or 16 channels, each of which comprises a simultaneous printing of different electrical potentials transmitted by a standardized pair of electrodes.

Brain electrical activity recorded by the EEG is evaluated according to the frequency, amplitude, and form of brain wave tracings. The frequency of brain waves is measured in cycles per second (c/s), 1 Hz corresponding to 1 c/s. In a normal adult during the awake state, frequencies range from 8 Hz to 13 Hz. Such frequencies constitute an alpha rhythm. Frequencies from 4 Hz to 7 Hz are termed theta activity, and frequencies less than 4 Hz are termed delta activity. Brain rhythms that are faster than 14 Hz are called beta activity. The amplitude of the brain waves of a normal adult averages 50 μV to 70 μV, although extensive variation of voltage routinely occurs in normal persons. EEG activity of children and of adults during sleep states or in response to stimuli may show normal variations from the characteristic frequencies and amplitudes. Abnormal frequencies, forms, and amplitudes may occur secondary to various pathologic conditions including seizure disorders, metabolic disease, degenerative disease, inflammatory disease, a vascular lesion, and with toxic substances including drugs.

To enhance the ability of the EEG to diagnose brain disorders, certain techniques are used to exaggerate or elicit latent EEG abnormalities that are not evident in a routine tracing. Included among these techniques are the following:

1. Special placement of nasopharyngeal electrodes or sphenoidal electrodes enables the EEG to pick up abnormal electrical activity in the anterior temporal lobes that may otherwise be missed. This is impor-

tant in the diagnosis of temporal lobe epilepsy. In this disorder partial complex seizures often give rise to behavioral abnormalities.

2. Hyperventilation may elicit three per second spike-and-wave patterns that occur with petit mal epilepsy or other abnormal focal slow wave patterns.

3. Photic stimulation is a procedure wherein flashing lights emitted from strobes may evoke spike-and-slow-wave activity that is otherwise suppressed.

4. Drug activation is based on the principle that many medications, including enthylenetetrazol (Metrazol) and methohexital, enhance epileptiform activity. This technique is rarely used because of the side-effects of medication and the danger in precipitating a seizure.

5. Sleep deprivation or sedative-induced sleep both are used to reveal or enhance pathological spikes or EEG patterns not otherwise detected by routine EEG testing.

During the 1930s and 1940s the EEG was used principally to explore brain activity during conscious states. Loomis and colleagues (1935) were among the first to observe and report changes in EEG patterns during sleep. Sleep stages may be summarized as follows:

Stage 0: wakefulness with the eyes closed. EEG recordings are principally alpha waves (8 c/s to 12 c/s) with low voltage, mixed frequency activity.

Stage 1: the nonconscious state associated with sleep. EEG activity is beta (14 c/s to 30 c/s) and theta activity (4 c/s to 8 c/s). EEG voltage is relatively low, and sharp waves may be present at the vertex.

Stage 2: EEG tracings show prominent sinusoidal bursts of waves at 12 c/s to 14 c/s (called sleep spindles) and high-amplitude negative waves that are followed by positive activity (termed K-complexes). High-amplitude delta waves (0.5 c/s to 3.5 c/s) may also be found in stage 2. In the background are irregular theta waves.

Stage 3: delta waves constitute 20% to 50% of the EEG pattern. These waves have characteristically high amplitudes.

Stage 4: EEG pattern contains over 50% slow-wave sleep. Persons in stage 4 sleep have high thresholds of arousal, and if allowed to sleep after significant sleep deprivation, will show increases in the amounts of stage 4 sleep. Stages 1 through 4 sleep are collectively known as *non-REM (NREM) sleep.*

There are four to five periods of desynchronized sleep per night that are called rapid eye movement (REM) sleep. The total time taken up by REM periods is approximately 1½ hours, or about 20% of total sleep time. In humans, dreaming occurs predominantly during REM periods.

Although there is no specific EEG abnormality in schizophrenics, the percentage of diffusely abnormal EEGs is two to three times that found in the normal population. Included among abnormal EEG patterns in schizophrenic patients are the increased presence of delta activity, a reduction in stages 3 and 4 of sleep, and a reduction in REM sleep.

REM sleep is characterized by rapid, conjugate eye movements, irregularity in pulse rate, increased respiratory rate, and increased blood pressure. REM sleep also is accompanied by generalized muscular atony, which is interrupted by movements of small muscle groups, and in men, by full or partial penile erections. REM latency is defined as the time that elapses between the point at which a person falls asleep (stage 1 sleep) and the point at which he begins the first rapid eye movement phase of sleep. A shortened REM latency period (less than 20 minutes) has been proposed by many investigators as a biological marker for depression. In the absence of narcolepsy, a significantly increased number of patients with depression show short REM latency and concomitant cortisol hypersecretion as compared to a group of nondepressed patients. Because this feature is found in other pathological situations, it must be used in combination with other data to help establish a diagnosis of major depressive illness.

Recently, there has been an increased use of computers to enhance the utility of EEG diagnosis. A technique known as brain electrical activity and mapping (BEAM) employs the computer to process EEG and evoked potential data derived from 20 or more electrical leads. The computer transforms electrical data into multicolored maps of the brain, which can be applied to investigate a wide variety of psychiatric and neurologic conditions. These conditions include epilepsy, brain tumors, affective disorders, schizophrenia, and even dyslexia. Supporters of this new approach maintain that computed topographic mapping of electrophysiological data in psychiatry has an advantage over CT scans, PET scans, and cerebral blood flow studies in that the patient receives no radiation. At present, brain electrical activity mapping and other computer-assisted EEG technologies are principally used for research. Nevertheless, it is likely that with technological advances such techniques will have clinical applications in the near future.

Computed Tomography (CT)

Computed tomography (CT, formerly known as CAT, scan) of the brain is a method by which minute variations in the density of bone, cerebrospinal fluid, blood, vessels, and gray and white matter can be assessed by utilizing an X-ray source, computer processing, and photographic material. Many brain lesions larger than 1.5 cm in cross section can be visualized. In addition, ventricular size and displacement, hemorrhage, softened and edematous brain tissue, abscess, and other brain changes may be visualized upon CT. CT has been a revolutionary diagnostic procedure in neurology and is invaluable to psychiatry in the recognition of those mental disorders that may be related to brain disease. In addition, psychiatric investigators have utilized the CT in efforts to diagnose or to monitor the course of disorders traditionally considered to be psychiatric. Brain changes in patients with schizophrenia have been reported by numerous investigators. In 1976, it was reported that schizophrenics show enlargement of lateral ventricles when compared with control populations. It was later found that similar changes could be detected in other psychiatric disorders, which led to the questioning of the specificity of this finding in schizophrenia. Other studies used the ventricles-to-brain ratio (VBR), which measures the area of the body of the lateral ventricles divided by the area of the brain at the same level of the ventricles. Most controlled studies utilizing the VBR have reported larger lateral ventricular size in patients with schizophrenia. In addition, some researchers have reported the widening of cortical sulci in patients with schizophrenia, but other investigators have failed to show this phenomenon. Further studies have looked at cerebral asymmetries, and have found that whereas right-handed people usually show wider frontal lobes in the right hemisphere and wider occipital lobes in the left hemisphere, in schizophrenics this normal asymmetry is reversed. Other investigators have not been able to document this finding. Recently, Weinberger and associates reported atrophy of the cerebellar vermis in patients with schizophrenia, and this finding has been confirmed by other investigators. The structural brain abnormalities that have been shown on CT scan in patients with schizophrenia have been linked to the following clinical situations and findings: (1) a chronic debilitating course with poor response to treatment with antipsychotic medication; (2) a higher instance of extrapyramidal side-effects when treated with neuroleptics; (3) a preponderance of negative symptoms; (4) an increased incidence of suicide attempts; (5) an increase in the percentage of first degree family members who have a history of schizophrenia.

CT also has been utilized to document brain changes in patients with affective disorders. However, the findings in this area are even more controversial and seemingly less specific than those found in schizophrenic patients. Numerous investigators have suggested that changes in ventricular size in both schizophrenic patients and patients with manic-depressive illness may relate to chronic treatment with antipsychotic and other psychotropic medications, and that the increased VBR in both categories of patients actually may be reversible. CT changes in patients with dementia have been reviewed in the assessment of regional cortical functioning (see Chap. 4). At present, CT changes in patients with major psychiatric disorders have more theoretical interest than diagnostic value. The authors believe that as techniques and technologies inevitably improve with CT and derivative analyses, this approach will provide useful data for the diagnosis and monitoring of major psychiatric disorders.

Magnetic Resonance Imaging (MRI)

Magnetic resonance imaging (MRI) promises to be a major advance over previous diagnostic techniques in achieving a highly defined image of the brain in living humans. MRI images of the brain are accomplished by placing the patient's head in an exceedingly powerful electromagnetic field, abruptly removing the magnetic force, and using sensors, a computer, and a monitor to organize subsequent electrical changes into images of brain structure. The electrical changes detected by MRI involve energy transfers of hydrogen protons of the body. The technique is valuable not only for revealing highly detailed images of fine structures of the brain, but also for providing such images of other organs throughout the body. In the brain, white and gray matter can be differentiated, and the presence of lesions can be detected more precisely with MRI than with any previous brain imaging technique. MRI is finding many uses in neurology as well as psychiatry. Its capacity to differentiate gray from white matter has enabled MRI to aid in establishing definitive diagnoses of such illnesses as multiple sclerosis. In addition, mass effects of tumors are better seen through MRI than through other procedures, but bone pathology and small calcifications are not, at this point, so effectively visualized as they are on CT scans. At the present time, the uses of MRI in the diagnosis and monitoring of psychiatric illnesses are being explored. Efforts are being made to substantiate brain changes that have been reported in schizophrenic populations and patients with affective illness upon CT scanning. Although there has not yet been a specific finding on MRI that is pathognomonic of a psychiatric illness, optimism for this procedure in the diagnosis of psychiatric illness is high. MRI has advantages over CT scan in that it is safer than CT scan, which uses ionizing radiation, and because its images derive from chemical interactions within tissues and therefore can provide information about energy transfers within the brain. CT scan relies only on two-dimensional anatomic features that are based upon the specific gravity of tissue. This advantage of MRI over CT provides the promise of the imaging of specific metabolic and neurotransmitter defects that occur in psychiatric disorders such as schizophrenia and major

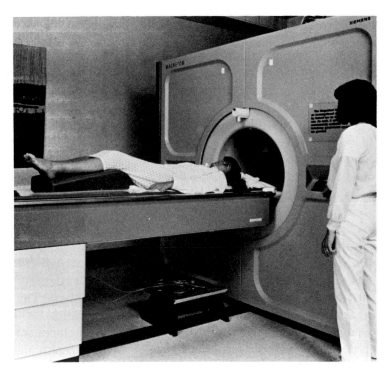

FIG. 3-2. MRI scanner in general hospital setting. (Photograph by Mike Murphy.)

affective illness. The constraints in the use of MRI involve the significant expense in setting up the instrument hardware, which requires huge magnets that must be shielded by massive structures, and secondly the time-consuming nature of the procedure. At the present time, for example, CT scans of the brain generally last 15 minutes, whereas MRI scans of the brain commonly take 1 hour to administer. Figure 3-2 shows an MRI apparatus in a general hospital setting.

Imaging Based on Brain Function: Positron Emission Tomography and Regional Cerebral Blood Flow

Positron Emission Tomography (PET)

Although laboratory diagnostic techniques have depended upon the capacity of a test to isolate brain lesions through structural alterations of the brain, newer diagnostic tests produce images through the measurement of brain function. Positron emission tomography (PET) makes use of the brain's specific and focalized utilization of glucose during times of brain activity. The theory underlying PET scan is that specific sets of neurons utilize increased amounts of glucose during times of increased activity. In this technique, radioactive deoxyglucose, or F-2-deoxy-2-fluoro-D-glucose (F-FDG), is injected into a vein of the patient. The patient is then placed into a device that can measure the presence, in a highly specific and localized fashion, of F-FDG in the brain. These data are translated through the use of computers and imaging devices into detailed and specifically colored images of brain function. In this fashion, parameters of selective functioning of the brain can be detected to correspond with neuroanatomical regions of approximately 0.5 cm. With this technique, specific changes in brain functioning have been documented in "normal patients" who are asked to perform specific tasks. By comparing normative values of localized brain functions during specific activities with the values of patients with psychiatric disorders, investigators have documented reproducible, nonspecific changes in patients with schizophrenia and major affective illness. Thus far, in assessing schizophrenic patients with PET scans and comparing them to control populations, the major finding has been reduced metabolism in the anterior cortex relative to the posterior cortex in the schizophrenic patient. Other studies have shown lower metabolic ratios in central gray matter on the left side, which includes the left anterior caudate nucleus, globus pallidus, thalamus, and even parts of the internal capsule and ventricles. Investigators have also found higher metabolism of glucose in the left hippocampus and hypothalamus. Although these data are preliminary and need to be reproduced in other schizophrenic patients as well as tested in other diagnostic populations, they suggest that schizophrenics have abnormalities both at cortical and subcortical levels of neural activity. The lower metabolic activities that have been found in schizophrenics upon PET evaluation have led to speculation that the condition may, in part, explain problems that many schizophrenics have with social judgment and impulse control. Because the PET procedures are in their infancy, and because such tests are exceedingly expensive to administer and involve risks of exposing patients to radioactivity, the value of the PET scan in diagnosing and monitoring psychiatric illnesses is presently limited to research. However, as the PET scan becomes refined and less invasive, this novel technique will likely lead to newer technological developments with important clinical value for psychiatry. In neurology at the present time, clear and specific increases in regional glucose utilization during seizures can be documented using PET technology, and investigators are attempting to use the PET scan to detect metabolic derangement, which can distinguish Alzheimer's disease from benign senescence.

Cerebral Blood Flow (CBF)

Cerebral blood flow (CBF), also called in the literature regional cerebral blood flow (RCBF), makes use of measured changes in blood flow in specific areas of the brain, both in function and in dysfunction. Although there have been many techniques for measuring CBF, presently the most useful and least invasive technique involves the inhalation of radioactive xenon (^{133}xenon). Cerebral blood flow is calculated by measuring sequential changes as the freely diffusible radioisotopes are cleared from the brain. Scintillation detectors are utilized to record the progressive decline in radioactivity over the scalp, which gives a measurement of regional cerebral blood flow. In studying the schizophrenic population, most investigators have found reduced CBF values for all brain regions. The reduction in gray matter perfusion is more extensive, according to several studies, in anterior brain regions, particularly on the left side. Investigators have also studied CBF in patients with depression and alcoholism. These two groups, as a whole, also show significant reduction in cerebral perfusion. Because such studies are in their infancy, these findings remain controversial and are not consistently reproducible. Cerebral blood flow changes in dementia have been evaluated more extensively, with most studies showing global reductions in brain blood flow and metabolism in patients with dementias. An exciting potential for CBF in psychiatric research is in the study of the regional effects of psychotropic agents on the brain. At present, CBF studies in psychiatry and neurology are limited to research uses.

THE RISK-BENEFIT RATIO OF LABORATORY TESTING

As with any other procedure in medicine, biological and laboratory testing in psychiatry has risks as well as benefits. The principal psychological risk of these tests is that the patient or his family will misunderstand the role and impact of the test in the overall diagnostic and treatment regimen. For example, a depressed patient, aware that his dexamethasone suppression test is "positive," might erroneously believe his overall problem to be his "hormones." Such a patient may prefer biological explanations of his problems and seize upon every opportunity to deny the existence of the psychological component of his illness. This patient may believe medication to be the sole treatment necessary to reverse his hormonal problem, and thereby "cure" his depression. Such an attitude significantly interferes with the psychiatrist's ability to initiate individual psychotherapy, family interventions, and other supportive therapies that ultimately may have greater impact than medication on the long-term treatment of the patient's depression. The psychiatrist should communicate to both the patient and his family that biologic and other laboratory evaluations in psychiatry are merely adjuncts that are not in themselves therapeutic, and that the return to normal of clinical laboratory values does not necessarily imply a recovery from the psychiatric disorder. The reverse is also true: a severely depressed patient with a normal DST may feel that solely psychological treatments will prove beneficial, and therefore will refuse antidepressant treatment.

A second risk is that clinical problems may be *elicited* during the actual administration of clinical laboratory tests. Psychiatrists, like other physicians, often are not aware of the physical and psychological stresses to which their patients are subjected during the administration of laboratory tests. Some clinicians are unaware that CT scans of the brain require the patient to be immobilized, and his head inserted into a complex and formidable-looking machine—often in a room devoid of other persons and of familiar, comforting objects such as pictures or furniture. A patient with a paranoid psychosis requires prior explanations by the psychiatrist (and perhaps even "field trips," with the psychiatrist accompanying the patient to the site of the laboratory test) to gain his cooperation. The patient may find it comforting to have his psychiatrist either in the room, when possible, or outside the room while a test is being performed.

The potential benefit of each test should be weighed against the physical pain or discomfort inherent in a particular laboratory evaluation. For example, many of the more recent biological tests in psychiatry require that venipuncture be repeated many times during the course of the patient's evaluation and treatment. We do not believe that there are any "routine" laboratory tests; clinical judgment must always be employed in deciding whether or not to order a test. For example, information derived from a lumbar puncture may certainly be of value in diagnosing a patient with extensive psychomotor retardation. However, if the patient has a long history of schizophrenia, is receiving high doses of chlorpromazine, exhibits mask-like face, cogwheeling, and other extrapyramidal features, it is far more likely that his motor problems are related to parkinsonian side-effects from medication or to catatonia, than they are to a life-threatening, infectious process that may be diagnosed from analyzing samples of the cerebrospinal fluid. In such a case it is likely that the psychiatrist, exercising good clinical judgment, may forego subjecting the patient to the immobilization by staff members and to the discomfort of a spinal tap.

All experienced clinicians recognize that mistakes occur involving laboratory tests. Such mistakes include problems in securing biological samples from a patient (such as contaminations or insufficient quantities); logistical problems (such as placing a label with a name of one patient on the test tube containing a sample from another); and actual human and mechanical errors in the analysis of the sample. Therefore, the clinician should be cautious not to overreact in his communication of any test result to a patient. Later, if there are conflicting data, the patient may develop understandable mistrust of and resistance to the entire evaluation process and treatment plan. Finally, some clinicians may use testing to avoid contact with the patient. These clinicians may seek to save time that is necessary in securing the requisite psychiatric history, or even, unconsciously, to avoid what for them may be unpleasant or unsettling symptomatologies in the patient.

SUGGESTED READING

Andreasen NC, Olsen SA, Dennert JW, et al: Ventricular enlargement in schizophrenia: Relationship to positive and negative symptoms. Am J Psychiatry 139:297, 1982

Andreasen NC, Smith MR, Jacoby CG, et al: Ventricular enlargement in schizophrenia: Definition and prevalence. Am J Psychiatry 139:292, 1982

Ariel RN, Golden CJ, Bert RA, et al: Regional cerebral blood flow in schizophrenics. Arch Gen Psychiatry 40:258, 1983

Bassuk EL, Schoonover SC, Gelenberg AJ: The Practitioner's Guide to Psychoactive Drugs. New York, Plenum, 1983

Besson JAO, Corrigan FM, Foreman EI, et al: Differentiating senile dementia of Alzheimer type and multi infarct dementia by proton NMR imaging. Lancet, Vol 2, p 789, Oct. 1, 1983

Buchsbaum MS, Ingvar DH, Kessler R, et al: Cerebral glucography with position tomography, use in normal subjects and in patients with schizophrenia. Arch Gen Psychiatry 39:251, 1982

Carrol BJ, Feinberg M, Greden JF, et al: A specific laboratory test for the diagnosis of melancholia. Arch Gen Psychiatry 38:15, 1981

Cooper TB, Carrol BJ: Monitoring lithium dose levels: Estimation of lithium in blood and other body fluids. J Clin Psychopharmacol 1:53, 1981

DeMyer MK, Hendrie HC, Gilmor RL, et al: Magnetic resonance imaging in psychiatry. Psychiatr Annals 15(4):262, 1985

Extein I, Pottash ALC, Gold MS, et al: Changes in TSH response to TRH in affective illness. In Post RM, Ballenger JC (eds): Neurobiology of Mood Disorders. Baltimore, Williams & Wilkins, 1984

Farkas T, Wolfe AP, Jaeger J: Regional brain glucose metabolism in chronic schizophrenia—A positron emission transaxial tomographic study. Arch Gen Psychiatry 41:293, 1984

Freeman LM (ed): Freeman and Johnson's Clinical Radionuclide Imaging, 3rd ed. New York, Grune & Stratton, 1984

Gold MS, Kronig MH: Comprehensive thyroid evaluation in psychiatric patients. In Hall RCW (ed): Handbook of Psychiatric Diagnostic Procedures, Vol 1. Jamaica, NY, Spectrum Publications, 1984

Gur RE: Positron Emission Tomography in Psychiatry Disorders. Psychiatr Annals 15 (4):268, 1985

Gur RE, Skolnick BE, et al: Brain function in psychiatric disorders: I. Regional cerebral blood flow in medicated schizophrenics. Arch Gen Psychiatry 40:1250, 1983

Gur RE, Gur RC, Skolnick BE, et al: Brain function in psychiatric disorders: III. Regional cerebral blood flow in unmedicated schizophrenics. Arch Gen Psychiatry 42:329, 1985

Hall RCW, Beresford TP: Handbook of Psychiatric Diagnostic Procedures Vol 1 and 2. Jamaica, New York, Spectrum Publications, 1984

Halsted JA, Halsted CH: The Laboratory in Clinical Medicine: Interpretation and Application, 2nd ed. Philadelphia, WB Saunders, 1981

James AE, Price RR, Rollo FD, et al: Nuclear magnetic resonance imaging: A promising technique. JAMA 247:1331, 1982

Kautzky R, Zulch KJ, Wende S, et al: Neuroradiology: A Neuropathological Approach. New York, Springer–Verlag, 1982

Kupfer DJ: REM latency: A psychobiological marker for primary depressive disease. Biol Psychiatry 11:159, 1976

Lassen NA: Cerebral blood flow determined by radioactive diffusible tracers in special regard to the use of xenon-133. In Passonneau JV, Hawkins RA, Lust WD et al (eds): Cerebral Metabolism and Neural Function. Baltimore/London, Williams & Wilkins, 1980

Luchins DJ, Meltzer HY: A blind controlled study of occipital cerebral asymmetry in schizophrenia. Psychiatry Res 10:87, 1983

Mathew RJ: Cerebral blood flow in psychiatric disorders. Psychiatr Annals 15 (4):257, 1985

Mathew RJ, Duncan GC, Weinman ML, et al: A study of regional cerebral blood flow in schizophrenia. Arch Gen Psychiatry 39:1121, 1982

Morihisa JM (ed): Brain Imaging in Psychiatry. Washington, D. C., American Psychiatric Press, 1984

Morihisa JM: Computerized topographic mapping of electrophysiologic data in psychiatry. Psychiatr Annals 15 (4):250, 1985

Morihisa JM, Duffy FH, Mendelson WB, et al: The use of brain electrical mapping (BEAM) as an exploratory technique to delineate regional differences between schizophrenic patients and control subjects. In Flor-Henry P, Gruzelier J (eds): Laterality and Psychopathology. New York, Elsevier, 1983

Morihisa JM, Duffy FH, Wyatt RJ: Brain electrical activity mapping (BEAM) in schizophrenic patients. Arch Gen Psychiatry 40:719, 1983

Nasrallah HA, Coffman JA: Computerized tomography in psychiatry. Psychiatr Annals 15 (4):239, 1985

Nasrallah HA, McCalley-Whiters M, Pfohl B: Clinical significance of large cerebral ventricles in manic males. Psychiatry Res 13:155, 1984

Phelps ME: The biochemical basis of cerebral function and its investigation in humans with positron CT. Proceedings of the American Psychiatric Association 137th Annual Meeting, Los Angeles, May 5–11, 1984

Risberg J, Gustafson L, Prohovnik I: rCBF measurements by [133]xenon inhalation: Applications in neuropsychology and psychiatry. Prog Nucl Med 7:82, 1981

Rumack BH, Peterson RG: Clinical toxicology. In Doull J, Klaassen CD, Amdur MO (eds): Toxicology: The Basic Science of Poisons, 2nd ed, pp 667–696. New York, Macmillan, 1980

Sachar EJ: Endocrine abnormalities in depression. In Paykel ES (ed): Handbook of Affective Disorders. New York, Guilford Press, 1982

Spar JE, Gerner R: Does the dexamethasone suppression test distinguish dementia from depression? Am J Psychiatry 139:238, 1982

Sramek JJ, Baumgartner WA, Tallos JA, et al: Hair analysis for detection of phencyclidine in newly admitted psychiatric patients. Am J Psychiatry 142:950, 1985

Svirbely J: Toxicology and therapeutic drug monitoring (TDM). In Kaplan LA, Pesce AJ (eds): Clinical Chemistry: Theory, Analysis and Correlation, pp 1327–1390. St Louis, CV Mosby Company, 1984

Task Force on the Use of Laboratory Tests in Psychiatry: Tricyclic antidepresants—blood level measurements and clinical outcome: An APA task force report. Am J Psychiatry 142(2):155, 1985

Tsai L, Nasrallah HA, Jacoby CG: Hemispheric asymmetry in schizophrenia and mania: A controlled study and a critical review. Arch Gen Psychiatry 40:1286, 1983

Weinberger DR, DeLisi LE, Perman GP, et al: CT scans in schizophreniform disorder and other acute psychiatric patients. Arch Gen Psychiatry 39:778, 1982

Williams H: Textbook of Endocrinology, 6th ed. Philadelphia, WB Saunders, 1981

Winek CL: Drug and Chemical Blood-Level Data. Pittsburgh, PA, Fisher Scientific, 1985

4

Evaluation of Regional Cortical Functioning

Frontal Lobes 125
  Psychological Changes 125
    Social and Behavorial Changes 125
    Affective Changes 126
    Intellectual Changes 126
  Neurological Changes 128
  Laboratory Tests 128

Temporal Lobes 129
  Language Disturbances in Temporal Lobe Impairment 129
    Clinical Types of Aphasia 130
      Global Aphasia 130
      Broca's Aphasia 130
      Wernicke's Aphasia 131
      Conduction Aphasia 132
      Anomic Aphasia 132
  Affective Changes in Temporal Lobe Impairment 135
  Perceptual Changes in Temporal Lobe Impairment 135
  Memory Disturbances in Temporal Lobe Impairment 135

Parietal Lobes 137

Occipital Lobes 138

Diffuse Cortical Impairment 138
  Delirium 139
  Dementia 139
  Pseudodementia 140

In the evaluation of cortical impairment, the psychiatrist focuses his attention chiefly on assessing the cerebral cortex, where lesions may give rise to changes in behavior, emotions, and cognition. This is in contrast to the neurologist, who is more likely to concentrate on impairment of sensory and motor functions as revealed by the neurological examination.

A comprehensive study of psychological and emotional problems is difficult without an understanding of cortical functions and dysfunctions. The importance of this is obvious when one understands the incidence of damage to cortical regions from trauma, stroke, tumor, and toxicities. Each year in the United States there are over 1 million new cases of brain injury. The incidence of traumatic brain injury in the United States is 180 per 100,000 population, and this is approximately one-half the incidence of schizophrenia. Stroke, which often affects the cortical regions of the brain, is the fourth most costly of all illnesses, behind cancer, injuries from automobiles, and heart disease. Cortical injury invariably leads to psychiatric changes. These

TABLE 4-1. Architectonic Areas

Brodmann Areas	Gross Landmarks	Function, Known or Assumed
3-1-2-5	Postcentral gyrus	General sense
7	Anterior parietal area	Sensory association
4*	Precentral gyrus	Motor
6*	Posterior frontal area	Motor organization
8	Superior frontal gyrus	Contains major part of frontal eye field
17	Occipital pole, calcarine fissure	Visual
18-19	Surround 17	Visual association, automatic eye motor
41	Superior temporal gyrus, floor lateral fissure	Auditory
42	Surrounds 41	Auditory association
44	Inferior frontal gyrus, pars triangularis (Broca's convolution)	Motor speech on left in right-handed subjects, and vice versa
23-24	Gyrus cinguli	Erotic experience
9-10-45	Anterior frontal lobe	Planning, foresight

* 4 and 6 on medial check of hemisphere (superior frontal gyrus, sulcus cinguli, supplementary motor).

(Adapted from Elliott HC: Textbook of Neuroanatomy. Philadelphia, JB Lippincott, 1969. Reprinted with permission.)

changes may result from the neuronal lesion per se, or may be a psychological reaction to the traumatic event and disability, or, most commonly, they may be a combination of both. In the following section, emotional and behavioral disabilities secondary to cortical lesions will be discussed. Table 4-1 describes the respective functions of the specific cortical areas.

FRONTAL LOBES

Psychological Changes

The prefrontal and frontal regions of the cortex are especially vulnerable to traumatic injury resulting from automobile, occupational, and home accidents, and an ever-increasing number of athletic injuries. Apart from motor functions, the frontal lobes of the cortex are involved in the regulation of social behavior, the expression of emotion, and in cognition. The ability to focus, to concentrate, to attend, to reason, to use logic, to employ judgment, to abstract, to utilize concepts, and to carry out higher intellectual functions such as planning for the future depend on intact frontal lobe function. Damage to the frontal cortex may result in exacerbation of pre-existing characterologic or personality traits, as well as in the initiation of prominent symptoms in the following areas.

Social and Behavioral Changes

With injury to the frontal cortex, prominent pre-existing behavioral traits such as disorderliness, suspiciousness, argumentativeness, disruptiveness, and anxiousness become more pronounced. The patient may exhibit a lack of interest in social interactions and show apathy, which may include a global lack of concern for the consequences of his behavior. Some patients may show uncharacteristic lewdness with loss of social graces and inattention to personal appearance and hygiene. Intrusiveness, boisterousness, increased volume of speech, and pervasive profanity characterize some patients with frontal cortical impairment. Also present may be increased risk taking, unrestrained drinking of alcoholic beverages, indiscriminate selection of foods, and gluttony. An example is the patient with advanced Alzheimer's syndrome who removes all the desserts from a tray that is being circulated at the dinner table and then begins to gorge himself. Patients may also exhibit impulsivity and distractibility. Patients with severe frontal lobe damage may be unable to attend to a conversation, because they are distracted by and react to background stimuli, such as the sound of a radio in another room or the sight of a person walking by the window, or an internal stimulus, such as modest hunger, the desire for a cigarette, or the need to urinate. Occasionally, extensive deterioration of personal hygiene to the point of urinary and fecal incontinence may develop with extensive prefrontal cortical damage.

Affective Changes

Affective changes in a patient with frontal cortex injury include apathy, indifference, and shallowness. Thus, the patient with chronic prefrontal cortical damage is usually disinterested and withdrawn. However, he may intermittently show extreme lability of affect with irritability, manic states, and dyscontrol of rage and violent behavior. For example, a patient may exhibit profuse sobbing over a mildly sentimental event on a television program, or may shout and throw things when told that he is not allowed to smoke a cigarette in his bed. Manic-depressive illness and recurrent unipolar depressions are aggravated by prefrontal lesions. Investigators also have documented that major depressive episodes may occur *de novo* subsequent to injury to the prefrontal cortex.

Intellectual Changes

The intellectual changes that result from lesions in the prefrontal cortex involve reduced capacity to utilize language, symbols, and logic. Patients may express themselves with simple, short sentences in the same fashion as a young child or as a person learning a new language. The ability to use mathematics, to calculate, to process abstract information, and to reason is compromised. In diffuse lesions, the patient's ability to focus, to concentrate, or to be oriented to time and place also may be impaired.

The diagnosis of damage to prefrontal lobes of the cortex depends upon both the history and the mental status examination. Decreased attention and motivation, the slowing of mental processes, decreased ability to concentrate or to carry out planned activity, impulsivity, and impairment in social judgment, particularly with loss of concern over the consequences of lewd or aggressive actions, should raise the clinician's suspicion of frontal lobe lesions.

Neuropsychological testing on the Comprehensive and the Similarities subtests of the Wechsler Adult Intelligence Scale-Revised (WAIS-R) is useful in the assessment of prefrontal lobe changes. Examples of comprehensive subtest questions similar to that in the WAIS-R include the following: (1) Why do people take baths? (2) What are some reasons that many foods need to be refrigerated? (3) Why should people obey traffic signs? The following question is an example of verbal concept formation similar to that on the WAIS-R: How are the following items alike? (1) Roses and orchids; (2) Golf club and tennis racket; (3) Car and bicycle. Reasoning may be tested using the verbal and pictoral absurdity section from the Stanford–Binet test. In the assessment of verbal reasoning, the patient may be asked to tell an examiner what is foolish about a sentence. Examples of test statements are similar to the following: (1) A man lost both of his legs in an accident. Now he gets more tired riding his bicycle; (2) The mother cat gave birth to three kittens and two puppies; (3) The survivors of the airplane crash were buried the following day.

The use of proverbs to test frontal lobe functioning is commonly utilized by mental health professionals, but investigators have demonstrated this method's poor reliability in detecting deficits in abstract thinking. Some researchers suggest that fewer than 25% of adults without brain damage are able to comprehend fully and respond abstractly to proverbs. Furthermore, because during the course of chronic illnesses many patients may be asked the same proverb on numerous occasions, the clinician may be testing the temporal lobe's capacity for memory more than the frontal lobe's capacity to reason abstractly. Many of the common proverbs involve shared social and cultural values. Such proverbs are often bewildering to people from differing cultures and backgrounds, and therefore, are an inexact measure of their cognitive abilities. Nevertheless, by carefully choosing a proverb to match the patient's intelligence and cultural background and by utilizing unfamiliar proverbs for patients who have had extensive previous mental status testing, proverbs may add other data that suggest frontal lobe damage. The following are examples of common parables and sayings: (1) It is better to extend a hand than to throw a fist; (2) Penny wise and pound foolish; and (3) A bird in hand is worth two in the bush. The use of proverbs to detect subtle deficiencies in social judgment or in abstract reasoning may be more difficult in patients with more advanced educational backgrounds. A proverb that we invented for such purposes is: "People do not look in your window when it's raining outside." An abstract, nonconcrete, not overpersonalized response to this parable would be, "When a person has troubles of his own, he is less likely to look for the problems of other people." A concrete interpretation typical of a patient with frontal lobe disease would be, "Rain makes windows steam up so that it is impossible to look through them." A response that is too subjective and would suggest oversuspicion and possible paranoia would be, "Psychiatrists have no right prying into the business of innocent people." (A more extensive review of neuropsychological testing is found in Chap. 5.)

Neurological Changes

Patients who have severe frontal lobe atrophy, such as may be seen in tertiary syphilis or in advanced Alzheimer's disease, may show motor abnormalities upon neurological examination. Gait disturbances in the form of short, hesitant steps with imbalance and decreased capacity to make postural adjustments are common. The patient's speech may be slow and dysarthric. Pathological reflexes such as the sucking, the grasping, the snout, and palmomental reflexes may be present. As the disease advances, incontinence of urine resulting from decreased cortical inhibitory control of the urinary sphincter is common.

Laboratory Tests

Laboratory testing may or may not show decreased size of frontal cortical areas, widened sulci in this region, and slower, higher amplitude waves on the EEG.

Studies of schizophrenic patients with computed tomography (CT scan) have shown changes in the frontal cortex of patients with chronic schizophrenia. Investigators also have reported laterality shifts and hemispheric asymmetries of function in patients with chronic schizophrenia. For example, in normal right-handed persons, usually there is a wider frontal lobe in the right hemisphere and a wider occipital lobe in the left hemisphere. However, this normal asymmetry has been reported to be reversed in schizophrenic patients. Although some reports have confirmed this finding, other reports have not. Many studies have shown sulcal widening on CT scan of the frontal lobes of patients with chronic schizophrenia, and this is generally regarded as evidence of cortical atrophy. In studies of schizophrenic patients using cerebral blood flow technology, investigators have shown reduced frontal and increased occipital–temporal flows at rest. The recent testing of schizophrenic patients with positron emission tomography (PET scan) shows hypofrontality or a decreased metabolic functioning in the frontal lobes in those patients with advanced illness. Investigators believe that problems such as lability and poor capacity to utilize abstract reasoning (characteristics of the chronic schizophrenic patient) may be related to biologic changes in the frontal cortical area.

TEMPORAL LOBES

The main functions of the temporal cortex are the regulation of language, affect, perception, and memory. As opposed to the prefrontal cortex, laterality—or variance in the regulatory function between the right and left cortical regions—is significant. Trauma, stroke, tumor, seizure disorders, and chronic degenerative diseases are the most common causes of lesions in the temporal region.

Language Disturbances in Temporal Lobe Impairment

Although speech and language are complex functions requiring intactness of many areas of the brain, the mental representation of language lies predominantly in the temporal cortex and in the posterior inferior region of the frontal cortex known as Broca's area. *Aphasia* is defined as a language disturbance resulting from a brain lesion. The term does not refer to motoric irregularities of speech or articulation, but rather to true linguistic dysfunction such as in syntax, comprehension, or the capacity to choose words. In most right-handed persons, aphasias are usually due to lesions in the left hemisphere; however, in left-handed persons, where approximately 50% have right cortical dominance and 50% have left cortical dominance, aphasia may be the result of lesions in either the right or left hemisphere. Clinically, it has been found that patients whose affective disorders are treated with nondominant unilateral electroconvulsive therapy (ECT), in which stimulating electrodes are placed on the side of the scalp that is opposite to the hemisphere controlling language, have fewer side-effects involving memory and language. However, it is important to note that spacial disturbances may be increased with such placement.

Language disturbances are viewed conceptually in many different ways. Deficits in language may be classified by the fluency or the nonfluency of speech. In nonfluent aphasias, the rate of output of words is decreased to fewer than 50 per minute. Obvious effort is required for the patient to initiate speech or thoughts. Therefore, spontaneity of expression is significantly reduced. Also, in nonfluent aphasias, the inflections and rhythms of speech are altered, and lengths of phrases tend to be shortened with an increased predilection for nouns and monosyllabic verbs. In fluent aphasias, speech expression is unaltered, whereas comprehension is impaired. Spontaneous speech may be increased dramatically. Logorrhea, jargon, neologisms, and paraphasias are typically present.

Defects in articulation with intact intellectual functions, normal comprehension, and memory are not aphasias but dysarthrias or anarthrias. Disturbances of speech due to problems with the larynx or its enervation or to problems of respiration are called *aphonias* or *dysphonias*.

Clinical Types of Aphasia

Precisely, *aphasia* connotes a complete loss in the capacity to communicate through language. True aphasias are rare, and the term *dysphasia* is more accurate in describing the typical impairment of language secondary to neurological lesions. Nevertheless, we use the term *aphasia* to connote dysphasia in keeping with the conventional use in medicine.

GLOBAL APHASIA

Global aphasia is the result of an extensive lesion of the cerebral cortex that usually involves the entire left temporal area and includes portions of the parietal and frontal lobes. Patients with global aphasia are not able to articulate, to comprehend, or to repeat speech. Such patients may produce repetitive, stereotyped sounds but are unable to form comprehensible words. They can neither read nor write. Because comprehension is impaired, patients with global aphasia are unable to carry out even the most simple commands. The most common lesion associated with global aphasia is the occlusion of the left internal carotid or of the middle cerebral artery, the latter of which nourishes most cortical areas involved in language. Hemorrhages, tumors, and other lesions may also give rise to this syndrome.

BROCA'S APHASIA

There is considerable variation in the language deficits commonly grouped under the name *Broca's aphasia*. In general, patients with Broca's aphasia comprehend both spoken and written language, whereas verbal expression is severely impaired. Nevertheless, all patients with aphasia have some problems with comprehension, so the term *expressive aphasia* (used by some interchangeably with Broca's aphasia) may be misleading. In the mildest form of Broca's aphasia, patients speak slowly and laboriously and use mainly nouns and verbs. Enunciation, intonation, accentuation, and phrasing are severely impaired. The patient often appears tortured by the strain to extract the proper word. At the same time, however, the comprehension of patients with Broca's aphasia is, for the most part, spared. They are able to understand and to respond to uncomplicated spoken and written language, but they cannot fully comprehend complicated or abstract data. In addition, most patients with Broca's aphasia have difficulties communicating in writing. Not infrequently, a lesion in the temporal lobe that results in Broca's aphasia also causes a paralysis of the right side of the face, the right arm and the right leg. Although writing to aural dictation is not possible, patients are still capable of copying words and letters from visual presentations. The most frequent cause of Broca's aphasia is an obstruction in the upper main division of the middle cerebral artery. Because this vascular event is usually of rapid onset, etiologic diagnosis is rarely a problem for the clinician. More insidious onsets of Broca's aphasia can occur with tumor, multiple small infarcts, and with etiologies that lead to more difficult diagnostic challenges.

An excellent way to test for Broca's aphasia is to have patients repeat phrases or sentences. The phrase "no ifs, ands, or buts," or the appellation "Methodist Episcopal" is often utilized for this test. Because patients with Broca's aphasia have difficulty naming objects correctly but little difficulty in recognizing objects, the examiner might point to his stethoscope, watch, or belt buckle, and ask the patient to name those items. Should the patient be unable to name the objects, the examiner then might ask the patient to point to his own nose, to the examiner's shoe, or to the door. Patients with mild Broca's aphasia should be able to carry out the latter, simple recognition task without difficulty.

WERNICKE'S APHASIA

Patients with *Wernicke's aphasia* are often referred directly to a psychiatrist with a misdiagnosis of schizophrenia, because their presenting symptoms involve impairments of speech, language, and behavior. Wernicke's is a fluent aphasia in which the speech is well articulated, has proper tonality, and appears spontaneous and effortless. The central problem of patients with Wernicke's aphasia is the incapacity to comprehend what they hear and, often, what they see. Their language is replete with jargon, disconnected ideas, neologisms, and paraphasias. A neologism is a word invented by the patient that is not part of the language. Paraphasia is the use of words that are either malformed or are incorrectly substituted for other words. The result is that the patient with Wernicke's aphasia appears unaware of his deficit, and speaks with proper inflections, articulation, and cadence, but his language content is largely incomprehensible.

The second major feature of a patient with Wernicke's aphasia is the incapacity for auditory comprehension. They are unable to repeat, to read, to write, to understand simple commands, or even to follow their own speech. The cortical lesion involved in Wernicke's aphasia is in the posterior perisylvian region of the temporal lobe. Occasionally, contiguous portions of the parietal lobe are also involved. The source of the lesion is usually an embolic occlusion of the lower division of the left middle cerebral artery. Thrombosis or hemorrhage also may give rise to Wernicke's aphasia.

There is only a superficial similarity between the disorganized language production of a patient with severe schizophrenia and the language of a patient with Wernicke's aphasia. A history of a rapid onset of the language disorder, without the prodrome and social isolation common in schizophrenia, is helpful in establishing a diagnosis. The nonagitated schizophrenic is usually able to respond to simple verbal commands such as "Point to the pencil" or "Sit down in the red chair," whereas the patient with Wernicke's aphasia will be bewildered by such directions. Naming, reading, repetition, and writing are almost always preserved in the schizophrenic patient, whereas the patient with Wernicke's aphasia is unable to accomplish such tasks. Disconnected ideas, loose associations, and word salad in the schizophrenic patient are secondary to ideational confusion, as opposed to the focal lesions in language centers of the temporal–parietal cortex in the patient with Wernicke's aphasia. The latter patient sometimes develops reactive psychological symptoms including hallucinations, paranoia, and affective changes. In such instances, a careful history, as well as confirmatory laboratory data on EEG, CT scan, MRI, and neuropsychologic testing are essential.

CONDUCTION APHASIA

Conduction aphasia may arise from lesions in either the temporal or parietal lobes. The speech is fluent, and the patient can comprehend both spoken and written language. However, the patient is unable to repeat words, name objects, or express himself in writing. The ability to write with good penmanship is preserved. The importance of conduction aphasia is that it involves specific fiber bundles in the arcuate fasiculus or the connecting fibers between the temporal, parietal, and frontal lobes. Highly specific combinations of language function and dysfunction help to localize lesions that may be too small to be revealed on standard laboratory testing. The usual cause of a conduction aphasia is an embolus in either the posterior temporal or the ascending parietal branch of the middle cerebral artery. Trauma, neoplasm, or other vascular disease also can produce this syndrome.

ANOMIC APHASIA

The patient with *anomic aphasia* has difficulty in naming objects. The speech is fluent, but there are pauses in which the patient gropes for words or substitutes synonyms or phrases that convey the meaning of the word the patient cannot produce. The patient is able to understand both written and spoken language with full comprehension and has full capacity for repetition. The patient who has difficulty naming a series of familiar objects often refers to their function in lieu of their names. If asked to point to an object that is named by the examiner, the patient has no difficulty in complying. Anomic aphasias occur in a wide variety of illnesses and from lesions in multiple locations in the temporal and parietal cortex. Anomic aphasia may be one of the earliest symptoms of Alzheimer's disease, and it is also common in multi-infarct dementia. Table 4-2 summarizes an approach of Sir

---

TABLE 4-2. *Questions Used in the Diagnosis of Aphasia*

1. Is the patient right- or left-handed, and if the latter, did he write with the right hand? Is there any family history of left-handedness? Does he kick a ball with the right foot for preference? Does he "take aim" using his right eye?

2. What was his state of education as regards reading, writing, and foreign tongues?

3. Does he understand the nature and uses of objects, and can he understand pantomine and gesture, or express his wants thereby?

4. Is he deaf? If so, to what extent and on one or both sides?

5. Can he recognize ordinary sounds and noises?

6. Can he comprehend language spoken? If so, does he at once attempt to answer a question?

7. Is spontaneous speech good? If not, to what extent and in what manner is it impaired? Does he make use of wrong words, recurring utterances, or jargon?

8. Can he repeat words uttered in his hearing?

9. Is the sight good or bad; is there hemianopsia, or papilloedema?

10. Does he recognize written or printed speech and obey a written command? If not, does he recognize single words, letters, or numerals?

11. Can he write spontaneously? What mistakes occur in writing? Is there paragraphia? Can he read his own writing some time after he has written it?

12. Can he copy written words, or from printed to printing? Can he write numerals or perform simple mathematical calculations?

13. Can he read aloud?

14. Can he name at sight words, letters, numerals, and common objects?

15. Can he write from dictation?

16. Can he match an object with its name, spoken or written, when a series of objects and names are simultaneously presented?

(Adapted from Brain's Clinical Neurology, 6th ed. Revised by Sir Roger Bannister, New York, Oxford University Press, 1985)

TABLE 4-3. Clinical Characteristics of Aphasias

Type	Verbal Output	Repetition	Comprehension	Naming	Associated Signs*	Lesion
Broca	Nonfluent	Impaired	Normal	Marginally impaired	RHP, apraxia of the left limbs and face	Left posterior inferior frontal
Wernicke	Fluent	Impaired	Impaired	Impaired	±RHH	Left posterior superior temporal
Conduction	Fluent	Impaired	Normal	Impaired (paraphasic)	±RHS, apraxia of all limbs and face	Left parietal
Global	Nonfluent	Impaired	Impaired	Impaired	RHP, RHS, RHH	Left frontal temporal parietal
Anomic	Fluent	Normal (anomic)	Normal	Impaired	None	Left posterior inferior temporal, or temporal–occipital region
Transcortical motor	Nonfluent	Normal	Normal	Impaired	RHP	Left medial frontal or anterior border zone
Sensory	Fluent	Normal	Impaired	Impaired	±RHH	Left medial parietal or posterior border zone
Mixed (isolation)	Nonfluent	Normal	Impaired	Impaired	RHP, RHS	Left medial frontal parietal or complete border zone

* RHP, right hemisparesis; RHH, right homonomous hemianopsia; RHS, right hemisensory defect

(Reprinted by permission of the publisher from Kandel ER, Schwartz JH: Principles of Neural Sciences, p 595. Copyright 1981 by Elsevier Science Publishing Co., Inc.)

Roger Bannister for evaluating a patient for aphasic symptomatology. Table 4-3 outlines clinical features of the commonly occurring aphasias.

Affective Changes in Temporal Lobe Impairment

The inferior division of the middle cerebral artery serves the temporal–parietal cortex, and it is highly susceptible to occlusion secondary to embolus and other cerebral vascular accidents. There is a high incidence of affective changes following cerebral vascular accidents in the temporal lobes. Robinson and Price reviewed 103 clinic patients to assess depressive illness after a stroke. Their study, conducted over a 12-month period, revealed that almost one third of the patients were depressed at the time of their initial evaluation, and of these, two thirds remained depressed when reevaluated 8 months later. In other studies, as many as 45% of stroke victims have a significant depression.

Perceptual Changes in Temporal Lobe Impairment

Excitatory lesions of the temporal region can produce deja vu phenomena, which is the vivid sensory experience in which a new situation is regarded as a repetition of a previous experience. In addition, excitatory lesions such as those initiated by seizure disorders or by tumor may result in visual, auditory, olfactory, and gustatory hallucinatory experiences. It has been postulated that lesions in the nondominant temporal lobe may commonly result in depression, irritability, and dysphoria, whereas lesions in the dominant temporal lobe result in aphasias, amnesias, and learning deficits.

Memory Disturbances in Temporal Lobe Impairment

Although the temporal lobes are vital for the retention of learned experiences, all other regions of the cortex are also involved in this function. Memory may be divided into the following functions:

1. *Registration* involves the utilization of perceptual capacities to process the environment. Alertness, attention, concentration, and sensory intactness are required for the registration component of memory to function. Certain impairments of the sensory apparatus lead to

a clouding of the sensorium that is seen in deliria, dementia, and other confusional states.

2. In the *retention* stage, organized sensory and ideational data are stored within the brain for later utilization.

3. *Recall* is the capacity to reproduce stored data, or return such data to the conscious mind. Amnesia, which is impairment of memory, may be of either psychological or organic origin. In *retrograde amnesia,* memory is impaired for varying periods of time prior to the onset of illness. The extent of pretrauma memory loss depends on the nature of the lesion in the brain. *Anterograde amnesia* is the impaired ability to lay down and to store new memories for the period that is subsequent to the onset of the illness. In most organic illness, anterograde amnesia is more prevalent and disabling than retrograde amnesia. When memory impairment persists beyond several weeks, the patient often confabulates. Confabulation is the fabrication of stories to compensate for data that either were not stored or cannot be recalled.

Remote memory may be evaluated by asking the patient to recite information that was learned in the past, such as former addresses, telephone numbers, simple multiplication tables, nursery rhymes, and common songs. *Short-term memory* is defined as the capacity to retain new material, through concentrated effort, for duration of at least 30 minutes. Short-term memory can be tested by having a patient recall a series of specific memory pairs from the Wechsler Memory Scale. The patient is instructed to listen carefully as the examiner reads aloud a list of word pairs. After a pause of 5 seconds, the psychiatrist then reads to the patient one word from each pair in random order, and the patient attempts to recall each co-word. The patient is given three trials to learn the word pairs. The patient is then tested on his ability to retain the newly learned material. Because the test has been standardized over thousands of normal subjects, this technique is preferred to the more traditional task of having the patient attempt to remember three or four random words provided by the examiner. The list of memory pairs from the Wechsler Memory Scale as well as the scoring of this test is summarized in Appendix 5-7 of Chapter 5.

Immediate retention. The Wechsler Memory Scale recommends the following procedure for the evaluation of immediate retention: Randomly select a series of four digits and ask the patient to repeat these digits. In each successive step add one more digit to a new random series of digits until the patient either fails twice in succession for that number of digits or accurately repeats a series of eight digits. The same procedure is then repeated, asking the patient to repeat the digits backwards to a maximum number of seven digits. The range of normal performance is six to eight digits forward and four to seven digits in reverse. Impaired memory is not the only cause of subnormal performance on the digit span. Performance anxiety may result in an apparent incapacity on this test. Residual impairment in patients with minimal brain dysfunction (MBD), dyslexia, or other learning disabilities may take the form of reversal of digits, and of particular difficulty in repeating digits backwards. If the patient's performance on digit span tests is impaired, careful questioning may reveal the true source of the problem. The anxious patient can concentrate in situations where he does not feel under stress. Such a patient will report no difficulty, for example, in repeating a new telephone number that he just read. The patient with adult residua of a learning disability is usually aware of making mis-entries in his checkbook or of frequently dialing the wrong telephone number as the result of reversing digits. This trait may be found in bright and successful people.

PARIETAL LOBES

The parietal regions of the cortex are involved in the perception of touch, pain, temperature, proprioception, stereognosis, spatial relations, body awareness, facial recognition, and the coordination of complex motor activity (idiokinetic activities). The comprehension of the grammatical and syntactical components of language is a function of the dominant parietal lobe, as is the utilization of numbers, mathematics, and calculation. Because the sensory, perceptual, and cognitive impairments that result from parietal lobe lesions are unlikely to be confused with functional psychiatric illness, we will not review the detailed testing for parietal lobe dysfunction. An exception is the patient who denies profound illness (anosognosia) and neglects bodily parts or environmental objects on his left side as a result of a lesion in the nondominant parietal lobe. The patient who does not recognize the presence of the left side of his body because of right parietal lesions may be thought erroneously to have a dissociative reaction, conversion reaction, or even a somatic delusion. Capgras' syndrome occurs when a patient has the delusional conviction that other persons in his environment have replaced important familiar people. This delusion of doubles almost always occurs in patients who are suffering from paranoid psychosis and has been thought, since the description of the syndrome in 1923, to be secondary to a functional disorder. However, it has been found, that the belief that close friends or relatives are imposters can also occur in patients with nondominant parietal lesions, and this etiology must be evaluated in all patients with this symptomatology.

OCCIPITAL LOBES

The occipital lobes are largely involved with visual function. With bilateral lesions in the occipital lobes, rarely is there an entire loss of sight. In this situation, visual imagination and visual imagery in dreams are preserved. Infrequently, lesions in occipital lobes may produce visual symptoms that are misdiagnosed to be hysterical. Anton's syndrome, or visual anosognosia, is the denial of blindness in patients who obviously cannot see. Such patients behave as though they are able to see, and, for example, when ambulating often collide dangerously with objects. The patients may explain away their symptoms with excuses such as "The lights are too dim in this room" or "I forgot my glasses." Such a denial of blindness may be misperceived as having a functional etiology. Rather, the syndrome is the result of lesions that extend beyond the striate occipital cortex and involve visual association areas. Neuropsychological and neurophysiological testing are indicated when evaluating such symptoms.

DIFFUSE CORTICAL IMPAIRMENT

Diffuse impairment of the cortex may give rise to global cognitive abnormalities, which are categorized in DSM III under Delirium and Dementia. Mental status changes associated with delirium and dementia reflect a final common pathway of dysfunction and may be secondary to a wide variety of both reversible and irreversible etiologies. In similar fashion, depression may be caused by many disorders affecting the central nervous system. The symptoms of depression commonly include profound cognitive impairments, which may be misdiagnosed as dementia or other organic brain syndromes. In elderly populations, it is estimated that 5% of persons aged 65 years and older and 20% of those 80 years and older have dementia. When cognitive changes secondary to depression are misdiagnosed to result from organic brain syndrome, the patient may be deprived of effective somatic treatment of his depression. He may also be removed from a supportive, familiar home environment to be placed in a facility, such as a nursing home or a state psychiatric hospital, which can aggravate the depression. For these reasons we have chosen to highlight the clinical features of delirium, dementia, and pseudodementia, while emphasizing that the clinical evaluation of patients with such syndromes requires the comprehensive assessment approach presented in this textbook.

Delirium

In delirium, there is a clouding of consciousness or a diminished capacity to perceive and sustain attention to environmental stimuli. There may be disorientation, memory impairment, incoherent speech, irritability, changes in sleep and activity patterns, and perceptual disturbances including hallucinations. The clinical features in delirium develop over a short period of time and tend to fluctuate in severity.

DSM III defines intoxication as the development of a substance-specific syndrome that follows the recent ingestion and the presence in the body of that substance. Among the maladaptive behaviors that occur secondary to the effects of the substance on the central nervous system are impaired judgment, belligerence, poor job performance, disturbed social functioning, and failure to meet family or occupational responsibilities.

Dementia

Dementia is distinguished from delirium by the absence of a clouding of consciousness. In dementia there are memory impairment and the loss of intellectual capacities of such severity as to interfere with social or occupational functioning. Additional features of dementia may include diminished capacity for abstract thinking, impaired social judgment, and other disturbances of higher cortical function, such as aphasias, and the inability to accomplish complex motor activities despite an intact neuromuscular system. As with delirium, in dementia there is evidence from the history, physical examination, or laboratory data that an organic factor is etiologically related to the mental disturbance.

For many years dementia was considered, by definition, irreversible. Consistent with the views of researchers and clinicians who treat patients with dementia, DSM III redefines the term to include symptoms and etiologies that, in fact, are reversible. Various investigators now subcategorize dementias as those that are either reversible or irreversible, or treatable or nontreatable. While recognizing certain value to each method of subcategorization, we believe that the concepts of "irreversible" or "nontreatable" may be misleading and, in fact, deleterious to the patient with dementia. For all patients with dementia there are multifarious psychosocial and somatic interventions that, although they may not reverse the cognitive, intellectual, or other neurological impairments, nonetheless will improve functioning and reduce stress. Concepts such as "irreversible" or "nontreatable" may discourage both the patient's physician and his support group from attempting such interventions. Our preference is to subcategorize dementias into etiologic categories and conditions: (1) toxic; (2) traumatic; (3) infectious; (4) idiopathic; (5) neoplastic; (6) nutritional; (7) collagen, vascular, and autoimmune; (8) congential and hereditary; (9) endocrine; (10) vascular; (11) metabolic; and (12) degenerative.

Pseudodementia

A subgroup of seriously depressed patients, often elderly, may be misdiagnosed to have dementia because of their complaint of memory impairment, difficulty in thinking and concentrating, and an overall reduction in performance. Such patients may also perform poorly on neuropsychological testing and have altered mental states in areas of orientation, judgment, and insight. Investigators such as Wells have coined the term *pseudodementia* to describe the condition in which cognitive deficits are secondary to depression. On formal mental status, patients with pseudodementia show variability of performance and response as opposed to the pervasively poor performance of patients with dementia. With pseudodementia, the disturbance of mood impairs motivation; therefore, encouragement and assistance from the examiner may result in improved intellectual functioning, memory, and orientation.

Some psychiatrists believe that a positive therapeutic response to antidepressant medication supports the diagnosis of pseudodementia, while an unusual sensitivity to the side-effects of antidepressant medication is more likely in patients with brain injury. For example, if a patient with a major depressive episode becomes sedated and confused on very low doses of an antidepressant such as desipramine that has relatively few anticholinergic side-effects, the clinician should suspect an underlying organic etiology.

In depressed elderly patients who show impairment in intellectual capacities and memory, the differential diagnosis between dementia and pseudodementia may be difficult. In such patients, the use of electroconvulsive therapy may not only be therapeutic but also diagnostic. Patients whose apparent dementia clears with a course of electroconvulsive therapy along with an improvement in mood are suffering from a primary affective illness. However, patients who, with the first few treatments, become more confused, disoriented, and unable to maintain their personal hygiene may have an underlying organic impairment that is etiologically related to their clinical features of dementia. For the patient who has both depression and dementia, the aware clinician will utilize nondominant, unilateral ECT with pulsatile currents and increase the interval to 3 to 4 days between treatments. Utilizing fewer treatments in the entire course results in an amelioration of depressive symptoms without further aggravation of the dementia.

TABLE 4-4. Clinical Features Differentiating Pseudodementia from Dementia

Pseudodementia	Dementia
1. Symptoms of short duration suggest pseudodementia	1. Symptoms of long duration suggest dementia
2. Patients usually complain much of cognitive loss	2. Patients usually complain little of cognitive loss
3. Patients' complaints of cognitive dysfunction usually detailed	3. Patients' complaints of cognitive dysfunction usually imprecise
4. Patients usually communicate strong sense of distress	4. Patients often appear unconcerned
5. Memory loss for recent and remote events usually equally severe	5. Memory loss for recent events more severe than for remote
6. Memory gaps for specific periods of events common	6. Memory gaps for specific periods unusual*
7. Attention and concentration often well preserved	7. Attention and concentration usually faulty
8. "Don't know" answers typical	8. "Near miss" answers frequent
9. Patients emphasize disability	9. Patients conceal disability
10. Patients make little effort to perform even simple tasks	10. Patients struggle to perform tasks
11. Patients highlight failures	11. Patients delight in accomplishments, however trivial
12. Patients do not try to keep up	12. Patients rely on notes, calendars, etc. to keep up
13. Marked variability in performing tasks of similar difficulty	13. Consistently poor performance on tasks of similar difficulty
14. Affective change often pervasive	14. Affect labile and shallow
15. Loss of social skills often early and prominent	15. Patients often retain social skills
16. On tests of orientation, patients often give "don't know" answers	16. On tests of orientation, patients mistake unusual for usual
17. Behavior often incongruent with severity of cognitive dysfunction	17. Behavior usually compatible with severity of cognitive dysfunction
18. Nocturnal accentuation of dysfunction uncommon	18. Nocturnal accentuation of dysfunction common
19. History of previous psychiatric dysfunction common	19. History of previous psychiatric dysfunction unusual

* Except when due to delirium, trauma, and seizures

(Reprinted with permission of the publisher from Wells CE, Duncan GW [eds]: Neurology for Psychiatrists, p 93. Philadelphia, FA Davis, 1980)

Finally, certain nonorganic psychological states can produce a false dementia or pseudodementia. In diagnostic conditions such as malingering, Ganser's syndrome, and the dissociative disorders, there may be the appearance of a diminution in intellectual abilities, memory impairment, decreased judgment, and other disturbances of higher cortical function. Careful history taking, combined with neuropsychological testing, a precise mental status examination, and laboratory testing aid in confirming a functional etiology. Table 4-4 summarizes the different clinical features of dementia caused by organic disease and pseudodementia caused by depression. (See Chap. 5 for additional discussion of this topic.)

SUGGESTED READING

Albert ML: Subcortical dementia. In Katzman R, Terry RD, Bick KL (eds): Alzheimer's Disease: Senile Dementia and Related Disorders. New York, Raven Press, 1978

Bannister R: Brain's Clinical Neurology. New York, Oxford University Press, 1985

Bear DM, Fedio P: Quantitative analysis of interictal behavior in temporal lobe epilepsy. Arch Neurol 34:454, 1977

Bear DM, Freeman R, Greenberg M: Behavioral alterations in patients with temporal lobe epilepsy. In Blumer D (ed): Psychiatric Aspects of Epilepsy. Washington, DC, American Psychiatric Press, 1984

Benton AL, Hamsher K des, Varney NR, et al: Contributions to Neuropsychological Assessment: A Clinical Manual. New York, Oxford University Press, 1983

Benson DF: Aphasia, Alexia and Agraphia: Clinical Neurology and Neurosurgery Monographs. Edinburgh, Churchill Livingstone, 1979

Benson DF: Subcortical dementia: A clinical approach. In Mayeux R, Rosen WG (eds): The Dementias. New York, Raven Press, 1983

Coyle JT, Price DL, Delong MR: Alzheimer's disease: A disorder of cortical cholinergic innervation. Science 219:1184, 1983

Craine ED: Pseudodementia: Current concepts and future directions. Arch Gen Psychiatry 38:1359, 1981

Cummings JL: Cortical Dementias. In Benson DF, Blumer D (eds): Psychiatric Aspects of Neurologic Disease, Vol 2. New York, Grune & Stratton, 1982

Cummings JL, Benson DF: Dementia: A Clinical Approach. Boston, Butterworth, 1983

Folstein MF, McHugh PR: Dementia syndrome of depression. In Katzman R, Terry RD, Bick KL (eds): Alzheimer's Disease: Senile Dementia and Related Disorders. New York, Raven Press, 1978

Geschwind N: Disconnection syndromes in animals and man. Part I: Brain 88:237, 1965; Part II: Brain 88:585, 1965

Jeste DV, Karson CN, Wyatt RJ: Movement disorders and psychopathology. In Jeste DV, Wyatt RJ (eds): Neuropsychiatric Movement Disorders. Washington, DC, American Psychiatric Press, 1984

Kandel ER, Schwartz JH: Principles of Neural Science. New York, Elsevier Science Publishers, 1981

La Rue A: Memory loss and aging: distinguishing dementia from benign senescent forgetfulness and depressive pseudodementia. Psychiatr Clin N Am 5:89, 1982

Lazare A: Conversion symptoms. N Engl J Med 305:745, 1981

Lezak MD: Neuropsychological Assessment, 3rd ed. New York, Oxford University Press, 1983

Luria AR: The Working Brain: An Introduction to Neuropsychology. Hough B (trans): New York, Basic Books, 1973

McAllister TW: Overview: pseudodementia. Am J Psychiatry 140:528, 1983

Pincus JH, Tucker GJ: Behavioral Neurology, 2nd ed. New York, Oxford University Press, 1978

Plum F: Dementia: An approaching epidemic. Nature 279:372, 1979

Reed SL, Small GW, Jarvick LJ: Dementia syndrome. In Hales RE, Frances AJ (eds): American Psychiatric Association Annual Review, Vol 4, pp 211–226. Washington DC, American Psychiatric Press, 1985

Robinson RG, Starr LB, Price TR: A two-year longitudinal study of mood disorders following stroke: prevalence and duration at six months follow up. Br J Psychiatry 144:256, 1984

Robinson RG, Lipsey JR, Bolla-Wilson K, et al: Mood disorders in left-handed stroke patients. Am J Psychiatry 142:1424, 1985

Stub RL, Black FW: The Mental Status Examination in Neurology. Philadelphia, FA Davis, 1977

Taylor MA: The Neuropsychiatric Mental Status Examination. New York, SP Medical and Scientific Books, 1981

Taylor MA, Sierles F, Abrams R: The Neuropsychiatric Evaluation. In Hales RF, Frances AJ (eds): American Psychiatric Association Annual Review, Vol 4, pp 109–141. Washington, DC, American Psychiatric Press, 1985

Waxman SA, Geschwind N: The interictal behavior syndrome of temporal lobe epilepsy. Arch Gen Psychiatry 32:1580, 1975

Wells CE: Dementia. Philadelphia, FA Davis, 1977

Wells CE, Duncan GW: Neurology for Psychiatrists. Philadelphia, FA Davis, 1980

Wells CE: Pseudodementia. Am J Psychiatry 136:895, 1979

Yudofsky SC: Section II Neuropsychiatry Editor. In Hales RE, Frances AJ (eds): American Psychiatric Association Annual Review, Vol 4, pp 101–225. Washington, DC, American Psychiatric Press, 1985

Yudofsky SC, Silver JM: Psychiatric Aspects of Brain Injury: Trauma, Stroke, and Tumor. In Hales RE, Frances AJ (eds): American Psychiatric Association Annual Review, Vol 4, pp 142–158. Washington, DC, American Psychiatric Press, 1985

Yudofsky SC: Malingering. In Kaplan HI and Sadock BJ (eds): Comprehensive Textbook of Psychiatry, Vol 2, pp 1862–1865. Baltimore, Williams & Wilkins, 1985

5

Psychological Testing and Psychiatric Rating Scales

Overview of Psychological Testing and Rating Scales 146
    Standardization 147
    Reliability 147
    Validity 148

Evaluation of Intelligence 148
    Wechsler Adult Intelligence Scale-Revised (WAIS-R) 149
    Wechsler Intelligence Scale for Children-Revised (WISC-R) 151

Personality Tests 151
    Projective Personality Tests 151
        The Rorschach Personality Test 151
        Thematic Apperception Test (TAT) 153
        Projective Drawings 154
    Nonprojective Personality Tests 155
        The Minnesota Multiphasic Personality Inventory (MMPI) 155

Neuropsychological Tests and Assessment 157

Clinical Application of Psychological Testing Batteries 159
    Assessment of Cognitive Functioning in the Elderly 159
    Assessment of Brain Function 160
        Halstead–Reitan Neuropsychological Battery 160
        Luria–Nebraska Neuropsychological Battery 164

Psychiatric Rating Scales 165
    Self-Report Questionnaires 166
        Self-Report Symptom Inventory-Revised (SCL-90-R) 166

Naturalistic Observation Scales   167
   Nurse's Observation Scale for Inpatient Evaluation (NOSIE-30)   167
   Overt Aggression Scale (OAS)   169
Interview Assessment Scales   170
   Hamilton Rating Scale for Depression (HAMD)   170
   Schedule for Affective Disorders and Schizophrenia (SADS)   171
   Personality Disorder Examination (PDE)   176
   Structured Clinical Interview for DSM-III-R (SCID)   177

Appendix 5-1. Beck Depression Inventory (BDI) (Short Form)   190
Appendix 5-2. Global Assessment Scale (GAS)   192
Appendix 5-3. Hamilton Anxiety Rating Scale (HAMA)   195
Appendix 5-4. Hamilton Rating Scale for Depression (HAMD)   197
Appendix 5-5. The Mini-Mental State Examination   200
Appendix 5-6. Overt Aggression Scale (OAS)   203
Appendix 5-7. Wechsler Memory Scale: Form I (WMS)   206

OVERVIEW OF PSYCHOLOGICAL TESTING AND RATING SCALES

Psychological tests and psychiatric rating scales are widely used for a variety of clinical assessments of the patient. Included are tests for intelligence and cognitive functioning; brain disorders; personality organization; and psychodynamic evaluation of unconscious conflicts. Other tests and batteries of psychological tests and rating scales are designed to measure specific symptom clusters and general levels of adaptive functioning.

There has been a reduction in the use of psychological testing as part of the standard psychiatric evaluation in most teaching centers during the past 30 years. It is our view that this phenomenon is, in part, the result of the introduction of specific rating scales that are used to quantify psychological impairment. Such instruments now enjoy a widespread popularity to the extent that one cannot understand most clinical research papers without a familiarity with the more commonly utilized rating scales. It is for that purpose that the currently popular scales will be reviewed in this chapter.

Another reason for the relative decline in the use of comprehensive psychological testing in academic settings is that during the Sixties and Seventies most American-trained psychiatrists received intensive training in psychodynamic psychiatry during their residencies. Consequently, these clinicians are capable of making an in-depth psychodynamic assessment of their patients—a role once performed largely by clinical psychologists. Also, the time-consuming aspects of a comprehensive personality evaluation may be viewed as unwarranted in the light of the trend towards brief inpatient psychiatric hospitalization and outpatient treatments.

It is not our view that psychological testing is any less useful than it was in the past; it is only performed less routinely. In fact, one of the shortcomings of the current trend towards the use of rating scales stems from their very specificity. Comprehensive psychological evaluation can uncover trends or psychopathology that the psychiatrist has missed in his own evaluation. Scales such as the SADS-Lifetime are supposed to address this problem, but they still measure a rather limited range of intellectual and personality functioning when compared with a battery of tests that might include, for example, the WAIS-R, MMPI, TAT, Sentence Completion, and Rorschach Tests.

Most psychologists are aware of and make the important distinction between *psychological testing* and *psychological assessment*. Psychological assessment should be performed by a clinically trained psychologist, but tests can be administered by a person with minimal training. The interaction between psychologist and patient plays a significant role in the quality of test data elicited, as well as in their interpretation.

Standardization

Psychological tests must be standardized, valid, and reliable. *Standardization* is a process by which a relatively controlled sample of a patient's responses or behavior may be compared with normative data of a specifically chosen, larger, reference sample. To secure reliable and valid data, it is necessary to control and standardize the fashion in which questions are asked, observations are made, and data are scored and interpreted.

Reliability

Reliability as it relates to psychological testing and to rating scales is the consistency with which subjects are discriminated from one another. In more simple terms, reliability is the extent to which scores obtained by testing a patient on one occasion will be the same if that same person is reexamined by the same test on a different occasion. Because no test is capable of absolute consistency, there is an acceptable range of error that takes into consideration random fluctuations expected in an individual's score. Test–retest reliability is determined by first administering a test and then readministering the test on another occasion. A reliability coefficient is then calculated by correlating the scores for the same person on the two different administrations. If the correlations are high, the results of the test are less likely to be secondary to random fluctuations in the state of mind of the person tested or in the testing environment. With a high reliability coefficient, one can be more confident that any differences in scores are due to actual changes in the responses being measured.

Validity

Validity is the capacity of a specific test to measure what it purports to measure. In general, a test is neither valid nor invalid; rather, it has a variety of "validities" for different purposes. For example, a test may be valid for discriminating among patients during acute episodes of their illness, but may have little predictive ability regarding their level of functioning or symptoms 6 months later. Selection of any psychological test or rating procedure should be based upon the evidence of the validity of that procedure for its chosen purpose.

EVALUATION OF INTELLIGENCE

A precise definition of intelligence is the subject of significant controversy and disagreement. We believe intelligence to be a conceptual construct—that is, a human invention—that has both utilitarian advantages and serious dangers of misinterpretation and abuse. Most definitions of intelligence involve an individual's capacity to (1) adapt to his environment and to new situations; (2) learn from experience; (3) pursue goal-related activities; (4) utilize abstract thinking, including concepts and symbols; and (5) solve problems by using personal insight. As with most conceptual inventions, theory and definition are intertwined. For example, some psychologists view intelligence through a "learning theory approach," in which the ability and capacity to acquire new data and to change with experience are measures of intellectual functioning. Neurobiologists, on the other hand, may seek to understand intelligence mechanistically by striving to reduce the components of intelligence to molecules and physical properties of matter. Developmental theories of intelligence such as that of Piaget postulate that intelligence develops in certain stages, and therefore must be understood against the background of complex psychosocial processes. Finally, psychometric properties of intelligence derive from differences in individuals that are revealed when standardized tests are administered and readministered to large numbers of people. Conclusions about intelligence from psychometric testing rely not only upon standardized methods of collecting data, but upon complex mathematical methods of analyzing multiple factors.

Wechsler Adult Intelligence Scale-Revised (WAIS-R)

Currently, the most widely used individual intelligence test is the Wechsler Adult Intelligence Scale-Revised (WAIS-R). WAIS-R is an achievement test, although it is often misunderstood as a test of intellectual potential. The WAIS-R is divided into verbal and performance scales and takes into account the age of the subject being tested, with nine separate age norms, ranging from 16 years to 75 years of age. The verbal scale measures the following: the ability of the patient to work with abstract symbols; his verbal memory capacity; his verbal fluency; and the amount and degree of benefit that the patient has received from his educational background. The verbal scale consists of six subtests to measure information, digit span, vocabulary, arithmetic, comprehension, and similarities. Information testing on the Wechsler Verbal Scale rates such areas as the general fund of the patient's information, his intellectual curiosity, and his alertness to the everyday world. The digit span component of the verbal scale measures concentration, attention, short-term or immediate auditory memory, and the capacity to shift thought patterns. The vocabulary section is a test of accumulated verbal learning, and focuses on language usage and concept formation. Vocabulary is thought to be the most reliable verbal subtest and is also considered the best single indicator of general intelligence. The arithmetic section of the WAIS-R involves concentration and attention, reflects school learning, and measures the capacity to abstract, to reason, and mental alertness in general. The comprehension section of the WAIS-R tests not only social judgment and the ability to adapt when presented with novel problems, but it also is a reflection of the patient's conscience development. Finally, the similarities subtest reflects the patient's associative ability, his capacity for logical and abstract reasoning, and his ability to form and to utilize verbal concepts. People who score low on this section often have concrete, rigid, literal, or inflexible thinking. The performance scale has subtests for picture completion, picture arrangement, block design, object assembly, and digit symbol. The performance section measures a patient's overall ability to integrate perceptual stimuli with motor responses. It involves awareness of environmental detail, the perception of the whole in relation to its parts, and the ability to differentiate the essential from the nonessential. The capacity for sustained effort, for concentration, and for nonverbal concept formation is measured by the block design subtest. The object assembly subtest measures visual–motor organization and the ability to place familiar objects together in familiar configurations or groupings. The digit–symbol component of the performance scale measures visual–motor speed and coordination through the ability to learn an unfamiliar task. The ability to shift from task to task in the digit–symbol component of the performance scale is a measurement of mental flexibility.

The WAIS-R measures a person's score on this particular test as compared with the performances of others in his age group. Meaningful comparisons can also be drawn between persons of different ages. The score, which utilizes standard deviations, is reported in points called *intelligence quotient* (IQ). The IQ is a specific sample of a patient's intellectual performance at a fixed point in time. It does not necessarily measure a person's innate capacity. Persons with an IQ score of 130 or above are considered to have very superior intellectual performance; scores of 120 through 129 are classified superior; 110 through 119, high average; 90 through 109, average; 80 through 89, low average; 70 through 79, borderline; and 69 and below are considered mentally retarded. The WAIS-R measures intellectual functioning specific to the time in which the patient is being tested, and changes of more than 10 points over time are uncommon. The WAIS-R and the WISC-R provide three separate IQ scores: a full scale IQ, a verbal IQ, and a performance IQ. In addition to correlations made on subtest scores, interpretations are also made through consideration of scores and discrepancies on the overall verbal and performance IQs. For example, action-oriented people usually score significantly higher on performance subtests than on verbal subtests. Patients with psychoses tend to score higher on verbal tests than on performance tests. Digit span tests are often the lowest in psychotic persons, and this is thought to reflect the patient's distractibility, poor concentration, and inability to differentiate between essential and nonessential details. The clinical utility of the WAIS-R is controversial in that some critics maintain it has inherent cultural and socioeconomic biases. The subtests of the WAIS-R that are affected by speed, such as object assembly and digit symbol, may be greatly influenced by psychomotor retardation. An excellent general principal is that it is best to do intelligence testing when the subject is out of the acute phase of his illness. Proponents of the test believe that it is highly useful for testing general information, abstract and symbolic logic, attention and focusing capacity, and social sensitivities. Scatter patterns on subtest scores may reflect intellectual impairment as well as personality features. The WAIS-R is useful clinically to describe "cognitive style" and current level of functioning. Some psychologists believe the test is valuable in deriving hypotheses about psychodynamics and for elucidating thought disorders.

Wechsler Intelligence Scale for Children-Revised (WISC-R)

In 1949, Wechsler developed an intelligence scale for children ages 6 years through 16 years. The Wechsler Intelligence Scale for Children (WISC) utilizes easier items specifically designed for children. This scale was standardized on 2200 white American boys and girls, and in 1967, was revised (WISC-R) to provide a more accurate reflection of modern youths. The WISC-R also was standardized to take into consideration representatives of minority groups and children from lower socioeconomic levels. The Wechsler Preschool and Primary Scale of Intelligence (WPPSI) was introduced to measure the intelligence of preschool-age children and children ranging in age from 4 years to 6-1/2 years.

PERSONALITY TESTS

Projective Personality Tests

As with definitions of intelligence, there are also many definitions of and conceptual models for personality. The construction of personality tests is based on theoretical and hypothetical preferences. Projective personality tests strive to measure a person's psychological status by assessing his personal responses to ambiguous, vague, or unstructured stimuli or instructions. Through his own subjective and personal reaction to standardized stimuli, the subject reveals meaningful data related to his psychological strengths and frailties. Certain tests are designed to evoke strong emotional responses in the subject to facilitate the projective process.

The Rorschach Personality Test

The Rorschach Personality Test (an inkblot test) is the best known and most frequently used projective test. It is composed of a standard set of ten amorphous inkblots that serve as the stimuli for associations. The patient is shown ten rectangular cards, five of which have colors and five of which are not colored. He is then instructed to look carefully at the cards, one at a time, and to report what each looks like or of what it reminds him. The patient is encouraged to be thorough and to take as long as he wishes in responding. Once a person has exhausted his spontaneous responses related to a particular card, the examiner may ask focused questions related to the more important aspects of the subject's response. More scientific publications are devoted to the Rorschach Test than to all other projective tests combined. Although the Rorschach Test is relatively simple to administer, its scoring is complex and requires extensive experience to interpret. In the past, the Rorschach Test has been used to differentiate between various diagnostic populations, such as between schizophrenic patients and patients with personality disorders. Proponents of the test also claim that it is useful for bypassing the patient's conscious resistance, revealing data related to unconscious processes and conflicts. It has also been used to gain basic information about the patient's emotions, cognitive style, and perceptual organization. Scoring and interpretation of the Rorschach Test are based on theories and recommendations advanced by Herman Rorschach in his original paper on the subject in 1921. Details such as whether a patient responds to the whole inkblot or a small detail within the blot are examined and interpreted. The content of a patient's response is also considered to be highly revealing. For example, whether the responses reflect human concerns or behaviors as opposed to those of nonhuman animals are noted and interpreted. In addition, responses that involve human movement, animal movement, and that consider color are also observed, scored, and interpreted. The manner in which a patient responds to color may be interpreted as a reflection of his emotional state. An illustration of a response of a schizophrenic patient to a Rorschach card might be the following:

> I see a monster which is half man and half tree. The bottom part of his body has turned into a tree trunk with legs that look like roots that sink into the ground. It seems like the ground is made up of a mixture of blood clots and dirt. The man appears like he has the eyes of Pudgey. The man's nose is missing and blood is coming out of the hole where his nose used to be. The picture frightens me because it reminds me of being left alone in my backyard when I was little.

An analysis of this patient's response might discuss his problem with ego boundaries and body image. The preoccupation with deterioration, the preponderance of unpleasant imagery, and the blending of human body parts with inanimate objects and animal body parts are more common responses for schizophrenic patients than for patients with other disorders. The fact that the patient did not reveal to the examiner that "Pudgey" was a dog that he had when he was 8 years old displays highly personalized and autistic thought processes, which are also common in the schizophrenic patient. The overall bizarre nature of the patient's response indicated poor reality testing. When accompanied by themes of castration (the loss of the objects, nose, blood, etc.) and transformation (the changing of the man into a tree), this reflects paranoia and confused sexual identification, which are also common in the responses of schizophrenic patients.

Interpretations of a patient's response relate to theoretical and conceptual

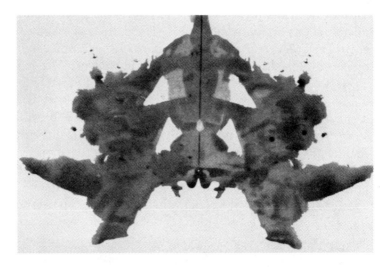

FIG. 5-1. Rorschach Inkblot Test, plate 1. (Reprinted by permission. Hans Huber, Bern, Switzerland)

preferences of the examiner. Attempts have been made by numerous investigators to standardize the scoring and interpretation of responses to the Rorschach Test. Despite attempts at standardization, the Rorschach Test interpretation is highly influenced by the skill and subjective impressions of the examiner. Proponents of the test feel that it is a highly valid and reliable tool. Such areas as the patient's defensive style, unconscious psychodynamic conflicts, impulse control, gender identification, psychosexual level, and responses to stress may be probed by the Rorschach Test. Issues such as ego boundaries and psychotic distortions may also be assessed. Criticism of the Rorschach Test and other personality tests stems from their widespread misuse for diagnostic purposes, despite the fact that they are more appropriate for psychodynamic assessment. Critics of the test believe that personality tests are not reliable, especially if one uses evidence of validity agreement with good clinical diagnoses that take into account symptoms, prior course, response to treatment, and follow-up data. Most personality tests provide "state" measurements rather than "trait" measurements; therefore, they may be misleading if used for diagnostic purposes. Figure 5-1 is plate 1 of the Rorschach Test.

Thematic Apperception Test (TAT)

In the thematic apperception test (TAT), the patient is asked to view, one at a time, pictures selected from a wide variety of scenes, including one blank card. Most of the pictures are clear representations of individuals involved in ambiguous dramatic situations. The patient is asked to make up a story about each picture that explains what is happening in the picture, how the scene developed, and what its outcome will be. The patient is asked to disclose his feelings related to the picture and to predict an outcome of the dramatic situation. In theory, the patient will identify with a figure in the scene and project his "inner" feelings, thoughts, and conflicts through his story. The scoring and interpretation of the TAT is intricately related to the theories of personality of Henry Murray, who developed the test in 1938. His aim was to use the test as "a method of revealing to the trained inter- preter some of the dominant drives, emotions, sentiments, complexes, and conflicts of personality. Special value resides in its power to expose underly- ing inhibited tendencies which the subject is not willing to admit, or cannot admit because he is unconscious of them." The scoring of the TAT centers around Murray's theoretical concepts of human needs, which include those needs motivated by (1) the desire for power, property, prestige, knowledge, or creative achievement; (2) affection, admiration, sympathy, love, and de- pendence; (3) the desire for freedom, change, excitement, and play; and (4) miscellaneous needs including such things as blame avoidance, harm avoid- ance, passivity, and rejection. He also postulated the term *press*, or environ- mental pressures and stimuli that elicit certain behaviors or needs in the patient such as deprivation, alien situations, coercion and restraint, hostile and aggressive environments, danger, injury, and death. The TAT is scored and interpreted in a variety of ways, many of which are also directly related to Murray's theories of personality. Proponents of the TAT believe that the test is an easy to administer and nonstressful projective measurement of the patient's personality and underlying conflicts. Critics believe that the ef- forts to quantify the test fall far short of ideal, and that the TAT is too dependent upon the nonobjective interpretations of the psychologist. Crit- ics also believe that the test is too derivative of theories of Murray that have not been adequately validated or extensively accepted by academic or clini- cal communities. Figure 5-2 is card 12F of the TAT.

Projective Drawings

In this category of projective testing, the patient reveals unconscious feel- ings, conflicts, attitudes, and reactions in their drawings. The most com- monly used test in this category is the Draw-A-Person test (DAP), in which the patient is requested to make three drawings: one of a man, one of a woman, and one of himself. In the House–Tree–Person test, (HTP) the patient first is asked to draw these objects with a pencil, later is questioned about his drawings, and thereafter is asked to draw the same objects with different colored crayons. A variation of this test has the patient draw a

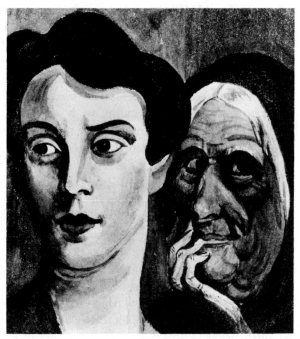

FIG. 5-2. Thematic Apperception Test. (Reprinted by permission of the publishers from Henry A. Murray, Thematic Apperception Test, Cambridge, MA: Harvard University Press, Copyright 1943 by the President and Fellows of Harvard College, © renewed 1971 by Henry A. Murray)

single picture that includes a house, a tree, and a person. The Draw-A-Family Test (DAF) requires the patient to draw his family in an activity. Projective drawing tests are interpreted utilizing a wide variety of theoretical approaches and observational consideration. Such issues as organization, symmetry, perspective, detail, color, shading, content, omissions, arrangements, and continuity of figures, motion, boundaries, and test behavior are assessed. Analyses similar to those described earlier for interpretation of the Rorschach Test are employed. Many clinicians find these tests to be useful because of the relative ease with which they may be administered and because patients tend to find them less stressful than more detailed and structured tests. The tests are criticized by others because of problems related to their standardization, reliability, and validity. Furthermore, some psychologists feel that these tests depend too much on the individual's artistic talent.

Nonprojective Personality Tests

The Minnesota Multiphasic Personality Inventory (MMPI)

The Minnesota Multiphasic Personality Inventory (MMPI) is a nonprojective personality test that has broad use in both clinical assessment and research. The MMPI was first published in the early Forties. Its purpose was "to provide an objective assessment of some major personality characteristics that affect personal and social adjustment." The MMPI is designed to be used for patients who are 16 years of age or older, who have a minimum of sixth-grade education, who are literate, and who have an IQ above 80. The test is composed of 550 declarative statements that the patient is asked to apply to himself by responding with a "true," "false," or "I cannot say" answer. As distinct from most of the tests reviewed in this chapter, psychologists or other highly trained professionals are not required to administer the MMPI. Often the test is given by clerks, technicians, or unskilled hospital personnel, and the scoring may also be accomplished by minimally trained personnel or by computer. The most common version of the MMPI is the "group" booklet form, which is accompanied by a two-sided answer sheet that can be scored by a computer. In the average patient, the test requires approximately 2 hours to take. A short form is available that may be completed in approximately half of this time. Responses are organized so that a patient is rated using nine clinical axes: hypochondriasis, depression, hysteria, psychopathic deviation, masculinity–femininity, paranoia, psychoasthenia (indecision, fears, obsessions), schizophrenia, and hypomania. As with other self-report inventories, many criticisms center around the capacity or willingness of a person to respond with honesty, accuracy, and objectivity. To address this issue, an L scale—occasionally referred to as the lie scale—attempts to measure deliberate simulation, carelessness, or gross eccentricity in the patient's responses. Once the data are collated, a skilled professional examines them to generate hypotheses about the patient. Interpretations of MMPI data require a high level of clinical skill, which must include a sound knowledge in psychopathology to complement a substantive knowledge about the individual patient that is gained from history and mental status examination. Computers are being used increasingly to generate "readouts" of MMPI test responses, but such reports are limited to standard, programmed interpretations. Therefore, many researchers and educators in the area of psychological testing believe that, despite the extensive use of computer interpretations of MMPI, this approach is far inferior to clinical judgment and human interpretation.

Today the MMPI is used to aid in differential diagnosis, as a generalized screening device for school and industry, and for research purposes. The advantages of the MMPI as a personality test are that it can be administered and scored easily. Therefore, it can be used as a screening device with minimal expenditure of a professional's time. Proponents of the test state that it may be used to identify personality characteristics in psychiatric populations, to establish psychiatric diagnoses, and for delineating psychodynamics. Proponents of the MMPI maintain that the extensive data base that has been accumulated on vast numbers of people with varying problems adds to the validity of the test. Critics of the test have raised major questions regarding its validity for the purposes listed, including its failure to consider sufficiently the social or cultural background of the patient and its omission of categories related to such vital areas as substance abuse. Critics of the MMPI also emphasize the trend towards the test being interpreted by computers or by persons with little or no clinical training. These critics maintain that when the MMPI is interpreted in this fashion, the diagnostic and prognostic conclusions are formulaic, nonspecific, and invalid. Occasionally these reports may even be mistaken by the patient or his family to be even more accurate because of the role of the computer.

NEUROPSYCHOLOGICAL TESTS AND ASSESSMENT

In the past several years psychiatrists have made increased use of specialized psychological tests for the diagnosis and localization of brain dysfunction. It is our opinion that this rapidly advancing area provides exciting new opportunities to expand the clinical usefulness of psychological testing. Neuropsychological tests, like other current neurodiagnostic techniques such as the PET scan and cerebral blood flow testing, are able to document brain damage by measuring functional brain capacities. Tests have been devised to isolate discrete deficits to provide data for localizing brain lesions. A significant percentage of the cortex—approximately 75%—does not relate to perceptual or motor functions, but rather to complex integrative, cognitive, and behavioral processes. (See Chap. 4.) Many brain lesions give rise to subtle behavioral and emotional changes long before more obvious sensory and motor impairments emerge. It is now recognized that such illnesses as multiple sclerosis, Parkinson's disease, Huntington's chorea, and others that have been more commonly associated with motor and sensory dysfunction also have significant cognitive and emotional disturbances as persistent features. Such symptoms as weakness, lethargy, decreased ability to concentrate, decreased motivation, and affective changes are common to major psychiatric and neurological illnesses.

Neuropsychological tests are helpful in isolating those persons with major psychiatric illnesses who also are afflicted with brain disorders. Many tests have been devised to measure specific brain functions, and batteries of these tests are often combined to help arrive at specific neuropsychiatric diagnoses. Among the areas of brain functioning tested are: (1) *Memory*. The Wechsler Memory Scale comprises seven tests that measure personal and current information, orientation to time and place, mental control, logical memory, digit span, immediate visual memory, and paired associated verbal learning. Other tests measure immediate, short-term, recent, and remote memory, and temporal orientation. The seven components of the Wechsler Memory Scale as well as the scoring and interpretation of this test are summarized in Appendix 5-7. (2) *Intelligence.* As discussed earlier, intelligence tests can measure the brain's capacity for learning new skills and for adaptation. Therefore, such tests as the WAIS-R may also be considered neuropsychological tests. (3) *Judgment and social capacity* can be evaluated by such instruments as the Vineland Social Maturity Scale or the WAIS-R. (4) *Perception and perceptual motor capacity.* Tests to measure these functions must sensitively measure the brain's capacity to perceive and to apply perceptions motorically. The best known of these tests is the Bender visual–motor gestalt test. In this test, the patient is asked to reproduce nine geometric figures supplied by the examiner. The patient is allowed to copy the nine figures with the nine designs remaining in view. (See Fig. 5-3). This test reflects the patient's capacity to attend to and visualize the figure, and the patient's capacity to transform a mental representation into motoric activity that results in the reproduction of the figures. Specific brain lesions result in specific incapacities reflected in the reproduction of the Bender

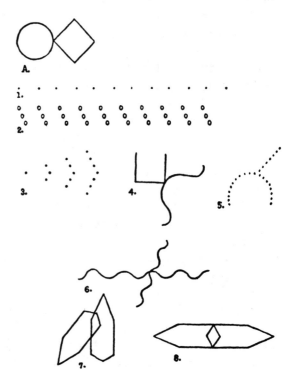

FIG. 5-3. Bender visual–motor gestalt test. (From the Bender Visual Motor Gestalt Test published by the American Orthopsychiatric Association, © 1938)

gestalt figures. (5) *Speed and coordination.* Such tests can quantify reaction times of sensory motor activities. The tests also are useful in measuring the capacity for fine motor coordination, rhythm, and complex constructional capacities. The Purdue Pegboard tests and finger-tapping tests are examples of tests of speed and coordination. (6) *Sensory capacity.* The Tactile Performance test reflects the patient's capacity to recognize objects while blindfolded, to place objects into appropriate receptacles, and to draw objects from memory. Sensory tests can measure tactile perception, fine discrimination, and fine motor coordination, and can discriminate between lesions involving visual and tactile areas of the cortex. (7) *Language.* Language function tests, such as the Token Test of DeRenzi and Vignolo, the Boston Aphasia Battery, and abstractions tests are used to diagnose the lesions in the cortex that result in aphasias. Highly focused neuropsychological tests are designed to localize the precise area of the cortex that results in the impaired language function. For example, the Token Test of DeRenzi and Vignolo uses 20 tokens that have either of two shapes, circles or rectangles. The tokens come in two sizes (big and little) and five colors (white, red, yellow, blue, and green). The test consists of 62 oral commands delivered in five sections of increasing complexity. The test measures the patient's capacity to comprehend the names of the tokens, as well as to understand the verbs and prepositions in the instructions. This test is considered to be a sensitive measurement of receptive dysphasia. (A more complete discussion of aphasias is found in Chap. 4.) (8) *Mental flexibility.* New scales and tests have been devised to measure the capacity of an individual to change his mind, and make rational shifts based on new data. These tests employ complex computer graphics and computer programs that modify the test depending on the response of the patient.

Specific batteries of neuropsychological tests such as the Halstead–Reitan neuropsychological examination and the Luria–Nebraska neuropsychological examination are used for screening purposes. These batteries are discussed later in this chapter.

CLINICAL APPLICATION OF PSYCHOLOGICAL TESTING BATTERIES

Assessment of Cognitive Functioning in the Elderly

An example of current use of batteries of psychological tests is that advocated by Albert (1984) in the assessment of cognitive functioning in an elderly patient. The neuropsychological testing of the elderly comprises five

(*Text continues on p. 162.*)

TABLE 5-1. Assessment of Cognitive Functioning in the Elderly Patient

Attention	Language	Memory	Visiospatial Ability	Conceptualization
NORMAL AGING				
Digit span forward intact; problems with switching attention	Problems with naming objects (can describe function or purpose of object, however)	Problems with abstract and logically disconnected material between tasks	Intact	Intact
DELIRIUM				
Impaired severely (but fluctuations common)	Intact	Difficulty assessing this function relating to patient's problems with attention	Intact	Difficulty assessing this function relating to patient's problems with attention
Distractability				
Disruptions on tasks involving continuous performance				

160

DEPRESSION				
Inconsistency of performance	Intact	Complains of memory difficulties, but formal testing shows intact memory capacity	Intact	Slight impairment related to motivation and negativistic thinking
Highly dependent on motivation				
DEMENTIA				
Intact in early stage	Severe problems with naming	Delayed recall impaired dramatically	Often highly impaired	Significant impairment
Forward digit span intact in early stages	Neologisms	Immediate and remote recall often spared in the early phase	Special problems related to perseveration (figures repeat or overlap)	Concrete interpretation of proverbs
Problems with reverse digit span	Confabulation			Perseverative responses
				Self-referential

Adapted from Albert M: Assessment of cognitive function in the elderly. Psychosomatics 24, No. 4:310, 1984 basic areas of mental function: attention, language, memory, visiospatial ability, and conceptualization.

With this assessment, the effects of normal aging, delirium, depression, and dementing disorders such as Alzheimer's disease are differentiated. Multifactorial tests such as the Wechsler Adult Intelligence Scale and short, quick mental status tests such as the Mental Status Questionnaire are used to mark the presence of a dysfunction, but they have limited benefit in describing the nature and extent of the dysfunction revealed. Among the tests recommended are the Wechsler Memory Scale, the Boston Naming Test, the Dementia Rating Scale, and the Delayed Recognition Span Test. The elderly patient with dementia generally experiences memory testing as the most stressful task in a neuropsychological examination, and special care should be taken in choosing memory tests so that the patient's optimal capacity may be revealed. Care should be taken so that (1) the task instructions are clearly understood; (2) the response required is a simple one; (3) the task has a game-like quality that makes it appealing and nonthreatening; (4) subjects are not openly confronted with their failures, such as by being drilled on the words they have missed; (5) numerous alternative forms of the task can be administered easily on repeated occasions; and (6) the task permits detailed tracking and quantification of memory ability. Table 5-1 displays cognitive function and dysfunction in the elderly patient with normal aging, delirium, depression, and dementia.

Assessment of Brain Function

Halstead–Reitan Neuropsychological Battery

The two most commonly utilized neuropsychological test batteries are the Halstead–Reitan neuropsychological battery and the Luria–Nebraska neuropsychological battery. The Halstead–Reitan battery originally was developed and validated by Halstead, and later was modified to be utilized for individual patients by Reitan. This battery may be used as a general screening approach to assess the effects of brain damage. As with any psychological test, the motivation, emotional status, and physical condition of the patient as well as the competence of the examiner are important for reliable and valid results. There are three separate Halstead–Reitan neuropsychological batteries: for adults, for adolescents and grade-school children, and for young children. Each battery includes 14 separate tests in addition to an aphasia and constructional praxis test with 31 separate items. Commonly, these batteries are used in conjunction with the Wechsler Intelligence Scale as well as the MMPI. The average time required to administer the tests to a reasonably healthy adult is approximately 4 or 5 hours. The adult neuropsychological battery includes the following tests. (1) *The Halstead Category Test* is a learning test to measure current learning skills, abstract concept formation, and mental efficiency. (2) *The Tactile Performance Test* assesses tactile capacity as well as motor speed and psychomotor coordination. The patient is blindfolded and attempts to place various blocks in the appropriate holes in a board as rapidly as possible. (3) *The Rhythm Test* requires the patient to identify 30 rhythmic beats presented on a tape recorder. The patient's task is to identify pairs of rhythmic beats as either the same or different. The score is scaled based on the number of a correct identifications, with one being the best and ten being the worst possible scaled score. It measures nonverbal auditory perception as well as attention and concentration. (4) During the *Speech–Sounds Perception Test,* the patient is presented with 60 nonsense words played on a tape recorder. The patient is required to identify written representations of the spoken nonsense words. This test measures auditory–verbal perception. (5) The *Finger Oscillation Test* measures the patient's capacity to depress a lever with his index finger as rapidly as possible. The score for each hand is measured, and right-hand and left-hand performances are compared. (6) The *Strength of Grip Test* employs a hand dynamometer to measure the strength for each hand. The test is also used to compare right-sided function with left-sided function. (7) The *Sensory–Perceptual Examination* involves the application of equal bilateral stimuli to specific areas of the body to determine how the patient perceives either or both stimuli. These stimulations may be either tactile, auditory, or visual, and often are used to measure parietal functioning. (8) The *Trail Making Test* involves the connection of numbered or lettered circles with a pencil according to specific instructions by the examiner. Part A consists of 25 circles randomly distributed over an 8 1/2 inch × 11 inch sheet of white paper. Within each circle is a number from 1 to 25. The patient is instructed to connect as rapidly as possible the circles with a pencil in numerical order. The score is the total time it takes for the patient to complete the test, including the time spent to correct errors. Part B of the test consists of 25 circles either numbered 1 to 13 or lettered A to L. The patient's task is to connect the circles in an order that alternates between numbers and letters, such as 1–A–2–B–3–C, and so on. Again, this score is the time required for the patient to complete the test. In addition to testing concentration and attention, this test also measures visual scanning and the patient's ability to utilize symbols and to follow rational sequences. (9) *Tactile, visual, and auditory testing* is done in a similar fashion to that performed on the standard neurologic examination. However, the sensory tests on neuropsychological batteries are structured and scored by standardized techniques. (10) The *Tactile Finger Localization Test* employs light touch applied to each finger of each hand. The patient is asked to close his eyes and identify which finger is touched. In addition to testing the spinothalamic tracks, this test may be used to evaluate specific temporoparietal function. (11) In the *Tactile Form Recognition Test*, the patient is asked to place one hand through a hole in a board. Into that hand is introduced one of four forms: a square, a cross, a triangle, or a circle. The patient, who cannot see the object, is then asked to identify it by pointing with the other hand to the shape on a board that corresponds to the form presently being grasped. (12) The modified *Halstead–Wepman Aphasia Screening Test* involves several tasks for the patient including copying, naming, spelling, identifying, and repeating. The procedure evaluates language ability, including the ability to read, to repeat spoken language, and to compute.

The Halstead–Reitan battery tests a broad range of neuropsychological functions. Specific deficits in function that are revealed on several subtests help to isolate and localize the anatomical lesion. For example, test results that would suggest left hemisphere lesion would be (1) impairments of items on the verbal test of the WAIS resulting in a verbal IQ lower than the performance IQ; (2) impairments in verbal items on the modified Halstead–Wepman Aphasia Screening Test; (3) poor right-hand performance on the Tactile Finger Localization test with normal left-hand performance. Test results indicating a lesion in the right hemisphere might include the following: (1) impaired ability to draw on the Modified Halstead–Wepman Aphasia Screening Test; (2) poor left-hand performance on the Rhythm Test with intact right-hand functions on the test; (3) impaired left-handed performance on the Strength of Grip Test with preserved right-handed strength; and (4) poor left-hand performance on the Tactile Finger Localization and Tactile Form Recognition Tests with normal right-hand function. An example of results on the Halstead–Reitan neuropsychological battery that might indicate a more focused left parietal lobe deficit would include (1) right-sided sensory losses; (2) deficits on the digit span, arithmetic, and block design subtests of the WAIS; (3) poor performance on the Trail Making Test; and (4) aphasic symptoms, which could include the inability to name objects, dyslexia and other reading deficits, dysgraphia, and problems with arithmetic. (A more extensive discussion of the evaluation of the cortical function is included in Chap. 4.)

Luria–Nebraska Neuropsychological Battery

A second battery of neuropsychological tests that has been widely used and accepted is the Luria–Nebraska neuropsychological battery. The standardized version consists of 269 items, each of which is administered separately and represents a specific aspect of function. The items vary in complexity, degree of difficulty, mode of answering (*i.e.,* motoric, speech, multiple choice), and the amount of time allowed for response. Ten major areas of neuropsychological performance are explored: motor skills; rhythmic and pitch abilities; tactile abilities; expressive and receptive speech skills; reading, writing, and arithmetic skills; memory skills; visual–spatial skills; and intellectual ability. Advantages of this battery over the Halstead–Reitan battery are that it takes less time to administer (approximately 2 1/2 hours) and that it allows the examiner to divide general cortical functions into both specific skills and deficits.

PSYCHIATRIC RATING SCALES

Several investigators have drawn a distinction between rating scales and behavior inventories or behavior checklists. These investigators believe that rating scales require the rater to make judgments or form impressions about a patient's state of mind or the severity of his symptoms, whereas checklists report only the presence or absence of certain observable or measurable qualities of the patient's behavior. We have chosen not to make such a distinction in the following discussion, because the differentiation has not been generally accepted by the psychometricians who develop or the researchers who use rating scales. Psychiatric rating scales are most often used to document and measure the severity of specific psychiatric conditions as well as to measure changes in the patient's clinical state at a particular time. Utilizing quantifiable measurements, psychiatric rating scales may be used to record the response of the patient to treatment, for either clinical or research purposes. Standardization in administering the test and in collecting, scoring, and interpreting data is an essential element of psychiatric rating scales. Because psychiatric rating scales measure psychological status at a specific time, *change* in a patient's condition is established by administering the scale under conditions similar to the initial evaluation. Rating scales are usually categorized by the manner in which the data are collected. For example, certain rating scales require the patient to complete self-report questionnaires. Other rating scales use professionals who observe and make ratings of patients in specific settings, such as on an inpatient unit. The most commonly utilized method in rating scales is for a professional rater to interview a patient, and then complete the specific scale. A major advantage of the interview method is that it permits the interviewer to interact with a patient to enhance the patient's motivation and compliance as well as to gain information from the process of the rater/patient interaction. Recently, computer programs have been designed to administer and score rating scales.

Self-Report Questionnaires

A major advantage of the self-report questionnaire is the saving of professional time and expense. Nevertheless, there are important limitations of self-report questionnaires in that the approach is not applicable to the agitated or psychotic patient, to patients who cannot read or understand the test, or to patients who are not motivated to cooperate. An extension of self-report questionnaires is those scales that are completed by other informants, usually family members or custodians. The advantage of this format is that data from the home or other outpatient settings may be secured. Problems related to informant reliability (*i.e.*, poor reality testing, low intelligence, lying, etc.) limit the approach for many research purposes.

Self-Report Symptom Inventory-Revised (SCL-90-R)

A commonly used example of a self-report questionnaire is the Self-Report Symptom Inventory-Revised (SCL-90-R), which was developed by Derogatis, Lipman, and Covi. This is a clinical rating scale oriented towards symptomatic behavior in psychiatric outpatients. The SCL-90-R is composed of 90 items reflecting nine primary symptom behaviors found in psychiatric outpatients. The primary symptom dimensions categorized are somatization; obsessive-compulsive; interpersonal sensitivity; depression; anxiety; hostility; phobic anxiety; paranoid ideation; and psychoticism. The patient is asked to read each of 90 symptoms carefully and to select one of the numbered descriptors that best reflects how much discomfort that particular symptom or problem had caused him during a discrete period of time (such as the past week or the past 2 weeks). For example, the patient is asked, "How much were you distressed by stomach pain?" and is given the following descriptors to choose from: 0—not at all; 1—a little bit; 2—moderately; 3—quite a bit; 4—extremely. Representative examples of other symptoms include: headaches; nervousness or shakiness inside; loss of sexual interest or pleasure; crying easily; pains in the lower back; feeling fearful; feeling inferior to others; trouble falling asleep; your mind going blank; a lump in your throat; having urges to break or smash things; feelings of worthlessness; having thoughts about sex that bother you a lot; never feeling close to another person; and feelings of guilt.

Because of the ease of administration as well as the wide range of symptoms reviewed in the SCL-90-R, the scale has found broad utilization as a general clinical screening device in numerous outpatient settings such as general psychiatric assessment and treatment services, emergency rooms, psychopharmacology clinics, and even substance abuse centers. It has also been utilized in nonpsychiatric settings such as counseling centers, student health facilities, medical clinics, cardiac rehabilitation units, and even executive health programs. It has been utilized to measure the outcome of procedures designed to alleviate both physical and psychological symptomatologies, such as the benefit of a comprehensive cardiac rehabilitation program for treating physical and psychological limitations following myocardial infarction. The SCL-90-R has also been used extensively as a research instrument, especially in treatment studies involving repeated assessments of broad symptom pictures across time. The relative ease of administration and the short time required to take the test allow repeated assessments without undue stress on patients and excessive utilization of resources. It is our belief that a major limitation of the SCL-90-R is its capacity to assess certain personality disorders. Specifically, very few items would be useful in making the diagnosis of dependent, narcissistic, borderline, or histrionic personality disorders. Also missing from the checklist are sufficient items related to manic symptomatology. Figure 5-4 is a sample of a page from the SCL-90-R. Examples of other self-report questionnaires commonly used include the Beck Depression Inventory (see Appendix 5-1), the Minnesota Multiphasic Personality Inventory, the Brief Symptom Inventory, and the Zung Self-Rating Scale, which focuses on depressive symptoms.

Naturalistic Observation Scales

Most naturalistic observation scales are designed for use in inpatient psychiatric facilities or in other restrictive settings. The scales allow the raters to be trained in assessing particular behaviors and for reliability assessments of the individual raters to be made. Importantly, naturalistic observation scales are less impressionistic and inferential than self-report questionnaires. Psychiatric rating scales utilizing naturalistic observations frequently limit ratings to highly specific aspects of behavior such as violence, withdrawal, or agitation.

Nurses' Observation Scale for Inpatient Evaluation (NOSIE-30)

A representative example of a naturalistic observation scale is the Nurse's Observation Scale for Inpatient Evaluation (NOSIE-30), which was devel-

SCL-90-R™

INSTRUCTIONS:

Below is a list of problems and complaints that people sometimes have. Please read each one carefully. After you have done so, please fill in one of the numbered circles to the right that best describes HOW MUCH DISCOMFORT THAT PROBLEM HAS CAUSED YOU DURING THE PAST WEEK INCLUDING TODAY. Mark only one numbered circle for each problem and do not skip any items. If you change your mind, erase your first mark carefully. Read the example below before beginning, and if you have any questions please ask the technician.

SEX

MALE ○

FEMALE ○

NAME: _____

LOCATION: _____

EDUCATION: _____

MARITAL STATUS: MAR___SEP___DIV___WID___SING___

DATE
MO	DAY	YEAR

ID. NUMBER

AGE

VISIT NUMBER: _____

EXAMPLE

HOW MUCH WERE YOU DISTRESSED BY:

	NOT AT ALL	A LITTLE BIT	MODERATELY	QUITE A BIT	EXTREMELY
1. Bodyaches	⓪	①	②	●	④

HOW MUCH WERE YOU DISTRESSED BY:

		NOT AT ALL	A LITTLE BIT	MODERATELY	QUITE A BIT	EXTREMELY
1. Headaches	1	⓪	①	②	③	④
2. Nervousness or shakiness inside	2	⓪	①	②	③	④
3. Repeated unpleasant thoughts that won't leave your mind	3	⓪	①	②	③	④
4. Faintness or dizziness	4	⓪	①	②	③	④
5. Loss of sexual interest or pleasure	5	⓪	①	②	③	④
6. Feeling critical of others	6	⓪	①	②	③	④
7. The idea that someone else can control your thoughts	7	⓪	①	②	③	④
8. Feeling others are to blame for most of your troubles	8	⓪	①	②	③	④
9. Trouble remembering things	9	⓪	①	②	③	④
10. Worried about sloppiness or carelessness	10	⓪	①	②	③	④
11. Feeling easily annoyed or irritated	11	⓪	①	②	③	④
12. Pains in heart or chest	12	⓪	①	②	③	④
13. Feeling afraid in open spaces or on the streets	13	⓪	①	②	③	④
14. Feeling low in energy or slowed down	14	⓪	①	②	③	④
15. Thoughts of ending your life	15	⓪	①	②	③	④
16. Hearing voices that other people do not hear	16	⓪	①	②	③	④
17. Trembling	17	⓪	①	②	③	④
18. Feeling that most people cannot be trusted	18	⓪	①	②	③	④
19. Poor appetite	19	⓪	①	②	③	④
20. Crying easily	20	⓪	①	②	③	④
21. Feeling shy or uneasy with the opposite sex	21	⓪	①	②	③	④
22. Feelings of being trapped or caught	22	⓪	①	②	③	④
23. Suddenly scared for no reason	23	⓪	①	②	③	④
24. Temper outbursts that you could not control	24	⓪	①	②	③	④
25. Feeling afraid to go out of your house alone	25	⓪	①	②	③	④
26. Blaming yourself for things	26	⓪	①	②	③	④
27. Pains in lower back	27	⓪	①	②	③	④
28. Feeling blocked in getting things done	28	⓪	①	②	③	④
29. Feeling lonely	29	⓪	①	②	③	④
30. Feeling blue	30	⓪	①	②	③	④
31. Worrying too much about things	31	⓪	①	②	③	④
32. Feeling no interest in things	32	⓪	①	②	③	④
33. Feeling fearful	33	⓪	①	②	③	④
34. Your feelings being easily hurt	34	⓪	①	②	③	④
35. Other people being aware of your private thoughts	35	⓪	①	②	③	④

Copyright © 1975 by Leonard R. Derogatis, Ph.D.

Please continue on the following page ▶

FIG. 5-4. Sample page from the SCL-90-R. (Copyright 1975 by Leonard R. Derogatis, Ph.D.)

oped by Honigfield, Gillis, and Klett. This instrument is a 30-item scale designed to measure a patient's strengths as well as his pathology through the assessment of inpatient behavior by skilled nursing personnel. The nursing staff is asked to rate behavior that has occurred "over the last three days only." This is done by rating behaviors as occurring (1) never, (2) sometimes, (3) often, (4) usually, or (5) always. Symptom items include statements such as the following: is sloppy; cries; shows interest in activities around him; refuses to do the ordinary things expected of him; refuses to speak; says he is no good; is slow moving and sluggish; keeps himself clean; laughs or smiles at funny comments or events. Ratings are made for such categories as social competence, social interests, personal neatness, depression, irritability, manifest psychosis, and psychomotor retardation. The uses of the NOSIE-30 are similar to those described for the SCL-90-R, but are for inpatients rather than outpatients. Advantages of the NOSIE-30 are its relative ease to teach to nursing personnel, the brief time required to fill out the form, and its coverage of a broad range of psychiatric symptomatologies. A disadvantage of this scale is its relative lack of sensitivity for quantifying severity of depression, violence, and anxiety.

Overt Aggression Scale (OAS)

An example of a naturalistic observation scale designed for sensitive measurement of specific symptomatologies is the Overt Aggression Scale (OAS) developed by Yudofsky, Silver, Jackson, and Endicott. This is to be used in inpatient settings, and it measures observable aggressive behaviors. The scale divides aggression into four categories: verbal aggression, physical aggression against objects, physical aggression against self, and physical aggression against other people. All aggressive behaviors that occur during a specific period of time (such as over a single nursing shift) are rated. The rater is guided in his assessment by representative examples of increasing severity such as those listed in the scale under Physical Aggression Against Other People: (1) makes threatening gesture, swings at people, grabs at clothes; (2) strikes, kicks, pushes, pulls hair of others (without injury to them); (3) attacks others causing mild–moderate physical injury (bruises, sprain, welts); and (4) attacks others causing severe physical injury (broken bones, deep lacerations, internal injury). To enhance the validity of the scale, an Intervention Check List rates the specific intervention utilized to address the aggressive incident. Examples of interventions include talking to the patient; immediate medication given by mouth; immediate medication given by injection; seclusion; restraints; and immediate medical treatment for the patient. The scoring of the OAS is accomplished by sophisticated computer programs capable of generating graphics, such as a graph of the patient's aggressive behaviors over an extended period of time, or graphs of the times of day when aggressive events occur. Advantages of the OAS are that it is easily taught to inpatient staff and requires only seconds to minutes to complete. Comparative studies have shown this scale to be far more sensitive for measuring aggression and changes in aggression than chart reviews, which previously were the standard method of quantifying aggression for research purposes. An important application of the OAS is its use in research to assess the effects of psychopharmocologic agents in the treatment of aggression. (The Overt Aggression Scale, its scoring, and interpretation are summarized in Appendix 5-6, p. 203.)

Other naturalistic observation rating scales include the Manic-State Rating Scale by Biegle, the Children's Behavior Inventory by Burdock and Hardesty, and the Performance Test of Activities of Daily Living (PADL) by Kuriansky and Gurland.

Interview Assessment Scales

Psychiatric rating scales that combine a clinical interview of the patient by a trained interviewer with the completion of a standardized rating scale have broad clinical and research utility. Often these scales are accompanied by extensive booklets that guide the rater specifically how to initiate the interview, what questions to ask, and appropriate follow-up responses to the patient's answers. Comprehensive booklets may include case vignettes and even videotapes to educate raters in administering the interview and to test for inter-rater reliability. In scales utilizing a structured interview, raters ask patients questions in a highly restricted, specific fashion. Structured interviews allow for research to be conducted in multiple centers while employing different teams of raters.

Hamilton Rating Scale for Depression (HAMD)

A well-known example of an interview assessment scale is the Hamilton Rating Scale for Depression (HAMD). This was developed to quantify the severity of depressive illness in a patient diagnosed to have depression and to show changes in the patient's clinical condition. The HAMD is not to be utilized as a diagnostic instrument. The test is a 21-item list of symptoms that are to be marked for severity (either 0 to 4 or 0 to 2) by a clinician on the basis on an interview and any other data that are available. Guidelines are provided to help the interviewer arrive at his rating. For example, under the symptom of suicide are 0 = absent, 1 = feels life is not worth living, 2 =

wishes he were dead or any thoughts of possible death to self, 3 = suicidal ideas or gestures, and 4 = attempts at suicide. In addition, the scale is highly dependent upon the skill and experience of the rater, and obtaining additional information from relatives, friends, nursing staff, and other sources is encouraged. Raters are trained by professionals with experience using the instrument, and training on more than a dozen patients is usually required before a rater becomes proficient in administering the test. Hamilton advised that, whenever possible, two interviewers should be present during the administration of the instrument. One interviewer should conduct the formal interview of the patient, and the second rater should ask supplementary questions at the conclusion of the first interview. Thereafter, both raters, without discussion between them, should independently record and calculate their scores. Hamilton felt that discrepancies of one point between the raters on any single item are of little consequence, but a difference of two points requires careful consideration before the validity of the particular rating is accepted. A difference of four points in the total score is the maximum allowable discrepancy. The HAMD has received broad use in both clinical and research settings for the quantification and measurement of change in the symptoms of depression. A common use of the scale is assessing the benefits of antidepressant agents and other approaches for the treatment of depression. (The Hamilton Rating Scale for Depression, its scoring, and interpretation are summarized in Appendix 5-4, p. 197.)

Schedule for Affective Disorders and Schizophrenia (SADS)

A second and more elaborate type of interview assessment scale is the Schedule for Affective Disorders and Schizophrenia (SADS) developed by Spitzer and Endicott. SADS is an example of a structured interview that is in the form of a large booklet designed as an interview guide for the evaluator. Some instruments provide the exact question to be asked in the order in which the patient is to be interviewed. Structured interviews are utilized almost exclusively for research purposes, and the intent of this format is to enhance reliability, especially when the instrument is being used for research conducted at multiple clinical sites. The two major sources of unreliability that lead to disagreement among clinicians on psychiatric diagnoses are criteria variance and information variance. Criteria variance refers to differences in the inclusion and exclusion criteria that clinicians use to summarize the patient data into psychiatric diagnoses. Information variance results when clinicians have different amounts or kinds of information about the patients.

The Schedule for Affective Disorders and Schizophrenia is available in three forms: the regular SADS, a lifetime version (SADS-L), and a version for measuring change (SADS-C). The SADS interview guide and rating form is composed of a 78-page booklet, and it is organized into two parts. Part 1 is designed to provide a detailed description of the patient's current episode or condition as well as his psychosocial functioning during the week prior to the interview. Part 1 can aid in arriving at a diagnosis and a prognosis, and in describing the phenomenology of the current episode of the illness. In addition, it is able to measure symptom change. Figures 5-5 and 5-6 illustrate two sample pages from part 1 of SADS. Part 2 of the SADS focuses primarily on historical information about past psychiatric disturbances. Figure 5-7 from part 2 of the SADS demonstrates how the critria for a given diagnosis, in this case alcoholism, are specified and documented. Both parts of the SADS may be administered in one sitting, with a short break after finishing

BEGINNING OF INTERVIEW AND RATINGS

The rater should first introduce himself to the subject and explain that the first part of the interview will focus on the subject's recent problems or difficulties and that some of the questions are standard questions that need to be asked of everyone who is interviewed. He should then obtain or confirm enough basic demographic information, such as age, marital status, and date admitted to the clinic or hospital, so that both the rater and the subject have an opportunity to orient themselves prior to beginning the interview.

The rater should then ask the subject to give an account of the history of the present illness in a brief unstructured interview which usually will last from 10 to 15 minutes. In addition to getting an overview of the kinds of difficulties that the subject has been having, the rater should obtain information necessary to rate the first 3 items (Classification of Current Condition, Duration, and Onset).

If a psychiatric patient: *I would like to hear about your problems or difficulties, and how they led to your coming to the (hospital, clinic).*

NOTES

If a patient refers to long-term difficulties: *What I would like to focus on now is what led to your coming here. Later I will be asking you about the past.*

If not a psychiatric patient: *I would like to hear about any problems or difficulties you are having in your life now.*

For all subjects: *When would you say you first noticed that something was wrong (this time)?*

How different has this trouble been from the way you were before or usually are?

How long was it from when you first noticed that something was wrong until you went to (treatment facility)?

Are you feeling better now or is it at its worst now?

If feeling better now: *How long has it been since you were (description of full-blown condition)?*

When did you last feel like your usual self for a couple of months?

Sample—Not for reproduction or clinical application

FIG. 5-5. Structured interview as initiated in SADS, part 1.

SADS

SCREENING ITEMS FOR MANIC SYNDROME

The next 5 items are screening items to determine the presence of manic-like behavior. If any of the items are judged present, inquire in a general way to determine how he was behaving at that time with such questions as, *When you were this way, what kinds of things were you doing? How did you spend your time?* Do not include behavior which is clearly explainable by alcohol or drug use.

If the subject has only described dysphoric mood, the following questions regarding the manic syndrome should be introduced with a statement such as: *I know you have been feeling (depressed). However, many people have other feelings mixed in or at different times so it is important that I ask you about those feelings also.*

Elevated or expansive mood and/or optimistic attitude toward the future which lasted at least several hours and was out of proportion to the circumstances.

Have (there been times when) you felt very good or too cheerful or high —not just your normal self?

If unclear: *Have you felt on top of the world or as if there was nothing you couldn't do?*

(Have you felt that everything would work out just the way you wanted?)

If people saw you would they think you were just in a good mood or something more than that?

(What about during the past week?)

			353
0	No information		
1	Not at all, normal, or depressed		
2	Slight, e.g., good spirits, more cheerful than most people in his circumstances, but of only possible clinical significance		
3	Mild, e.g., definitely elevated or expansive mood and overly optimistic which is somewhat out of proportion to his circumstances		
4	Moderate, e.g., mood and outlook are clearly out of proportion to circumstances		
5	Severe, e.g., quality of euphoric mood		
6	Extreme, e.g., clearly elated, exalted expression and says "Everything is beautiful, I feel so good"		

PAST WEEK 0 1 2 3 4 5 6   354

Less need for sleep than usual to feel rested (average for several days when needed less sleep).

Have you needed less sleep than usual to feel rested? (How much sleep do you ordinarily need?) (How much when you were [are] high?)

		355
0	No information	
1	No change or more sleep needed	
2	Up to 1 hour less than usual	
3	Up to 2 hours less than usual	
4	Up to 3 hours less than usual	
5	Up to 4 hours less than usual	
6	4 or more hours less than usual	

(What about during the past week?)

PAST WEEK 0 1 2 3 4 5 6   356

Unusually energetic (which lasted for at least several days), more active than usual without expected fatigue.

Have you had more energy than usual to do things?

(More than just a return to normal or usual level?)

(Did it seem like too much energy?)

		357
0	No information	
1	No different than usual or less energetic	
2	Slightly more energetic but of questionable significance	
3	Little change in activity level but less fatigued than usual	
4	Somewhat more active than usual with little or no fatigue	
5	Much more active than usual with little or no fatigue	
6	Unusually active all day long with little or no fatigue	

(What about during the past week?)

PAST WEEK 0 1 2 3 4 5 6   358

FIG. 5-6. Mental status information about manic symptomatology as elicited and documented in SADS, part 1. *(Continues on p. 174.)*

Increase in goal-directed activity as compared with usual level. Consider changes in involvement or activity level associated with work, family, friends, sex drive, new projects, interests or activities (e.g., telephone calls, letter writing).	0	No information	359
	1	No change or decrease	
	2	Slightly more interest or activity but of questionable significance	
Was there a time when you were more active or involved in things compared to the way you usually are?	3	Mild but definite increase in general activity level in one or a few areas, e.g., cleans house several times a day, more productive at work	
(What about your work, housekeeping, family, friends, sex, hobbies, new projects or interests?)	4	Moderate generalized increase in activity level involving several areas	
(How much of your day has been spent in this?)	5	Marked increase and almost constantly involved in numerous activities in many areas	
	6	Extreme, e.g., constantly active in a variety of activities from awakening till he goes to sleep	
(What about during the past week?)	PAST WEEK 0 1 2 3 4 5 6		360
Grandiosity. Increased self-esteem and appraisal of his worth, contacts, power or knowledge (up to grandiose delusions) as compared with usual level. Persecutory delusions should not be considered evidence of grandiosity unless the subject feels the persecution is due to some special attributes of his (e.g., power, knowledge, or contacts).	0	No information	361
	1	Not at all or decreased self-esteem	
	2	Slight, e.g., is more confident about himself than most people in his circumstances but of only possible clinical significance	
Have you felt more self-confident than usual?	3	Mild, e.g., definitely inflated self-esteem or exaggerates his talents somewhat out of proportion to circumstances	
(Have you felt that you are a particularly important person or that you had special talents or abilities?)	4	Moderate, e.g., inflated self-esteem clearly out of proportion to circumstances	
	5	Severe, e.g., clear grandiose delusion	
(What about special plans?)	6	Extreme, e.g., preoccupied with, or acts on the basis of, grandiose delusions	
(What about during the past week?)	PAST WEEK 0 1 2 3 4 5 6		362

CHARACTERISTICS OF BEHAVIOR AND IDEATION DURING A PERIOD WHICH MIGHT BE "MANIC"

☐ The 5 previous screening items were to determine the need for more exploration of a possible manic period. If all 5 screening items are rated 1 or 2, and there is no other evidence to suggest a manic period, the rater may check here and skip to Alcohol Abuse, page 23. If any of the 5 items are rated more than 2, the rater should complete this section, even if he is convinced that the subject did not have a manic period.

363*

Note: Some items are punched 1 when blank, b=1.

Sample—Not for reproduction

FIG. 5-6. *(Continued).*

part 1. In most circumstances the SADS evaluation should follow the initial clinical interview, or it may be given later when the patient is better able to provide accurate historical information.

The SADS interviewer is not limited by the data provided by the patient's responses to the structured interviews. The final rating will also be based on all other available sources of information, such as interviews with family members, reference to case records, and data provided by referring physicians. It is recommended that the interviewers for the SADS be highly trained in interviewing techniques as well as making judgments related to manifest psychopathology. In general, raters are limited to psychiatrists,

ALCOHOLISM

This section covers the details of alcohol use <u>up to the present</u>. The subject should be reminded of this. Sufficient information may already be available from the Part I interview to complete the screening items.

There are 2 criteria.

I At least 2 of the items 857 – 875:

	No info	No	Yes	

What have your drinking habits been like?

Was there ever a period in your life when you drank too much?..........................	X	1	2	857
Has anyone in your family – or anyone else – ever objected to your drinking?..	X	1	2	858
Was there ever a time when you often couldn't stop drinking when you wanted to?..	X	1	2	859

When you were drinking, how much did you drink?

☐ Ask additional questions if needed, then if no history suggestive of problems with alcohol, check here and skip to Drug Abuse or Dependence, page 57.   860

Was there ever a time when you frequently had a drink before breakfast?...........	X	1	2	861
Was there ever a time when, because of your drinking, you often missed work, had trouble on the job, or were unable to take care of household responsibilities (e.g., getting meals prepared, doing shopping)?...	X	1	2	862
Did you ever lose a job because of your drinking?...	X	1	2	863
Did you often have difficulties with your family, friends or acquaintances because of your drinking?...	X	1	2	864
Were you ever divorced or separated primarily because of your drinking?...........	X	1	2	865
Have you ever gone on a bender? [Definition: drinking steadily for 3 or more days more than a fifth of whiskey daily (or 24 bottles of beer, or 3 bottles of wine). Must have occurred 3 or more times.]..	X	1	2	866
Have you ever been physically violent while drinking? [Must have occurred on at least 2 occasions.]	X	1	2	867
Have you ever had traffic difficulties because of your drinking – like reckless driving, accidents, or speeding?...	X	1	2	868
Have you ever been picked up by the police because of how you were acting while you were drinking? [Examples: disturbing the peace, fighting, public intoxication. Do not include traffic difficulties.]	X	1	2	869
Have you often had blackouts? [Definition: memory loss for events that occurred while conscious during a drinking eposide.]	X	1	2	870
Have you often had tremors (that were most likely due to drinking)?.................	X	1	2	871
Have you ever had the DT's? [Definition: Confusional state following stopping drinking that includes disorientation and illusions or hallucinations.]...................	X	1	2	872

FIG. 5-7. Historical information about alcohol dependence is elicited and documented by SADS, part. 2. (*Continues on p. 176.*)

	No info	No	Yes	
Did you ever hear voices or see things that weren't really there, soon after you stopped drinking? [Hallucinations — must have occurred on at least two separate occasions.]	X	1	2	873
Have you ever had a seizure or fit after you stopped drinking? [In a non-epileptic.]	X	1	2	874
Did a doctor ever tell you that you had developed a physical complication of alcoholism, like gastritis, pancreatitis, cirrhosis, or neuritis? [Include good evidence of Korsakoff's Syndrome - chronic brain syndrome with anterograde amnesia as the predominant feature]	X	1	2	875

Has had at least 2 of the items 857 — 875: □ 1 No / 2 Yes   913

II Period of heavy drinking that lasted at least a month. □ 1 No / 2 Yes   914

→ Skip to Drug Abuse or Dependence, below.

Has met the 2 criteria for Alcoholism.......................... YES   915

Currently has a problem with alcohol.......................... YES   916

Age started drinking heavily.. ____   917–18

Age stopped drinking heavily (leave blank if drinking heavily within the last 6 months)................ ____   919–20

Sample—Not for reproduction

FIG. 5-7. *(Continued).*

clinical psychologists, or psychiatric social workers. The authors of the SADS advise that if other research personnel are used to administer the SADS, much more training with the instrument is generally necessary. An experienced and well-trained interviewer who is familiar with the SADS usually requires half an hour to 2 hours to complete the evaluation, depending upon the degree of disturbance of the patient. The SADS currently is used in a large number of studies to investigate a broad variety of research questions related to the genetics, psychobiology, response to treatment, and clinical description of mental disorders. It has particular value in collaborative research projects both in the United States and in Europe. An advantage of the SADS is its modern structure, which enables the conclusions to be consistent with the diagnostic categories included in the third edition of the American Psychiatric Association's *Diagnostic and Statistical Manual* (DSM III). Other interview assessment scales include the Hamilton Anxiety Rating Scale (HARS), the Mental Status Schedule (MSS), the Mental Status Examination Record (MSER), the Psychiatric Status Schedule (PSS), the Global Assessment Scale (GAS).

Personality Disorder Examination (PDE)

Until recently, rating scales in general and structured interviews in particular have provided inadequate coverage of personality disorders. The personality disorders are coded on axis II of the DSM-III-R classifications system, and include the following disorders: paranoid, schizoid, schizotypal, histrionic, narcissistic, antisocial, borderline, avoident, dependent, compulsive, passive-aggressive, and other. To address this deficiency, two new structured interviews that assess personality disorders have been developed and tested recently. The Personality Disorder Examination (PDE) by Loranger, Susman, Oldham, and Russakoff was designed to survey systematically the phenomenology and life experience relevant to the diagnosis of the personality disorders in the DMS-III-R. The test is not intended to be given to subjects under the age of 18 years, or to patients with psychoses, low intelligence, or substantial cognitive impairment. The PDE is administered in a single session lasting from 1 to 2 hours, and it is designed to be administered by an experienced clinician—either a psychiatrist, psychologist, or psychiatric social worker—who is familiar with the directions and scoring of the PDE. The examiner instructs the patient as follows: "The questions I'm going to ask concern what you are like most of the time. I'm interested in what has been typical of you throughout your adult life, and not just recently. But if you have changed and your answers might have been different at some time in the past, be sure to let me know." The questions are designed to flow in a natural sequence and are arranged under six headings: work, self, interpersonal relations, affects, reality testing, and impulse control. Each of the six sections is introduced by an open-ended inquiry that offers the subject an opportunity to discuss the topic in as much detail as he chooses. There are items that pertain to the subject's behavior during the interview, and certain of these questions are designed to provide a record of the subject's mental state during the examination. The examiner scores each item in the interview by assigning a zero if the behavior is absent, a 1 when it is present but of uncertain clinical significance, a 2 when it is present and clinically significant, and a question mark (?) when the subject fails to respond or it is not possible to classify the response. A scoring guide is provided to help select the appropriate score. Based on the patient's score, DSM-III-R criteria are either met or not met, and thereafter algorithms are applied to determine whether the subject fulfills DMS-III-R requirements for the personality disorders. Figure 5-8 demonstrates the assessment of affects by the PED utilizing the structured interview format, and Figure 5-9 is an example of the manner in which behavior is observed by the rater during the interview.

Structured Clinical Interview
for DSM-III-R (SCID)

The most recent and possibly the most innovative and far-reaching psychiatric rating scale is the Structured Clinical Interview for DSM-III-R (SCID). Developed by Spitzer and Williams in collaboration with a large array of

(Text continues on p. 181.)

Now I would like to ask you some questions about your feelings. Again I'm interested in the way you have been most of your life, and not just recently. If you have changed and are different from the way you used to be, please let me know.

How do you usually feel?

How do you usually feel deep down inside?

What problems do you have with your feelings?

Appears or claims to be indifferent to the praise and criticism of others	0 1 2 ?			*1068*
128. When some people are praised or complimented it seems to have no effect on them. Are you like that?	0 1 2 ?			
129. What about when you're criticized?	0 1 2 ?			
Feelings easily hurt by criticism or disapproval	0 1 2 ?			*1069*
130. Are your feelings easily hurt when people criticize you?	0 1 2 ?			
131. What about when someone disapproves of you or of something you've done?	0 1 2 ?			
Reacts to criticism with feelings of rage, shame, or humiliation (even if not expressed)	0 1 2 ?			*1070*
132. Do you usually have a strong reaction to criticism, so that you feel very ashamed or humiliated?	0 1 2 ?			
133. When you're criticized does it usually make you feel furious, even if you don't show it?	0 1 2 ?			

FIG. 5-8. Example of assessment of affect by PDE. (Reprinted with permission. Loranger AW, Susman VL, Oldham JM, et al: Personality Disorder Examination (PDE): A Structured Interview for DSM-III-R Personality Disorder. Version: May 15, 1985. White Plains, NY, The New York Hospital-Cornell Medical Center, Westchester Division)

Easily slighted and quick to react with anger or counterattack	0 1 2 ? *1071*
134. Are you easily slighted and quick to take offense?	0 1 2 ?
135. When you are slighted, do you get angry quickly?	0 1 2 ?
136. Are you too quick to fight back?	0 1 2 ?

Preoccupied with feelings of envy	0 1 2 ? *1072*
137. Do you often find yourself feeling envious of other people? (If yes) Is it hard for you to get rid of that feeling?	0 1 2 ?

Scoring

1. Present but of uncertain clinical significance
2. Present and clinically significant
? When the subject fails to respond or not possible to classify response
Sample—Not for reproduction

FIG. 5-8. *(Continued)*.

250. Dress inappropriate	0 1 2
251. Unkempt	0 1 2
252. Little or no variation in facial expression	0 1 2
253. Sad facial expression	0 1 2
254. Angry facial expression	0 1 2
255. Frightened or anxious facial expression	0 1 2
256. Appears "cold" and unemotional	0 1 2
257. Tearful	0 1 2
258. Fails to smile or laugh when expected	0 1 2
259. Smiles or giggles when subject is not humorous	0 1 2
260. Talks to self	0 1 2
261. Avoids eye contact	0 1 2
262. Peculiar mannerisms	0 1 2
263. Socially gauche or inappropriate	0 1 2
264. Seems uninterested in befriending or relating to examiner	0 1 2
265. Guarded or secretive	0 1 2
266. Hypervigilant	0 1 2
267. Suspicious	0 1 2
268. Reads hidden threatening meanings into benign remarks	0 1 2
269. Easily slighted and quick to react with anger or counterattack	0 1 2
270. Continually draws attention to self	0 1 2
271. Speaks with exaggeration or hyperbole	0 1 2

FIG. 5-9. Example of assessment of observed behavior during PDE interview. (Reprinted with permission. Loranger AW, Susman VL, Oldham JM, et al: Personality Disorder Examination (PDE): A Structured Interview for DSM-III-R Personality Disorder. Version: May 15, 1985. White Plains, NY, The New York Hospital–Cornell Medical Center, Westchester Division) *(Continues on p. 180.)*

272. Dramatic, expresses emotions in exaggerated manner   0 1 2
273. Appears overly concerned with physical appearance   0 1 2
274. Appears egocentric and self-indulgent   0 1 2
275. Distractible   0 1 2
276. Paces about room   0 1 2
277. Wrings hands or picks at clothing or body   0 1 2
278. Does not gesture, move or change position   0 1 2
279. Flirts or makes suggestive sexual remarks   0 1 2
280. Seductive clothes or posture   0 1 2
281. Appears shallow and lacking genuineness   0 1 2
282. Has irrational angry outburst or tantrum   0 1 2
283. Bangs fist in anger or frustration   0 1 2
284. Raises voice in anger   0 1 2
285. Becomes sulky   0 1 2
286. Without a good reason is critical of persons in positions of authority   0 1 2
287. Demanding   0 1 2
288. Speaks in a loud voice   0 1 2
289. Displays a prolonged reaction time in answering questions   0 1 2
290. Speaks softly   0 1 2
291. Speaks slowly   0 1 2
292. Voice trembles   0 1 2
293. Little or no variation in vocal pitch, volume, or inflection   0 1 2
294. Cracks jokes or makes witty remarks (infectious humor)   0 1 2
295. Makes silly remarks (noninfectious humor)   0 1 2
296. Brags or boasts   0 1 2
297. Makes sarcastic comments   0 1 2
298. Threatens to hit someone   0 1 2
299. Criticizes treatment or hospital   0 1 2
300. Constantly seeks reassurance, approval, or praise   0 1 2
301. Complains, directly or indirectly, about being unappreciated   0 1 2
302. Clings to examiner   0 1 2
303. Poverty of Speech   0 1 2
Spontaneous speech is absent, or rarely or ever provides more information than requested; frequently does not answer questions or replies are brief and not elaborated.
304. Poverty of Content of Speech   0 1 2
Replies are long enough but convey little or no information, because speech is vague, metaphorical, abstract, too specific or concrete.
305. Tangentiality   0 1 2
Spontaneous speech digresses and fails to return to the original goal; replies have no obvious relationship or are only remotely related to question.
306. Loose Associations   0 1 2
Speech fails to reach a goal or objective, or moves from one idea to another, which is either not obviously related or only obliquely or remotely related.
307. Incoherence   0 1 2
No logical or meaningful connection between words in same sentence, or violates rules of syntax or grammar beyond what might be expected due to education, intelligence, ethnicity, regionalisms, or second language.

FIG. 5-9. *(Continued)*.

308. Circumstantiality   0 1 2
Listener feels like telling speaker to get to the point, because
he includes many related but unnecessary details in arriving at
a goal.
309. Word Approximations (Metonyms)   0 1 2
Meaning is evident but word usage is unusual or bizarre, because words are used in idiosyncratic or unconventional ways
or as approximations of more exact ones.
310. Stilted Speech   0 1 2
Uses multisyllabic or uncommon words when shorter or more
common ones would do just as well, or frequently injects formal or overly polite expressions into conversation.

Sample—Not for reproduction

FIG. 5-9. *(Continued).*

psychometricians, theoreticians, clinicians, and other authorities on psychiatric diagnosis, the SCID is an instrument designed to enable a clinically
trained interviewer to make DSM-III-R diagnoses. Three versions of the
instrument are available. The SCID-P (Patient Version) is designed for subjects who are already identified as psychiatric patients. The SCID-NP (Nonpatient Version) is to be used in studies in which the subjects are not identified as being psychiatric patients, such as for community surveys, research
in primary care, or for family studies. Developed with support from the
Upjohn Company, the SCID-UP (Upjohn Version) was developed for use in a
multinational collaborative study of panic disorder. In addition, the SCID-II
is a structured clinical interview for DSM-III-R personality disorders (axis II
diagnoses).

Designed to help the clinician arrive at a rapid but valid DSM-III-R multiaxial diagnosis, the SCID is modeled on the clinical diagnostic interview. It
is intended to be utilized by mental health professionals who have experience in doing clinical interviews, a basic knowledge of psychopathology,
and a familiarity with the DSM-III-R. Utilizing the structured-interview
format, each axis I diagnostic category is systematically reviewed. At the
beginning of the interview, an overview of the present illness and past
episodes of psychopathology is obtained. The interview schedule has many
open-ended questions that encourage the subject to describe his symptoms
rather than solely to agree or not to agree that a symptom described by the
interviewer is present. The sequence of the questions is designed to approxi-
mate the differential diagnostic process of an experienced clinician, and the
interviewer is instructed to use all sources of information available about
the subject in making ratings. Such information might include referral notes
and observations of family members, friends, and other informants. The
interviewer is directed to "stick to the questions" as they are written, except for necessary minor modifications to take into account what the sub-

(Text continues on p. 186.)

Chief Complaint
What led to your coming here (this time)? (What's the major problem you've been having trouble with?)

Onset of Present Illness (Including Prodrome)
When did this all begin? (When did you first notice that something was wrong?)

Were you your usual self before that?
 If unclear: What made you come for help now?

New SXS or Recurrence?
Is this something new or a return of something you had before?

Environmental Context and Possible Precipitants of Present Illness
What was going on in your life when this began?

Did anything happen or change just before all this started?

Course of Present Illness
After it started, what happened next? (Did other things start to bother you? What effect did it have on you?)

Since this began, when have you felt the worst?
 If more than a year ago: In the last year, when have you felt the worst?

Treatment of Present Illness
Note the types of treatment providers contacted, treatments received, and whether they helped: Did you go to anyone for help? (What treatment did you receive? Did it help?)

Other Problems
Has anything else been bothering you?

What's your mood been like?

How much have you been drinking (alcohol) since this all began?

Have you been taking any drugs? (What about marijuana, cocaine, other street drugs?)

How has your physical health been?

Previous Treatment for Emotional Disorders
(Before this time . . .)

Have you ever seen anybody for emotional or psychiatric problems?
 If yes: What was that for?

(Before this time . . .)

Have you ever been a patient in a psychiatric hospital?
 If yes: What was that for?
 If gives an inadequate answer, challenge gently: E.g., Wasn't there something else?
 People usually don't go to psychiatric hospitals just because they are tired or nervous.

Sample—Not for reproduction

FIG. 5-10. SCID-P. Chief complaint and history of present illness. (Reprinted with permission. Spitzer RL, Williams JBW, Biometrics Research Department, New York State Psychiatric Institute, New York, NY)

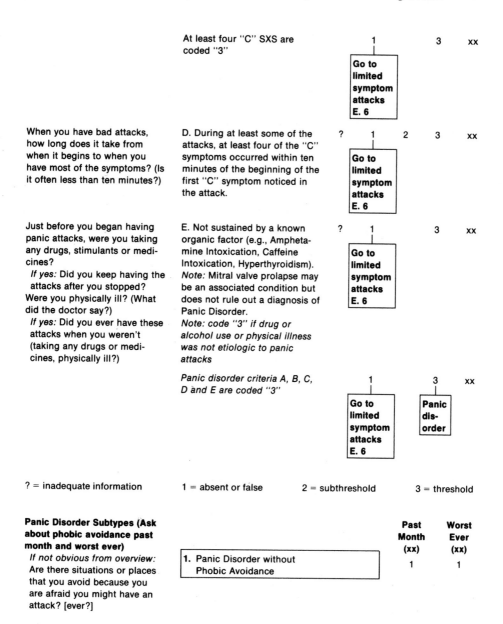

At least four "C" SXS are coded "3"

    1   3   xx

Go to limited symptom attacks E. 6

When you have bad attacks, how long does it take from when it begins to when you have most of the symptoms? (Is it often less than ten minutes?)

D. During at least some of the attacks, at least four of the "C" symptoms occurred within ten minutes of the beginning of the first "C" symptom noticed in the attack.

?   1   2   3   xx

Go to limited symptom attacks E. 6

Just before you began having panic attacks, were you taking any drugs, stimulants or medicines?
If yes: Did you keep having the attacks after you stopped?
Were you physically ill? (What did the doctor say?)
If yes: Did you ever have these attacks when you weren't (taking any drugs or medicines, physically ill?)

E. Not sustained by a known organic factor (e.g., Amphetamine Intoxication, Caffeine Intoxication, Hyperthyroidism).
Note: Mitral valve prolapse may be an associated condition but does not rule out a diagnosis of Panic Disorder.
Note: code "3" if drug or alcohol use or physical illness was not etiologic to panic attacks

?   1   3   xx

Go to limited symptom attacks E. 6

Panic disorder criteria A, B, C, D and E are coded "3"

    1   3   xx

Go to limited symptom attacks E. 6

Panic disorder

? = inadequate information   1 = absent or false   2 = subthreshold   3 = threshold

---

Panic Disorder Subtypes (Ask about phobic avoidance past month and worst ever)
If not obvious from overview: Are there situations or places that you avoid because you are afraid you might have an attack? [ever?]

	Past Month (xx)	Worst Ever (xx)
1. Panic Disorder without Phobic Avoidance	1	1

FIG. 5-11. SCID-P. Criteria for panic disorder. (Reprinted with permission. Spitzer RL, Williams JBW, Biometrics Research Department, New York State Psychiatric Institute, New York, NY) *(Continues on p. 184.)*

(Tell me all the things you avoid, or can only do by forcing yourself?) (What about going out of the house alone, being in crowds or certain public places like tunnels, bridges, buses or trains?) (How often do you go outside of your house alone?) (Do you often need a companion?) (What effect does avoiding these situations or places have on your life?)	2. Panic Disorder with Limited Phobic Avoidance (significant phobic avoidance or endurance despite intense anxiety)			2		2
	3. Panic Disorder with Agoraphobia (generalized travel restrictions, often needs a companion away from home, or markedly altered life style)			3		3

If no panic attacks during last 6 months specify: (No current panic attacks)
Coded in chronology section below

Chronology

If unclear: During the past month, have you had any panic attacks (even little ones), or worried a lot that you might have one, or have you avoided situations or places because you were afraid you might have one?	Has had some symptom(s) of Panic Disorder during past month	?	1	3	xx
When did you last have (any SX of panic disorder)?	Number of months prior to interview when last had a symptom of Panic Disorder	—	—	—	xx xx xx
If unclear: During the past month, how many panic attacks have you had?	Has met symptomatic criteria for Panic Disorder during past month, i.e., at least 3 panic attacks	?	1	3	xx

? = inadequate information   1 = absent or false   2 = subthreshold   3 = threshold

During the past five years, how much of the time have you been bothered by (*panic attacks, persistent fear of having an attack, or phobic avoidance*)?	Duration in months during past five years that any symptoms of Panic Disorder were present	—	—		xx xx
How old were you when you first started having a lot of panic attacks (or worried all the time that you might have one)?	Age at onset of Panic Disorder (at least three attacks over a three week period or one or more attacks followed by persistent fear of having another attack)	—	—		xx xx

? = inadequate information   1 = absent or false   2 = subthreshold   3 = threshold

FIG. 5-11. *(Continued).*

Obsessive Compulsive Personality Disorder	Obsessive Compulsive Personality Disorder Criteria					
	Perfectionism and inflexibility as evidenced by at least 5 of the following:					
Do you have a hard time expressing tender feelings?	(1) restricted expression of warm and tender emotions	?	1	2	3	xx
How often do you give presents or do favors for other people? *If not often:* Why?	(2) lack of generosity in giving time, money or gifts when no personal gain is likely to result	?	1	2	3	xx
Do you ever have trouble finishing something because you can't get it just right?	(3) perfectionism that interferes with task completion, e.g., unable to complete a project because one's own standards are not met	?	1	2	3	xx
Do you often get so involved with the details of something that you lose sight of the big picture?	(4) preoccupation with details, rules, lists, order, organization, or schedules to the extent that the major point of the activity is lost	?	1	2	3	xx
Do you get upset when other people don't do things exactly the way you want them done?	(5) stubborn insistence that others submit to precisely his or her way of doing things	?	1	2	3	xx

Go to passive aggress. P. 7

Are you so devoted to your work that there is hardly any time left for friends or just doing things that are fun?	(6) excessive devotion to work and productivity to the exclusion of leisure activities and friendships (not accounted for by obvious economic necessity)	?	1	2	3	xx

? = inadequate information   1 = absent or false   2 = subthreshold   3 = threshold

Is it hard for you to make decisions?	(7) indecisiveness: decision-making is either avoided, postponed, or protracted, e.g., the individual cannot get assignments done on time because of ruminating about priorities	?	1	2	3	xx

FIG. 5-12. SCID-II. Criteria for obsessive-compulsive personality. (Reprinted with permission. Spitzer RL, Williams JBW, Biometrics Research Department, New York State Psychiatric Institute, New York, NY) (*Continues on p. 186.*)

Do you have trouble throwing things out because they might come in handy some day? (How many of these things do you find that you actually use later?)	(8) unable to discard worn out or worthless objects even when they have no sentimental value	?	1	2	3	xx
Are you often bothered when you see people breaking rules or doing things that are legally or morally wrong?	(9) overly conscientious, scrupulous, and inflexible about matters of morality (not accounted for by cultural or religious identification)	?	1	2	3	xx
	At least five SXS are coded "3"		1	2	3	xx

obsessive compulsive P.D.

? = inadequate information   1 = absent or false   2 = subthreshold   3 = threshold

Sample—Not for reproduction.

FIG. 5-12. *(Continued).*

ject has already said, or to request elaboration or clarification. Interviewers are told, "Don't make up your own questions because you think you have a better way of getting at the same information. A lot of care has gone into the exact phrasing of each question. If you think you have a better way of phrasing the question, let us know." However, interviewers are also encouraged to ask additional clarifying questions such as, "Can you tell me more about that?" or "What do you mean exactly by . . .?"

The scoring and to some extent the interpretation of the SCID are based on criteria used to establish DSM-III-R diagnoses. Each diagnostic criterion is coded as either "question mark (?)," "1," "2," or "3." The question mark indicates the need for additional information—added from another source or from the subject in a subsequent interview—to arrive at a valid conclusion whether this criterion is present. The rating "1" refers to whether symptoms described in a criterion are clearly absent (e.g., no loss of weight or appetite) or if a criterion statement is clearly false. The rating of "2" refers to a "subthreshold" situation in which the threshold for the criterion is almost, but not quite, met—such as a subject who is being evaluated for depression and who reports a loss of interest in some activities but not the required "nearly all activities" that are necessary to establish the criterion. A rating of "3" refers to the clinical situation in which the threshold for a diagnostic criterion is met or exceeded, such as a subject who reports being severely depressed for many months.

Once the structured interview of the SCID is completed, the interviewer completes a summary score sheet that indicates the extent to which criteria for DSM-III-R disorders are met. Figure 5-10 demonstrates how the chief complaint and present illness components of the psychiatric history are obtained on the SCID-P; and Figure 5-11 shows how criteria for panic are elicited and rated on the SCID-P. Figure 5-12 demonstrates the evaluation of obsessive-compulsive personality disorder by the SCID-II.

The chapter appendices summarize the purpose, method of administration, scoring, and interpretation of seven of the most frequently used psychiatric rating scales. These scales have been selected because of their brevity and the relative ease in which they may be administered in the clinical setting.

SUGGESTED READING

Albert M: Assessment of cognitive function in the elderly. Psychosomatics, 25, No. 4:310, 1984

Anastasi A: Psychological Testing, 3rd ed. New York, Macmillan, 1976

Beck AT, Beamesderfer A: Assessment of depression: The depression inventory: Psychological measurements in psychopharmacology. In P Pichot (ed): Modern Problems in Pharmacopsychiatry, p 151. Basel, S Karger, 1974

Bender L: A Visual Motor Gestalt Test and Its Clinical Use. New York, American Orthopsychiatric Association, 1938

Benton AL, Hamsher K, Verney NR et al: Contributions of Neuropsychological Assessment. New York, Oxford University Press, 1983

Bigler ED: Diagnostic Clinical Neuropsychology. Austin, TX, University of Texas Press, 1984

Blumestein SE: Neurolinguistic disorders: Language–brain relationships. In Filskov SB, Boll TJ (eds): Handbook of Clinical Neuropsychology. New York, John Wiley & Sons, 1981

Carr AC: Psychological testing of personality. In Kaplan HI, Sadock BJ (eds): Comprehensive Textbook of Psychiatry/IV Vol 1. Baltimore, Williams & Wilkins, 1985

Colligan RC, Offord KP: Revitalizing the MMPI: The development of contemporary norms. Psychiatr Annals, 15, No. 9: 558, 1985

Comrey AL, Backer TE, Glaser EM: Sourcebook for Mental Health Measures. Los Angeles, Human Interactions Research Institute, 1973

Dahlstrom WG, Welsh GS: An MMPI Handbook: A Guide to Use in Clinical Practice and Research. Minneapolis, University of Minnesota Press, 1960

Dahlstrom WG, Welsh GS, Dahlstrom LE: An MMPI Handbook, Vol 1, Clinical Interpretation. Minneapolis, University of Minnesota Press, 1972

Dahlstrom WG, Welsh GS, Dahlstrom LE: An MMPI Handbook, Vol 2, Research and Applications. Minneapolis, University of Minnesota Press, 1975

De Renzi E, Vignolo LA: The Token Test: A sensitive test to detect receptive disturbances in aphasics. Brain 85:665, 1962

Derogatis LR: Manual for SCL-90. Clinical Psychometric Research. Baltimore, Johns Hopkins Press, 1977a

Derogatis LR: SCL-90: Administration, Scoring and Procedures Manual II. Clinical Psychometric Research. Baltimore, 1977b

Endicott J, Spitzer RL: Evaluation of Psychiatric Treatment: Psychiatric Rating Scales. Comprehensive Textbook of Psychiatry, Vol 3, Williams & Wilkins, Baltimore. pp 2391–2407, 1980

Endicott J, Spitzer RL: A diagnostic interview: the schedule for affective disorders and schizophrenia. Arch Gen Psych 35: 1978

Filskov SB, Boll TJ: Handbook of Clinical Neuropsychology. New York, Wiley-Interscience, 1981

Fitzbugh-Bell KB: Neuropsychological evaluation in the management of brain disorders. In Hendric HC (ed): Brain Disorders: Clinical Diagnosis and Management. The Psychiatric Clinics of North America, Vol 1. Philadelphia, WB Saunders, 1978

Folstein MF, Folstein SW, McHugh PR: Mini-Mental State: A practical method of grading the cognitive state of patients for the clinician. J Psychiatr Res 12:189, 1975

Golden CJ: Clinical Interpretation of Objective Psychological Tests. New York, Grune & Stratton, 1979

Golden CJ: Diagnosis and Rehabilitation in Clinical Neuropsychology. Springfield, Il, Charles C Thomas, 1978

Golden CJ, Hammeke T, Purisch A: Diagnostic validity of a standardized neuropsychological battery from Luria's neuropsychological tests. J Consult Clin Psychol, 48:1258, 1978

Golden CJ: Clinical Interpretation of Objective Psychological Tests. New York, Grune & Stratton, 1979

Groth-Marnat, G.: Handbook of Psychological Assessment. New York, Van Nostrand Reinhold, 1984

Halstead VC: Brain and Intelligence. Chicago, University of Chicago Press, 1947

Hamilton M: The assessment of anxiety states by rating. Br J Med Psychol 32:50, 1959

Hamilton M: A rating scale for depression. J Neurol Neurosurg Psychiatry 32:56, 1960

Lezak MD: Neuropsychological Assessment, 2nd ed. New York, Oxford University Press, 1983

Lezak MD: Neuropsychological Assessment, 3rd ed. New York, Oxford University Press, 1983

Loranger AW, Susman VL, Oldham JM et al: Personality Disorder Examination (PDE): A Structured Interview for DSM-III-R Personality Disorder. Version: May 15, 1985. White Plains, New York, The New York Hospital–Cornell Medical Center, Westchester Division, 1985

Lyerly SB: Handbook of Psychiatric Scales, 2nd ed. Rockville, MD, National Institutes of Mental Health, 1978

Maloney MP, Warde MP: Psychological Assessment: A Conceptual Approach. New York, Oxford University Press 1976.

Murray HA: Thematic Apperception Test Manual. Cambridge, MA, Harvard University Press, 1943

Osborne D: The MMPI in Psychiatric Practice. Psychiatr Annals 15, No. 9:534, 1985

Reitan RM: Investigation of the validity of Halstead's measure of biological intelligence. Arch Neurol Psychiatry 73:28, 1955a

Reitan RM: Validity of Rorschach Test as a measure of psychological effects of brain damage. Arch Neurol Psychiatry 73:445, 1955b

Reitan RM, Davison LA: Clinical Neuropsychology: Current Status and Applications. Washington, DC, Winston, 1974

Spitzer RL, Endicott J: Schedule for Affective Disorders and Schizophrenia. New York, New York State Department of Mental Hygiene, 1973b

Spitzer RL, Gibbon M, Endicott J: Global Assessment Scale. New York, New York State Department of Mental Hygiene, 1973

Spitzer RL, Williams JBW: Instruction Manual for the Structured Clinical Interview for DSM-III (SCID). New York, Biometrics Research Department, New York State Psychiatric Institute, 1985

Springer SP, Deutsch G: Left Brain, Right Brain. San Francisco, WH Freeman, 1981

Wechsler D: A standardized memory scale for clinical use. Psychol 19:87, 1945

Yudofsky SC: Section II: Neuropsychiatry, section ed. In Annual Review, Vol 4. Washington, DC, American Psychiatric Association Press, 1985

Yudofsky SC, Silver JM, Jackson W, et al: The overt aggression scale for the objective rating of verbal and physical aggression. Am J Psychiatry 143:1; 35–39, 1986

Zubin J, Eron LD, Schumer F: An Experimental Approach to Projective Techniques. New York, John Wiley & Sons, 1965

APPENDIX 5-1. BECK DEPRESSION INVENTORY (BDI) (SHORT FORM)

Purpose

The Beck Depression Inventory (BDI) is designed to help establish the existence of depression and to provide a guide to its severity.

Method

A questionnaire format is utilized in which the patient is asked to pick out one statement that best describes how he feels at that particular point in time.

Instructions

Instructions can be found on the inventory form, a portion of which is shown in the following illustration.

Name: _____ Date _____

Beck Inventory

On this questionaire are groups of statements. Please read the entire group of statements in each category. Then pick out the one statement in that group which best describes the way you feel today, that is, *right now.* Circle the number beside the statement you have chosen. If several statements in the group seem to apply equally well, circle each one.
Be sure to read all the statements in each group before making your choice.

A.
3 I am so sad or unhappy that I can't stand it.
2 I'm blue or sad all the time and I can't snap out of it.
1 I feel sad or blue.
0 I do not feel sad.

B.
3 I feel that the future is hopeless and that things cannot improve.
2 I feel I have nothing to look forward to.
1 I feel discouraged about the future.
0 I am not particularly pessimistic or discouraged about the future.

C.

3 I feel I am a complete failure as a person (parent, husband, wife).
2 As I look back on my life, all I can see is a lot of failures.
1 I feel I have failed more than the average person.
0 I do not feel like a failure.

D.

3 I am dissatisfied with everything.
2 I don't get satisfaction out of anything anymore.
1 I don't enjoy things the way I used to.
0 I am not particularly dissatisfied.

E.

3 I feel as though I am very bad or worthless.
2 I feel quite guilty.
1 I feel bad or unworthy a good part of the time.
0 I don't feel particularly guilty.

F.

3 I hate myself.
2 I am disgusted with myself.
1 I am disappointed in myself.
0 I don't feel disappointed in myself.

G.

3 I would kill myself if I had the chance.
2 I have definite plans about committing suicide.
1 I feel I would be better off dead.
0 I don't have any thoughts of harming myself.

H.

3 I have lost all of my interest in other people and don't care about them at all.
2 I have lost most of my interest in other people and have little feeling for them.
1 I am less interested in other people than I used to be.
0 I have not lost interest in other people.

I.

3 I can't make any decisions at all anymore.
2 I have great difficulty in making decisions.
1 I try to put off making decisions.
0 I make decisions about as well as ever.

J.

3 I feel that I am ugly or repulsive looking.
2 I feel that there are permanent changes in my appearance and they make me look unattractive.
1 I am worried that I am looking old or unattractive.
0 I don't feel that I look any worse than I used to.

K.

3 I can't do any work at all.
2 I have to push myself very hard to do anything.
1 It takes extra effort to get started at doing something.
0 I can work about as well as before.

L.

3 I get too tired to do anything.
2 I get tired from doing anything.
1 I get tired more easily than I used to.
0 I don't get any more tired than usual.

M.

3 I have no appetite at all anymore.
2 My appetite is much worse now.
1 My appetite is not as good as it used to be.
0 My appetite is no worse than usual.

Sample—Not for reproduction

Scoring

Directions for scoring can be found on the inventory form.

Interpretation

Because the maximum score for each item is 3, the maximum score for the entire scale is 39, which would be the maximum degree of depression measurable by this scale. The following chart is useful in estimating each level of depression.

Degree of Depression	Range of Scores
None or minimal	0–4
Mild	4–7
Moderate	8–15
Severe	16+

APPENDIX 5-2.   GLOBAL ASSESSMENT SCALE (GAS)

Purpose

The Global Assessment Scale (GAS) evaluates and rates overall psychosocial functioning (*i.e.*, reality testing, suicide or violent potential, daily living activities).

Method

Information from reliable source, such as the patient or his relatives, is elicited by a trained examiner, who makes ratings. Rating generally covers a specific time period to be assessed, such as the last week prior to the evaluation.

Instructions

Instructions can be found on the form. The GAS is shown on the opposite page.

Global Assessment Scale (GAS)

Robert L. Spitzer, M.D., Miriam Gibbon, M.S.W., Jean Endicott, Ph. D.

Rate the subject's lowest level of functioning in the last week by selecting the lowest range which describes his functioning on a hypothetical continuum of mental health-illness. For example, a subject whose "behavior is considerably influenced by delusions" (range 21-30), should be given a rating in that range even though he has "major impairment in several areas" (range 31-40). Use intermediary levels when appropriate (e.g., 35, 58, 62). Rate actual functioning independent of whether or not subject is receiving and may be helped by medication or some other form of treatment.

Name of Patient _____ ID No. _____ Group Code _____

Admission Date _____ Date of Rating _____ Rater _____ ____.

GAS Rating: _____

100 | 91	Superior functioning in a wide range of activities, life's problems never seem to get out of hand, is sought out by others because of his warmth and integrity. No Symptoms.
90 | 81	Good functioning in all areas, many interests, socially effective, generally satisfied with life. There may or may not be transient symptoms and "everyday" worries that only occasionally get out of hand.
80 | 71	No more than slight impairment in functioning, varying degrees of "everyday" worries and problems that sometimes get out of hand. Minimal symptoms may or may not be present.
70 | 61	Some mild symptoms (e.g., depressive mood and mild insomnia) OR some difficulty in several areas of functioning, but generally functioning pretty well, has some meaningful interpersonal relationships and most untrained people would not consider him "sick."
60 | 51	Moderate symptoms OR generally functioning with some difficulty (e.g., few friends and flat affect, depressed mood and pathological self-doubt, euphoric mood and pressure of speech, moderately severe antisocial behavior).
50 | 41	Any serious symptomatology or impairment in functioning that most clinicians would think obviously requires treatment or attention (e.g., suicidal preoccupation or gesture, severe obsessional rituals, frequent anxiety attacks, serious antisocial behavior, compulsive drinking, mild but definite manic syndrome).
40 | 31	Major impairment in several areas, such as work, family relations, judgment, thinking or mood (e.g., depressed woman avoids friends, neglects family, unable to do housework), OR some impairment in reality testing or communication (e.g., speech is at times obscure, illogical or irrelevant), OR single suicide attempt.
30 | 21	Unable to function in almost all areas (e.g., stays in bed all day) OR behavior is considerably influenced by either delusions or hallucinations OR serious impairment in communication (e.g., sometimes incoherent or unresponsive)or judgment (e.g., acts grossly inappropriately).
20 | 11	Needs some supervision to prevent hurting self or others, or to maintain minimal personal hygiene (e.g., repeated suicide attempts, frequently violent, manic excitement, smears feces), OR gross impairment in communication (e.g., largely incoherent or mute).
10 | 1	Needs constant supervision for several days to prevent hurting self or others (e.g., requires an intensive care unit with special observation by staff), makes no attempt to maintain minimal personal hygiene, or serious suicide act with clear intent and expectation of death.

(Reprinted with permission. Spitzer RL, Gibbon M, Endicott J, Biometrics Research Department, New York State Psychiatric Institute, New York, NY)

Scoring

Directions for scoring are given on the form.

Interpretation

91–100: Superior functioning in a wide range of activities; life's problems never seem to get out of hand; the patient is sought out by others because of his warmth and integrity. No symptoms.

81–90: Good functioning in all areas; many interests; socially effective; generally satisfied with life. There may or may not be transient symptoms and "everyday" worries that occasionally get out of hand.

71–80: No more than slight impairment in functioning; varying degrees of "everyday" worries and problems that sometimes get out of hand. Minimal symptoms may or may not be present.

61–70: Some mild symptoms (*e.g.*, depressive mood and mild insomnia) or some difficulty in several areas of functioning, but generally functioning pretty well; has some meaningful interpersonal relationships; and most untrained people would not consider him "sick."

51–60: Moderate symptoms or generally functioning with some difficulty (*e.g.*, few friends and flat affect, depressed mood and pathological self-doubt, euphoric mood and pressure of speech, moderately severe antisocial behavior).

41–50: Any serious symptomatology or impairment in functioning that most clinicians would think obviously requires treatment or attention (*e.g.*, suicidal preoccupation or gesture, severe obsessional rituals, frequent anxiety attacks, serious antisocial behavior, compulsive drinking, mild but definite manic syndrome).

31–40: Major impairment in several areas, such as work, family relations, judgment, thinking, or mood (*e.g.*, depressed woman avoids friends, neglects family, unable to do housework); or some impairment in reality testing or communication (*e.g.*, speech is at times obscure, illogical or irrelevant); or single suicide attempt.

21–30: Unable to function in almost all areas (*e.g.*, stays in bed all day); or behavior is considerably influenced by either delusions, hallucinations, or serious impairment in communication (*e.g.*, sometimes incoherent or unresponsive) or judgment (*e.g.*, acts grossly inappropriately).

11–20: Needs some supervision to prevent hurting self or others, or to maintain minimal personal hygiene (*e.g.*, repeated suicide attempts, frequently violent, manic excitement, smears feces); or gross impairment in communication (*e.g.*, largely incoherent or mute).

1–10: Needs constant supervision for several days to prevent hurting self or others; or makes no attempt to maintain minimal personal hygiene (*e.g.,* requires an intensive care unit with special observation by staff); or serious suicide act with clear intent and expectation of death.

APPENDIX 5-3.   HAMILTON ANXIETY RATING SCALE (HAMA)

Purpose

The Hamilton Anxiety Rating Scale (HAMA) evaluates the degree of anxiety and documents changes in anxiety in patients who already have been diagnosed to be suffering from anxiety.

Method

The scale is designed to be administered by the physician to the patient and to elicit the patient's objective responses. In clinical use, it is recommended to be administered before treatment is begun and periodically during treatment (*e.g.,* weekly for 4 weeks).

Instructions

Instructions for administering the HAMA are given on the form, which is illustrated here.

Scoring

Scoring for the HAMA can be found on the form.

Interpretation

This form is not to be utilized to establish a diagnosis of anxiety, but rather, to measure change in symptomatology. For example, if a patient were to have an initial score of 30, which would indicate a significant presence of anxiety, a score of 15 after 4 weeks of treatment would indicate a 50% improvement in the patient's symptomatology. This change could be inter-

Hamilton Anxiety Rating Scale

Patient's Name		Date of First Report	
Diagnosis		Date of This Report	
Current Therapy			

| Instructions | This checklist is to assist the physician in evaluating each patient with respect to degree of anxiety and pathological condition. Please fill in the appropriate rating. | 0 None
1 Mild
2 Moderate
3 Severe
4 Severe, grossly disabling |

Item		Rating	Item		Rating
Anxious Mood	Worries, anticipation of the worst, fearful anticipation, irritability.		Somatic (Sensory)	Tinnitus, blurring of vision, hot and cold flushes, feelings of weakness, picking sensation.	
Tension	Feelings of tension, fatigability, startle response, moved to tears easily, trembling, feelings of restlessness, inability to relax.		Cardiovascular Symptoms	Tachycardia, palpitations, pain in chest, throbbing of vessels, fainting feelings, missing beat.	
Fear	Of dark, of strangers, of being left alone, of animals, of traffic, of crowds.		Respiratory Symptoms	Pressure or constriction in chest, choking feelings, sighing, dyspnea.	
Insomnia	Difficulty in falling asleep, broken sleep, unsatisfying sleep and fatigue on waking, dreams, nightmares, night terrors.		Gastrointestinal Symptoms	Difficulty in swallowing, wind, abdominal pain, burning sensations, abdominal fullness, nausea, vomiting, borborygmi, loosness of bowels, loss of weight, constipation.	
Intellectual (Cognitive)	Difficulty in concentration, poor memory.		Genitourinary Symptoms	Frequency of micturition, urgency of micturition, amenorrhea, menorrhagia, development of frigidity, premature ejaculation, loss of libido, impotence.	
Depressed Mood	Loss of interest, lack of pleasure in hobbies, depression, early waking, diurnal swing.		Autonomic Symptoms	Dry mouth, flushing, pallor, tendency to sweat, giddiness, tension headache, raising of hair.	
Behavior at Interview	Fidgeting, restlessness or pacing, tremor of hands, furrowed brow, strained face, sighing or rapid respiration, facial pallor, swallowing, belching, brisk tendon jerks, dilated pupils, exophthalmos.		Somatic (Muscular)	Pains and aches, twitchings, stiffness, myoclonic jerks, grinding of teeth, unsteady voice, increased muscular tone.	
				Total Score	

Sample—Not for reproduction

(Reprinted with permission. Hamilton M, University of Leeds, Leeds, England)

preted as an indication of the efficacy of that specific treatment regimen. Individual items on the HAMA may be interpreted in similar fashion. For example, a patient with an original score of 4 on the insomnia item, who after 4 weeks of treatment was rated with a score of 0, also could be considered to have benefited from treatment.

APPENDIX 5-4. HAMILTON RATING SCALE FOR DEPRESSION (HAMD)

Purpose

The Hamilton Rating Scale for Depression (HAMD) quantifies the severity of depressive illness in a patient diagnosed to have depression and shows changes in this condition. The HAMD is not to be utilized as a diagnostic instrument.

Method

The scale is designed to be administered by trained professionals with experience using the instrument. Whenever possible, two interviewers should be present during the administration of the instrument. One interviewer should conduct the formal interview of the patient, and the second rater should ask supplementary questions at the conclusion of the first interview. Thereafter both raters, without discussion between them, should independently record and calculate their scores.

Instructions

Instructions for using the HAMD can be found on the form, as shown here.

Scoring

HAMD scoring is given on the form.

Interpretation

Although the form is not to be utilized to establish the diagnosis of depression, it is an excellent documentation of and measure of change in depressive symptomatology. For example, if a patient were to have an initial score of 53, which would indicate presence of significant depression, a score of 14 after 5 weeks of antidepressant treatment would indicate a marked improvement in the patient's symptomatology.

HAMILTON PSYCHIATRIC RATING SCALE FOR DEPRESSION

INSTRUCTIONS: *Code 01 under Sheet Number on GSS.*

For each item select the one "cue" which best characterizes the patient.

Be sure to record your answers in the appropriate spaces (positions 0 through 4), Columns 1–5, on the left half of the General Scoring Sheet.

See *Special Instructions* in Manual for Items 7, 16, 18, and 20.

Row 1 ::0:: ::1:: ::2:: ::3:: ::4::
2 ::0:: ::1:: ::2:: ::3:: ::4::
3 ::0:: ::1:: ::2:: ::3:: ::4::
4 ::0:: ::1:: ::2:: ::3:: ::4::
5 ::0:: ::1:: ::2:: ::3:: ::4::
6 ::0:: ::1:: ::2:: ::3:: ::4::
7 ::0:: ::1:: ::2:: ::3:: ::4::
8 ::0:: ::1:: ::2:: ::3:: ::4::
9 ::0:: ::1:: ::2:: ::3:: ::4::
10 ::0:: ::1:: ::2:: ::3:: ::4::
11 ::0:: ::1:: ::2:: ::3:: ::4::
12 ::0:: ::1:: ::2:: ::3:: ::4::
13 ::0:: ::1:: ::2:: ::3:: ::4::
14 ::0:: ::1:: ::2:: ::3:: ::4::
15 ::0:: ::1:: ::2:: ::3:: ::4::
16 ::0:: ::1:: ::2:: ::3:: ::4::
17 ::0:: ::1:: ::2:: ::3:: ::4::
18 ::0:: ::1:: ::2:: ::3:: ::4::
19 ::0:: ::1:: ::2:: ::3:: ::4::
20 ::0:: ::1:: ::2:: ::3:: ::4::
21 ::0:: ::1:: ::2:: ::3:: ::4::
22 ::0:: ::1:: ::2:: ::3:: ::4::
23 ::0:: ::1:: ::2:: ::3:: ::4::

Cols: 1   2   3   4   5

ROW NO.	Mark each item on left half of scoring sheet on row specified Use marking positions 0–4, columns 1–5
1	1. DEPRESSED MOOD (*Sadness, hopeless, helpless, worthless*) 0 = Absent 1 = These feeling states indicated only on questioning 2 = These feeling states spontaneously reported verbally 3 = Communicates feeling states non-verbally—i.e., through facial expression, posture, voice, and tendency to weep 4 = Patient reports VIRTUALLY ONLY these feeling states in his spontaneous verbal and non-verbal communication
2	2. FEELINGS OF GUILT 0 = Absent 1 = Self reproach, feels he has let people down 2 = Ideas of guilt or rumination over past errors or sinful deeds 3 = Present illness is a punishment. Delusions of guilt 4 = Hears accusatory or denunciatory voices and/ or experiences threatening visual hallucinations
3	3. SUICIDE 0 = Absent 1 = Feels life is not worth living 2 = Wishes he were dead or any thoughts of possible death to self 3 = Suicide ideas or gesture 4 = Attempts at suicide (*any serious attempt rates 4*)
4	4. INSOMNIA EARLY 0 = No difficulty falling asleep 1 = Complains of occasional difficulty falling asleep—i.e., more than ½ hour 2 = Complains of nightly difficulty falling asleep
5	5. INSOMNIA MIDDLE 0 = No difficulty 1 = Patient complains of being restless and disturbed during the night 2 = Waking during the night—any getting out of bed rates 2 (*except for purposes of voiding*)
6	6. INSOMNIA LATE 0 = No difficulty 1 = Waking in early hours of the morning but goes back to sleep 2 = Unable to fall asleep again if he gets out of bed

ROW NO.	Continue marking on left half of scoring sheet on row specified
7	7. WORK AND ACTIVITIES 0 = No difficulty 1 = Thoughts and feelings of incapacity, fatigue or weakness related to activities; work or hobbies 2 = Loss of interest in activity; hobbies or work—either directly reported by patient, or indirect in listlessness, indecision and vacillation (*feels he has to push self to work or activities*) 3 = Decrease in actual time spent in activities or decrease in productivity. In hospital, rate 3 if patient does not spend at least three hours a day in activities (*hospital job or hobbies*) exclusive of ward chores 4 = Stopped working because of present illness. In hospital, rate 4 if patient engages in no activities except ward chores, or if patient fails to perform ward chores unassisted
8	8. RETARDATION (*Slowness of thought and speech; impaired ability to concentrate; decreased motor activity*) 0 = Normal speech and thought 1 = Slight retardation at interview 2 = Obvious retardation at interview 3 = Interview difficult 4 = Complete stupor
9	9. AGITATION 0 = None 1 = Fidgetiness 2 = Playing with hands, hair, etc. 3 = Moving about, can't sit still 4 = Hand wringing, nail biting, hair-pulling, biting of lips
10	10. ANXIETY PSYCHIC 0 = No difficulty 1 = Subjective tension and irritability 2 = Worrying about minor matters 3 = Apprehensive attitude apparent in face or speech 4 = Fears expressed without questioning
11	11. ANXIETY SOMATIC 0 = Absent 1 = Mild 2 = Moderate 3 = Severe 4 = Incapacitating Physiological concomitants of anxiety, such as: Gastro-intestinal—*dry mouth, wind, indigestion, diarrhea, cramps, belching* Cardio-vascular—*palpitations, headaches* Respiratory—*hyperventilation, sighing* Urinary frequency Sweating

ROW NO.	Continue marking on left half of scoring sheet on row specified
12	12. SOMATIC SYMPTOMS GASTROINTESTINAL 0 = None 1 = Loss of appetite but eating without staff encouragement. Heavy feelings in abdomen 2 = Difficulty eating without staff urging. Requests or requires laxatives or medication for bowels or medication for G.I. symptoms
13	13. SOMATIC SYMPTOMS GENERAL 0 = None 1 = Heaviness in limbs, back or head. Backaches, headache, muscle aches. Loss of energy and fatigability 2 = Any clear-cut symptom rates 2
14	14. GENITAL SYMPTOMS 0 = Absent Symptoms such as: 1 = Mild *Loss of libido* 2 = Moderate *Menstrual disturbances*
15	15. HYPOCHONDRIASIS 0 = Not present 1 = Self-absorption (bodily) 2 = Preoccupation with health 3 = Frequent complaints, requests for help, etc. 4 = Hypochondriacal delusions
16	16. LOSS OF WEIGHT *Rate either A or B* A. When Rating By History: 0 = No weight loss 1 = Probable weight loss associated with present illness 2 = Definite (according to patient) weight loss 3 = Not assessed
17	B. On Weekly Ratings By Ward Psychiatrist, When Actual Weight Changes Are Measured: 0 = Less than 1 lb. weight loss in week 1 = Greater than 1 lb. weight loss in week 2 = Greater than 2 lb. weight loss in week 3 = Not assessed
18	17. INSIGHT 0 = Acknowledges being depressed and ill 1 = Acknowledges illness but attributes cause to bad food, climate, overwork, virus, need for rest, etc. 2 = Denies being ill at all
19	18. DIURNAL VARIATION A. Note whether symptoms are worse in morning or evening. If NO diurnal variation, mark none 0 = No variation 1 = Worse in A.M. 2 = Worse in P.M.

ROW NO.	Continue marking on left half of scoring sheet on row specified	ROW NO.	Continue marking on left half of scoring sheet on row specified
20	B. When present, mark the severity of the variation. Mark "None" if NO variation 0 = None 1 = Mild 2 = Severe	22	20. PARANOID SYMPTOMS 0 = None 1 = Suspicious 2 = Ideas of reference 3 = Delusions of reference and persecution
21	19. DEPERSONALIZATION AND DEREALIZATION 0 = Absent Such as: *Feelings* 1 = Mild *of unreality* 2 = Moderate *Nihilistic ideas* 3 = Severe 4 = Incapacitating	23	21. OBSESSIONAL AND COMPULSIVE SYMPTOMS 0 = Absent 1 = Mild 2 = Severe

Sample—Not for reproduction

(Reprinted with permission. Hamilton M, University of Leeds, Leeds, England)

APPENDIX 5-5.   THE MINI-MENTAL STATE EXAMINATION

Purpose

The Mini-Mental State Examination provides a quantitative assessment of the cognitive performance and capacity of a patient. The test is useful in quantitatively estimating the severity of cognitive impairment, and in serially documenting cognitive change.

Method

An interviewer is instructed first to make the patient comfortable, to establish rapport with the patient, and to avoid pressing the patient on items that the patient finds difficult while he asks a series of 11 questions. The examination generally requires 5 to 10 minutes to administer.

Instructions

ORIENTATION

1. Ask for the date. Then ask specifically for parts omitted (*e.g.,* "Can you also tell me what season it is?"). One point for each correct answer.
2. Ask in turn "Can you tell me the name of this hospital? (town, county, etc.)." One point for each correct answer.

REGISTRATION

Ask the patient if you may test his memory. Then say the names of three unrelated objects, clearly and slowly, about 1 second for each. After you have said all three, ask him to repeat them. This first repetition determines his score (0–3), but he should keep saying them until he can repeat all three, up to six trials. If he does not eventually learn all three, recall cannot be tested meaningfully.

ATTENTION AND CALCULATION

Ask the patient to begin with 100 and count backwards by 7. Stop after five subtractions (93, 86, 79, 72, 65). Score the total number of correct answers. If the patient cannot or will not perform this task, ask him to spell the word "world" backwards. The score is the number of letters in correct order (*e.g.,* dlrow = 5, dlorw = 3).

RECALL

Ask the patient if he can recall the three words you previously asked him to remember. Score 0–3.

LANGUAGE

Naming. Show the patient a wristwatch and ask him what it is. Repeat with a pencil. Score 0–2.

Repetition. Ask the patient to repeat the sentence after you. Allow only one trial. Score 0 or 1.

Three-Stage Command. Give the patient a piece of plain blank paper and repeat the command. Score 1 point apiece for each part correctly executed.

Reading. On a blank piece of paper print the sentence "Close your eyes." Print it in letters large enough for the patient to see clearly. Ask him to read it and do what it says. Score 1 point only if he actually closes his eyes.

Writing. Give the patient a blank piece of paper and ask him to write a sentence for you. Do not dictate a sentence; it is to be written spontaneously. It must contain a subject and verb and be sensible. Correct grammar and punctuation are not necessary.

"MINI-MENTAL STATE"

Maximum
Score	Score	

ORIENTATION

5   ( )   What is the (year) (season) (date) (day) (month)?

5   ( )   Where are we: (state) (county) (town) (hospital) (floor).

REGISTRATION

3   ( )   Name 3 objects: I second to say each. Then ask the patient all 3 after you have said them. Give 1 point for each correct answer. Then repeat them until he learns all 3. Count trials and record.

Trials

ATTENTION AND CALCULATION

5   ( )   Serial 7's. 1 point for each correct. Stop after 5 answers. Alternatively spell "world" backwards.

RECALL

3   ( )   Ask for the 3 objects repeated above. Give 1 point for each correct.

LANGUAGE

9   ( )   Name a pencil, and watch (2 points)
Repeat the following "No ifs, ands or buts." (1 point)
Follow a 3-stage command:
     "Take a paper in your right hand, fold it in half, and put it on the floor" (3 points)
Read and obey the following:

CLOSE YOUR EYES (1 point)

Write a sentence (1 point)
Copy design (1 point)
———————— Total score
ASSESS level of consciousness along a
continuum ————————————————————————

Alert	Drowsy	Stupor	Coma

Sample—Not for reproduction

Copying. On a clean piece of paper, draw intersecting pentagons, each side about 1 inch, and ask him to copy it exactly as it is. All ten angles must be present and two must intersect to score 1 point. Tremor and rotation are ignored.

Estimate the patient's level of sensorium along a continuum, from alert on the left to coma on the right.

Scoring

Scoring for the Mini-Mental State Examination can be found on the form, which is shown here.

Interpretation

A total possible score of 30; the mean score for patients with dementia was 9.7; for patients with cognitive impairment due to depression, the mean was 19.0; and for patients with an uncomplicated affective disorder or depression, the mean was 25.1. The mean score for normal persons was 27.6.

APPENDIX 5-6.   OVERT AGGRESSION SCALE (OAS)

Purpose

The Overt Aggression Scale (OAS) is an objective rating scale to measure the degree of aggressive behaviors in adults and children. The scale may be used to measure aggressive behaviors in a single patient over a prolonged period of time, to measure changes in aggressive behavior with the initiation of medications or therapy, or to document and record single aggressive episodes.

Method

Psychiatric staff or nursing personnel are trained to administer the scale. The scale has been used by family members of patients who demonstrate aggressive events. Ratings are made by checking off the appropriate items on the scale by observers of the aggressive event. An intervention scale is also present, which measures the specific intervention utilized for each specific aggressive event.

Instructions

Instructions for the OAS can be found on the form, which is shown here.

Scoring

The highest possible score for a single event as measured by the OAS is 26. The average score for a single aggressive event in a highly aggressive inpa-

Overt Aggression Scale (OAS)
Stuart Yudofsky, M.D., Jonathan Silver, M.D.,
Wynn Jackson, M.D., and Jean Endicott, Ph.D.

Identifying Data

Name of Patient _____ Name of Rater _____
Sex of Patient: 1—Male   Date ____/____/____ (mo/da/yr) (18-23)
       (17) 2—Female   Shift: 1-Night   2-Day   3-Evening
No aggressive incident(s) (verbal or physical) against self, others, or objects during the
shift ____ (check here)
       (25)

Aggressive Behavior
(check all that apply)

Verbal Aggression
____Makes loud noises, shouts angrily
(26)
____Yells mild personal insults, e.g.,
(27) "You're stupid!"
____Curses viciously, uses foul language in
(28) anger, makes moderate threats to
       others or self
____Makes clear threats of violence to-
(29) wards others or self, ("I'm going to kill
       you.") or requests to help to control
       self.

Physical Aggression Against Objects
____Slams door, scatters clothing, makes a
(30) mess
____Throws objects down, kicks furniture
(31) without breaking it, marks the wall
____Breaks objects, smashes windows
(32)
____Sets fires, throws objects dangerously
(33)

Physical Aggression Against Self
____Picks or scratches skin, hits self, pulls
(34) hair, (with no or minor injury only)
____Bangs head, hits fist into objects,
(35) throws self onto floor or into objects,
       (hurts self without serious injury)
____Small cuts or bruises, minor burns
(36)
____Multilates self, makes deep cuts, bites
(37) that bleed, internal injury, fracture,
       loss of consciousness, loss of teeth.

Physical Aggression Against Other People
____Makes threatening gesture, swings at
(38) people, grabs at clothes
____Strikes, kicks, pushes, pulls hair, (with-
(39) out injury to them)
____Attacks others causing mild–moderate
(40) physical injury (bruises, sprain, welts)
____Attacks others causing severe physical
(41) injury (broken bones, deep lacerations,
       internal injury)

Time incident began: ____ ____:____ ____ am   Duration of incident: ____ ____:____ ____ (hours:
              (42–45)   pm (46)   (47–50)   minutes)

(*Continues on p. 205.*)

Card No. _____
    (1–2)

Intervention
(check all that apply)

(51) _____None
(52) _____Talking to patient
(53) _____Closer observation
(54) _____Holding patient

(55) _____Immediate medication given by mouth
(56) _____Immediate medication given by injection
(57) _____Isolation without seclusion (time out)
(58) _____Seclusion

(59) _____Use of restraints
(60) _____Injury requires immediate medical treatment for patient
(61) _____Injury requires immediate treatment for other person

COMMENTS

To be completed by Research Staff: Pt.'s Hospital Chart No. __ __ __ __ __ __ __
Pt's Study No. __ __ __ __ __ __   Day of Study __ __ __   Study No. __ __
        (3–8)   (9–11)   (12–13)

Group Code __ __ __
      (14–16)

Sample—Not for reproduction

(New York State Psychiatric Institute and Department of Psychiatry, College of Physicians and Surgeons, Columbia University, New York, NY)

tient population is 6. This score was derived from analysis of 2000 aggressive events among chronically hospitalized inpatients at Creedmoor Psychiatric Center. This scale is used most often to measure total numbers of aggressive events as well as total scores of aggression over specific time periods, such as 1 month. Thus, changes in aggressive activity can be determined to monitor therapeutic interventions. If, for example, a patient's total aggressive score for 1 month were 66 with 11 individual aggressive outbursts, and with the institution of pharmacologic intervention, over the next month his total score were 20, with 5 events, one could conclude that both the total number and the intensity of events had been reduced, over that month, by over 50%. The OAS also has been used by inpatient staffs to document aggressive events in place of incident reports, which are more difficult to complete.

Interpretation

Scores may be obtained for the number of aggressive events, the severity of the aggressive events, the type of aggressive events (*i.e.*, physical aggression against self; physical aggression against others; physical aggression against objects; verbal aggression), and the nature of the interventions required.

APPENDIX 5-7.   WECHSLER MEMORY SCALE: FORM I (WMS)

Purpose

The Wechsler Memory Scale: Form I (WMS) provides a quantitative measurement of memory deficits in patients with specific organic brain injuries.

Method

The WMS is designed as a structured interview of the patient by a trained examiner.

Instructions

Instructions can be found on the form. (See following illustrations.)

WECHSLER MEMORY SCALE: FORM I

I.   *Personal and Current Information*

1. How old are you?
2. When were you born?
3. Who is President of the United States?
4. Who was President before him?
5. Who is Governor of (New York)?
6. Who is Mayor of this city?
   Scoring—Score 1 point for each item correctly answered.
   Maximum score—6.

II.   *Orientation*

1. What year is this?
2. What month is this?
3. What day of the month is this?

(Continues on p. 207.)

4. What is the name of the place you are in?
5. In what city is it?
Scoring—Score 1 point for each item correctly answered.
Maximum score—5.

III. *Mental Control*
1. Count backward from 20 to 1.
Say: "I want to see how well you can count backward from 20 to 1, like this—20, 19, 18—all the way back to 1." The examiner may repeat directions but gives no aid whatsoever during subject's effort. Record errors and time (in seconds). Time Limit 30".
Scoring—Score 2 credits if no error within time limit.
Score 1 credit if 1 error within time limit.
Score 1 credit extra for time if patient repeats correctly with no errors within 10".
(Spontaneous corrections not counted as errors.)
Maximum score—3.
2. "I want to see how quickly you can say the alphabet for me—A, B, C—go ahead!"
Record time and errors (in seconds). Time limit 30".
Scoring—Score 2 credits for no errors.
Score 1 credit for only 1 error.
Score 1 extra credit for no errors within 10".
Maximum score—3.
3. Counting by 3's.
I want to see how quickly you can count by 3's beginning with 1.
Like this—1, 4, 7. "Go ahead."
Stop subject when he reaches *40.* Record time and errors.
Time limit 45".
Scoring—Score 2 credits if no errors.
Score 1 credit if 1 error.
Score 1 extra credit if correctly given within 20".
Maximum score—3.
Maximum total score on 3 subtests—9.

IV. *Logical Memory* (Immediate recall)
"I am going to read to you a little selection of about 4 or 5 lines. Listen carefully because when I am through I want you to tell me everything I read to you. Are you ready?"
(Use the following selections.)

Memory Selection (A)
Anna Thompson/ of South/ Boston/ employed/ as a scrub woman/ in an office building/ reported/ at the City Hall/ Station/ that she had been held up/ on State Street/ the night before/ and robbed/ of fifteen dollars/. She had four/ little children/ the rent/ was due/, and they had not eaten/ for 2 days/. The officers/ touched by the woman's story/ made up a purse/ for her/.

Memory Selection (B)
The American/ liner/ New York/ struck a mine/ near Liverpool/ Monday/ evening/. In spite of a blinding/ snowstorm/ and darkness/ the sixty/ passengers, including 18/ women/, were all rescued/, though the boats/ were tossed about/ like corks/ in the heavy sea/. They were brought into port/ the next day/ by British/ steamer/.

After reading the first selection, say, "Now what did I read to you? Tell me everything and begin at the beginning." Record verbatim and score according to number of ideas as marked off in selection.
After first selection is completed, say, "Now I am going to read you another little selection and see how much more you can remember on this. Listen carefully." Examiner reads second selection and proceeds as before.
Final score is the *average* of number of ideas correctly reproduced on both passages.
Maximum Score—23.

V. *Digits Forward*
Say: "I want to see how well you can pay attention. I am going to say some numbers when I am through I want you to say them right after me. Listen." Begin with 4 digits forward, or at point where the patient will undoubtedly get series correct. Continue upward until both sets of a series are successively failed.

Digits Forward

6 4 3 9	4 2 7 3 1	6 1 9 4 7 3
7 2 8 6	7 5 8 3 6	3 9 2 4 8 7
5 9 1 7 4 2 3	5 8 1 9 2 6 4 7	
4 1 7 9 3 8 6	3 8 2 9 5 1 7 4	

Scoring—Score is maximum number of digits repeated correctly; for example, if subject repeats 5 digits on either of 2 trials, his score is 5.
Maximum score—8.

(Continues on p. 208.)

Digits Backward

Always begin with series of 3, after illustrating thus: "I want to see how well you can hold numbers in your mind. I am going to read to you a set of numbers and when I am through I want you to say them after me backward. For example: if I say 1, 9, 5, you should say (pause) 5, 9, 1." If subject does not get them correctly, say, "That was not quite right, you should have said . . . . Now listen again and remember, say them after me backward. Are you ready? Give following series. If subject gets first series of a set correctly, continue with next higher series; if he fails give second trial.

Digits Backward

2 8 3	3 2 7 9	1 5 2 8 6
4 1 5	4 9 6 8	6 1 8 4 3
5 3 9 4 1 8	8 1 2 9 3 6 5	
7 2 4 8 5 6	4 7 3 9 1 2 8	

Scoring—Score is maximum number of digits which subject can repeat backward: e.g., if subject repeats 4 digits backward his score is 4.

Maximum score—7.

N.B. If subject fails on repetition of 3 digits backward, he may be given 2 digits, and allowed a score of 2, if he passes either of 2 trials.

VI. Visual Reproduction

There are 3 cards with designs adopted from Army Performance tests and Binet:

Directions—The designs are given in order, (a), (b), (c).

Formula for (a) and (b): "I am going to show you a drawing. You will have just 10 seconds to look at it: then I shall take it away and let you draw it from memory. Don't begin to draw till I say 'go.' Ready?" After exposing card for 10 seconds say, "Now draw it, go."

Formula for (c): "Here is one that is a little harder. This card has 2 drawings on it. I want you to look at both of them carefully—again you will have only 10 seconds to look at the card, then I shall take it away and let you make both drawings; the one on the left side—here (pointing to space in which subject is to make drawing) and the right one—here (pointing). Ready?" Expose for 10", etc.

Scoring:

(a) 1. Two lines crossed, four flags 1
    2. Correctly facing one another 1
    3. Accuracy (lines nearly equal, nearly bisected, nearly at right angles; flags nearly square . . . 1
        Maximum score 3

(b) 1. Large square with two diameters. 1
    2. Four small squares within a large square. 1
    3. Two diameters in each small square 1
    4. Sixteen dots, each alone in a small square 1
    5. Accuracy of proportion (width of spaces around the four small squares between ¼ and ½ the width of the 16 smallest squares. 1
    6. If design is complete but with superfluous square or lines 3
        Maximum score 5

Score each design separately

(c-1) 1. Large rectangle with small rectangle inside 1
     2. All vertices of inner rectangle connected to vertices of larger rectangle 1
     3. Smaller rectangle correctly shifted to the right and approximately that of exposed figure 1
         Maximum score 3

(c-2) 1. Open rectangle with correct loop at each end 1
     2. Center and either left or right side correctly reproduced 1
     3. Figure correct except one of loop incorrectly reproduced 2
     4. Figure correctly reproduced and in approximate proportion 3
         Maximum score 3

Total maximum score on all figures 14

VII. Associate Learning

Say, "I am going to read to you a list of words, 2 at a time. Listen carefully because after I am through I shall expect you to remember the words that go together. For example, if the words were EAST—WEST; GOLD—SILVER; then when I would say the word EAST, I would expect you to answer (pause) WEST. And when I said the word GOLD you would, of course, answer (pause) SILVER. Do you understand?"

When patient is clear as to directions continue as follows: "Now listen carefully to the list as I read it." Read first presentation—METAL—IRON, BABY—CRIES, etc., at the rate of 1 pair every 2 seconds.

After reading the first presentation allow 5 seconds and test by presenting first recall list. Give first word of pair and allow a maximum of 5 seconds for response. If patient gives correct reply, say, "That's right," and proceed with the next pair. If patient gives incorrect reply, say, "No," supply the correct association, and proceed with the following words.

(Continues on p. 209.)

After the first recall has been completed allow a 10-second interval and give second presentation list proceeding as before.

Repeat a second time, making 3 presentations and recall tests in all.

Scoring: One credit for correct response if given within 5″. Get final score as follows: Add all credits obtained on *easy* associations in left-hand column[1] and divide score by 2. Add credits on *hard* association in right-hand column.[1] Total each column separately. Score on entire test is sum of both easy and hard association scores. Example: Sum of subject's credits on easy association 14; divide by 2; this makes subject's score on easy associations = 7. Sum of subject's credits on hard associations 6. Subject's total score on easy and hard associations 7 + 6 or 13.

The lists of words are:

First Presentation	Second Presentation	Third Presentation
Metal—Iron	Rose—Flower	Baby—Cries
Baby—Cries	Obey—Inch	Obey—Inch
Crush—Dark	North—South	North—South
North—South	Cabbage—Pen	School—Grocery
School—Grocery	Up—Down	Rose—Flower
Rose—Flower	Fruit—Apple	Cabbage—Pen
Up—Down	School—Grocery	Up—Down
Obey—Inch	Metal—Iron	Fruit—Apple
Fruit—Apple	Crush—Dark	Crush—Dark
Cabbage—Pen	Baby—Cries	Metal—Iron

First Recall	Second Recall	Third Recall
North	Cabbage	Obey
Fruit	Baby	Fruit
Obey	Metal	Baby
Rose	School	Metal
Baby	Up	Crush
Up	Rose	School
Cabbage	Obey	Rose
Metal	Fruit	North
School	Crush	Cabbage
Crush	North	Up

[1] Column indicated on record sheet. Examiners will find it convenient to use special record sheets available for the tests. These may be obtained from The Psychological Corporation, New York City.

Sample—Not for reproduction

(Wechsler D: A standardized memory scale for clinical use. Psychol 19:87, 1945. A publication of the Helen Dwight Reid Educational Foundation)

Scoring

1. Sum the subject's partial subtest scores as indicated on form.
2. To this total, which is the subject's raw score, add the constant assigned for the age group in which the subject falls, as given in Part A: Score Corrections for Age. This new total is the subject's weighted or corrected memory score.
3. Look up the equivalent quotient for this score on Part B: MQ Equivalents. The value found is the subject's MQ as corrected for age.
4. Example: A subject, age 42 years, makes a raw score of 64. In Part A, one finds that the bonus to be allowed is 40, which makes a corrected score of 104. In Part B, one finds the equivalent MQ to be 110.

PART A. Score Corrections for Age

Age	Add
20–24	33
25–29	34
30–34	36
35–39	38
40–44	40
45–49	42
50–54	44
55–59	46
60–64	48

Part B. MQ Equivalents

Corrected Score	Equivalent MQ	Corrected Score	Equivalent MQ	Corrected Score	Equivalent MQ
50	48	73	64	96	97
51	49	74	66	97	99
52	49	75	67	98	100
53	50	76	69	99	101
54	51	77	70		
55	52	78	72	100	103
56	52	79	73	101	105
57	53			102	106
58	54	80	74	103	108
59	55	81	76	104	110
		82	77	105	112
60	55	83	79	106	114
61	56	84	80	107	116
62	57	85	81	108	118
63	57	86	83	109	120
64	58	87	84		
65	59	88	86	110	122
66	59	89	87	111	124
67	60			112	126
68	61	90	89	113	129
69	62	91	90	114	132
		92	92	115	135
70	62	93	93	116	137
71	63	94	94	117	140
72	64	95	96	118	143

Interpretation

Wechsler attempted to utilize a numerical system of scoring similar to the IQ. Although numerous investigators have emphasized the shortcomings of this scoring system and have attempted to develop new scaling techniques and scoring combinations, the Wechsler Memory Scale is generally used and scored as initially proposed. For example, a patient whose MQ is 140 or above would be considered to have an outstanding memory capacity. An MQ in the range of 110 to 120 would be considered average. An MQ below 80 would indicate significant impairment of memory functioning.

6

DSM III Diagnosis and the Psychodynamic Case Formulation

Multiaxial Evaluation According to DSM III   214
  Axis I Diagnosis   215
  Axis II Diagnosis   215
  Multiple Diagnoses Within Axes I and II   216
  Axis III: Physical Disorders and Conditions   217
  Axis IV: Severity of Psychosocial Stressors   217
  Axis V: Highest Level of Adaptive Functioning in the Past Year   218

The Written Psychodynamic Case Formulation   219
  Description of the Patient   219
  The Present Illness   220
  Psychopathology   220
  Developmental Data   222
  Key Psychodynamics   223
    Theoretical Considerations   223
      The Model of Conflict   224
      The Id   224
      The Ego   224
        Ego Functions   225
          Defense Formation   228
          Regulation and Control of Drives, Affects, and Impulses   230
          Relationship to Others   230
          Self-Representation   231
          Stimulus Regulation   231
          Adaptive Relaxation in the Service of the Ego   232
          Reality Testing and Sense of Reality   232
          Synthetic Integrative Functioning   234
        Autonomous Ego Functions   234

      Ego Strength 235

      Developmental Aspects of Ego Functioning 235

          Imitation 236

          Identification 236

          Incorporation 237

          Introjection 237

          Projection 238

     The Superego 238

    Practical Considerations 239

     A Model of Symptom Formation 240

      The Role of Defense 240

      The Central Conflicts 241

      Developmental Deficits 243

  Diagnostic Classification 244

  Transference–Countertransference 244

  Therapeutic Formulation 245

    Goals of Treatment 245

    Motivation 246

    The Psychodynamic Life Narrative 246

  Prognosis 248

Appendix 6-1. Case Formulation 250

Appendix 6-2. Case Formulation 259

Appendix 6-3. Case Formulation 267

MULTIAXIAL EVALUATION ACCORDING TO DSM III

In its multiaxial approach, DSM III introduces new and useful dimensions to the concept of diagnosis. Some psychiatrists might consider the multiaxial diagnosis to be an adequate formulation of a case. Nevertheless, as the authors of DSM III point out, there is far more knowledge available and relevant for a comprehensive understanding of a patient, his problems, and an enlightened therapeutic approach than is encompassed in a five-axis DSM III diagnosis.

Few psychiatrists would claim to be interested solely in a patient's diagnosis. Even such decisions as whether to hospitalize a patient cannot be made exclusively on the basis of the diagnosis. Therefore, the second and major portion of this chapter is devoted to the additional elements that are encompassed in a more traditional psychodynamic case formulation. This more elaborate formulation not only enhances the clinician's understanding of the patient but also offers a rationale for treatment. Our viewpoint is based on psychodynamic principles derived from psychoanalytic theory.

These theories (as all theories) are incomplete; nevertheless, they are the best we have at the present time.

A major objective of DSM III is to establish a common diagnostic language based on descriptive criteria. DSM III attempts to avoid pathophysiology and psychodynamics in formulating diagnostic categories. DSM III also uses several dimensions, or axes, to enhance the scope and comprehensiveness of each patient's diagnosis.

Axis I includes clinical syndromes (mental disorders) and nonpsychiatric conditions that are a focus of attention or treatment.

Axis II comprises the personality disorders or specific developmental disorders. (Nonpathological personality types also may be coded on Axis II.)

Axis III includes concurrent physical disorders or conditions relevant to the understanding or treatment of the patients.

Axis IV, Severity of Psychosocial Stressors, codes the severity of a stressor judged to conribute to the current disorder.

Axis V records the highest level of adaptive functioning in the past year, and therefore provides an opportunity to rate certain aspects of the patient's ego strength.

Axis I Diagnosis

The Axis I diagnosis replaces the diagnostic categories of neurosis and psychosis, which have been used throughout American psychiatry. Historically, the psychotic disorders had been further subdivided into functional and organic psychoses. Axis I includes organic mental disorders; substance use disorders; schizophrenic disorders; paranoid disorders; psychotic disorders not elsewhere classified; affective disorders; anxiety disorders; somatoform disorders; dissociative disorders; psychosexual disorders; factitious disorders; disorders of impulse control; adjustment disorders; and psychological factors affecting physical condition.

Axis II Diagnosis

The Axis II diagnosis codes personality disorders and specific developmental disorders. Personality traits also can be listed as part of the Axis II diagnosis without using specific code numbers in instances where the number of traits is not sufficient to constitute a personality disorder. An understanding of the patient's personality type often is relevant in planning treatment and in obtaining a deeper understanding of the interplay between his personality type and his Axis I diagnosis, although connections are not made explicitly.

In spite of the attempt to correlate certain personality types with particular Axis I illnesses, there are major inconsistencies in the assignment of various personality disorders. Recent research has suggested that both schizophrenia and affective disorders may occur along spectra that extend to a corresponding character or personality disorder. On the affective spectrum, the condition that was formally called depressive personality is now referred to as dysthymic disorder and is classified under the affective disorders, an Axis I diagnostic classifications. Paradoxically, in an analogous situation, schizotypal personality, which is a condition believed to exist on a spectrum with schizophrenia, is classified on Axis II.

Multiple Diagnoses Within Axes I and II

DSM III states, "On both Axes I and II, multiple diagnoses should be made when necessary to describe the current condition. This applies particularly to Axis I, in which, for instance, an individual may have both a Substance Use Disorder and an Affective Disorder. It is possible to have multiple diagnoses within the same class. As an example, it is possible to have several Substance Use Disorders or, in the class of Affective Disorders it is possible to have Major Depression superimposed on Dysthymic Disorder or Bipolar Disorder superimposed on Cyclothymic Disorder. In other classes, such as Schizophrenic Disorders, however, each of the subtypes is usually exclusive."

DSM III continues, "Within Axis II, the diagnosis of multiple Specific Developmental Disorders is common. For some adults the persistence of a Specific Developmental Disorder in the presence of a Personality Disorder may require that both be noted on Axis II. Usually, a single Personality Disorder will be noted but when the individual meets the criteria for more than one, all should be recorded."

Although DSM III encourages multiple diagnoses, we caution the clinician to remember the medical principle of attempting to understand as many of the patient's symptoms as possible on the basis of a single condition or its complications. For example, depression, impulsivity, generalized anxiety, self-destructive behavior, and identity confusion can all be understood within the diagnosis of a borderline personality disorder. This principle does not mean that a patient cannot suffer from two or more conditions simultaneously.

DMS III states that "When an individual receives more than one diagnosis the principal diagnosis is the condition that was chiefly responsible for occasioning the evaluation or admission for clinical care. In most cases this condition will be the main focus of attention or treatment. The principal diagnosis may be an Axis I or an Axis II diagnosis. When an individual has both an Axis I and an Axis II diagnosis, the principal diagnosis will be assumed to be on Axis I unless the Axis II diagnosis is followed by the qualifying phrase (principal diagnosis)."

Axis III: Physical Disorders and Conditions

On Axis III, the clinician is expected to specify any current physical condition that is potentially relevant to the diagnosis or treatment of the patient. Important biological factors are to be considered here. In some cases the patient's psychiatric disease may be part of a medical illness or its sequelae. Examples are a case of dementia that is associated with Parkinson's disease, or an acute organic mental syndrome that is secondary to head trauma. In other situations, physical illness may serve as a psychological stressor. A major depression following a myocardial infarction is an example.

Axis IV: Severity of Psychosocial Stressors

With the exception of post-traumatic stress disorder, either chronic or delayed, most psychosocial stressors will have occurred within 1 year prior to the patient's present illness. It is in Axis IV and in the organic and the adjustment disorders that DSM III makes its most serious departures from an atheoretical model of the etiology of mental illness. DSM III states, "In some instances the stressor is the anticipation of a future event; for example the knowledge that one will soon retire." If the anticipation of retirement can be a stress, why not include the anticipation of college, of marriage, of graduation, of financial loss? How does the anticipation of a major life event such as retirement constitute a stress? DSM III attempts to provide a simple mechanical model of stress as an external event of measurable intensity that adversely affects the subject. In the instance of retirement, the stress would be the anticipated loss of the opportunity to feel needed or the fear of boredom associated with having no job and a lack of interesting hobbies. The DSM III view of stress stops at this level, because to go further requires a theoretical viewpoint that considers the deeper meaning of the stressful event. An example would be the case of paradoxical depression where a successful young physician became severely depressed and committed suicide shortly after he received a coveted promotion to chief resident. The role of the stress was great, but it made sense only if one understood its meaning to the patient. (For a further consideration of the subject of precipitating stress, please refer to Chap. 2.)

The clinician is asked to rate the patient's stress on a scale of 1 through 7. Although an attempt to quantify stress is reasonable, the clinician must remember that an arbitrary factor is introduced in this classification: there is no master list of human stresses. For example, almost everyone would agree that the death of a loved spouse is more stressful than the move to a new home, and most would concur that the occurrence of multiple stresses such as the development of cancer, the loss of a spouse, and the loss of a parent all in the same year constitutes an unusually heavy burden for any person. DSM III does not consider the personal significance of the stressors for the patient—a significant shortcoming, in our opinion.

Axis V: Highest Level of Adaptive Functioning in the Past Year

Axis V provides an opportunity for the clinician to rate on a scale of 1 through 7 the patient's highest level of adaptive functioning during the year prior to the onset of the patient's illness. This is important in establishing the goals of treatment and in estimating the patient's prognosis. According to DSM III, "Adaptive functioning is a composite of three major areas: social relations, occupational functioning, and the use of leisure time. These three areas are to be considered together, although there is evidence that social relations should be given greater weight because of their particularly great prognostic significance."

In considering the patient's social relations, the psychiatrist should pay particular attention to the role of persons closest to the patient. Usually, this includes immediate family members. The duration, depth, and quality of all close relationships should be considered. In evaluating occupational functioning, the psychiatrist should consider not only the patient's capacity to function at his job, but also the complexity of his work and his ability to perform without a significant level of subjective distress. Also included in the evaluation of adaptive functioning is the patient's ability to manage his personal affairs, to carry out his studies, maintain his home, pay his bills, or in general to fulfill the responsibilities appropriate to his age and role. The use of leisure time includes both recreational activities and hobbies. The clinician must consider not only the depth of the patient's involvement, but also the degree of pleasure derived. The patient's capacity to experience pleasure is an important factor in estimating prognosis. The severely depressed patient may not be able to provide accurate information concerning his ability to experience pleasure before his illness. In such instances it may be necessary to obtain additional data from significant others who knew the patient before he became ill.

THE WRITTEN PSYCHODYNAMIC CASE FORMULATION

The purpose of the written psychodynamic case formulation is to facilitate and broaden the clinician's understanding of the patient's personality structure and psychological conflicts, and to evolve an effective treatment plan with specific delineation both of goals and methods of treatment.

Such a formulation is useful whether the patient is to be treated with analytically oriented psychotherapy or supportive psychotherapy. Even decisions about whether to medicate or to hospitalize a patient can benefit from a thorough understanding of the balance of factors that caused the patient's illness at this particular time. The presence or absence of positive support systems in the patient's current life as well as his ego strength, reflected by his past successes and failures, all play a role in the formulation of a treatment plan.

A written case formulation is principally for the education of the clinician or for clinical case conferences. The thought and preparation involved in this exercise constitute an important learning experience for the student of psychiatry.

While a working, unwritten formulation is important, it runs the risk of being vague and incomplete. A written formulation forces one to review a case in depth, to organize and summarize information, thereby clarifying one's thinking about a case. Even an experienced therapist can benefit from this task in a confusing or difficult case. It is easier to prepare a lengthy document, but such records are rarely desirable in the patient's official hospital chart. To protect the patient's confidentiality, avoid including material such as the patient's name, address, schools attended, firms of employment, and street address.

Description of the Patient

The opening statement should provide the patient's age, sex, marital status, religious and ethnic background, occupation, current living situation (e.g., lives alone in a one-bedroom apartment; or lives with parents and younger brother in a three-bedroom suburban house), date of first appearance at the particular agency, and the chief complaint and its duration. This immediately orients the reader to the basic identifying data and provides a framework upon which subsequent data can be structured. The omission of one or more of these key facts in the opening sentence is frequently related to countertransference issues.

Following this, a brief description of the patient is presented. It should differ substantially from the stereotyped jargon that appears in the typical patient case history written by a medical student. Phrases such as "a well-developed, well-nourished white male" are of relatively little value, because these clichés lack the details that distinguish one person from another. A good description would enable the reader to identify the patient if he were to encounter him in a waiting room. The description should not merely include the patient's physical appearance, but also his typical dress, posture, gait, relatedness or lack thereof, and predominant moods and attitudes.

The Present Illness

The description of the present illness begins with the process that is believed to culminate in the chief complaint. It includes a brief discussion of the life situation in which the patient became symptomatic.

Some information should be provided about the stresses, both internal and external, that contribute to the understanding of why the patient's illness became apparent at this particular time.

The psychosocial or biological stressors may be acute or chronic, and are typically cumulative in their effects. Present the story chronologically, to achieve a sense of coherence. The details of the route of referral often provide clues into either the patient's unconscious expectations or unconscious motivation for treatment, or both. For example, the patient who seeks consultation with a psychoanalyst for his depression may be making a statement concerning his attitude about drug therapy.

The description of the present illness deals with the problems that the patient considers to be central; therefore, it is not appropriate to discuss all of his psychopathology in this section.

In most cases, the patient does have additional psychopathology that must be evaluated to make a complete formulation of the case and to develop a comprehensive treatment plan. This is covered in the next section.

Psychopathology

The clinician's description of the patient's psychopathology should reflect a picture of a person with an illness, and not the structure of a particular outline. To accomplish this task, it is necessary to group symptoms in a sequence that depicts the order of their importance to the patient, and to organize this section according to the chronology of their clinical presentation. The later sections on goals of treatment will be much easier to write if symptoms are listed numerically, so that it is clear exactly what the clinician considers to be the patient's problems. Inexperienced clinicians have great difficulty precisely defining the presenting symptoms. The task may be easier if one thinks of the patient's psychopathology as encompassing four basic categories.

1. *Behavioral disturbances* include character traits, interpersonal attitudes, and repetitive patterns of behavior that lead to some failure in adaptation.
2. *Cognitive disturbances* include disorders of awareness, attention, perception, memory, and all of the thought process disturbances described in the mental status.
3. *Emotional disturbances* include disturbances in mood and affective functioning. Anxiety, depression, mania, excessive anger, or diminished affect are considered under this heading.
4. *Physiological and somatic disturbances* are included in this category. The various somatoform disorders are described here.

Psychodynamically trained psychiatrists frequently confuse psychodynamic constructs with the patient's psychopathology. All psychodynamics should be placed in a later section of the case formulation. A general rule of thumb is that any statement containing an explanatory hypothesis or describing a mental mechanism or defense is psychodynamic, and therefore does not belong in this section. Psychopathology is phenomenologic (*i.e.*, simple descriptive psychiatry). Frequently, the novice clinician with a psychodynamic orientation feels that the patient's psychopathology began at about the age of 2 years, if not earlier, and will have difficulty distinguishing a present illness from the patient's total life development. Although there are situations in which such distinctions are difficult to make, it is generally possible to choose some point in time at which the patient's level of functioning began to deteriorate and when discrete psychiatric symptoms appeared.

Quotations from the patient are desirable in this section, particularly when they add to a picture of the patient. Begin with the problem that is most important to the patient. Making a correct diagnosis will be facilitated if, in organizing this section, psychopathology that has some common basis is grouped together. For example, if a patient reveals a number of obsessive symptoms, place them together in one section. Additional examples include behavior resulting from poor impulse control or low frustration tolerance, hysterical symptoms, organic symptoms, or paranoid symptoms. This principle would supersede the chronology principle if the two are in conflict. Those symptoms discussed in the section on present illness can simply be listed with a cross-referencing comment.

One of the most important elements of a case formulation is internal consistency. Each section should relate to every other section and to the same patient. If the initial description is of a patient with hysteric features, but the psychopathology portrays more obsessional symptoms, there is a strong likelihood that the clinician has misunderstood the patient. If the psychopathology is that of a borderline patient, then the other sections should also deal with typical borderline issues.

A question always arises about the psychopathology of which the patient is unaware or does not wish to change. Generally, but not always, these symptoms should be presented towards the end of this section, with the indication that the patient is not interested in treatment for these problems. Examples would include sexual deviations that the patient experiences as ego-syntonic, or almost any character pathology that the patient does not find distressing. An obvious exception would be the patient with denial of grossly maladaptive pathology as found in an organic mental syndrome. Prior treatment, medication, and so forth should be included at the end of the psychopathology section.

This organization keeps previous episodes of psychiatric disorder separate from the present illness and from the developmental data. When appropriate, it may be cross-referenced in the developmental data section.

Developmental Data

The developmental data section summarizes genetic, constitutional, familial, and environmental influences, as revealed in the history, as well as relevant medical and neurological deficits. The most important task in preparing this section is to organize and present a coherent chronological story of the patient's life.

The story begins with a description of the life situation into which the patient was born, and includes brief details about the background of both sides of the family. A discussion of the family members living in the home at the time of the patient's birth is significant, as are the socioeconomic circumstances of the family at that time. A brief description of the patient's mother and father, or parent surrogates, should appear at the beginning of this section.

While preparing a written formulation, the clinician may realize that major areas of the patient's life were not explored during the initial evaluation. The result is that the data necessary to prepare a psychodynamic formulation are missing at this point. There is a tendency for the therapist to disrupt the psychotherapy to take additional history. This results from the therapist's need to have a complete record. The fact that certain areas have been missed may itself provide important information. The patient may have neglected to mention significant material because of accompanying feelings of shame. In many instances, it is the patient's unconscious defenses that cause him to leave out crucial data. In still other situations, the missing data can also provide important clues about the transference, or countertransference blind spots, or inexperience on the part of the clinician.

To the extent the past history has relevance to the patient's current symptoms, the clinician will find himself directing the patient's discussion of his current problems back to missing material from his earlier life. If a detailed history is not secured during the initial months of psychotherapy, the therapist becomes immersed in the current events of the patient's life and may never obtain these data.

Certain historical information regularly is neglected by the inexperienced therapist. For example, a history of the patient's relationship with his siblings typically is omitted or minimized. A sexual history also is regularly omitted from the inexperienced interviewer's evaluation. Another area often neglected is the patient's religious upbringing. The later stages of the developmental section should be devoted to some description of the patient's adult life, marriages, and the like. In some cases it is more appropriate to discuss this material in the psychopathology section.

It is important to include data that document elements of health and normalcy (*i.e.*, ego strength). Statements concerning the duration, depth, and quality of the patient's relationships to others, his capacity for pleasure, and his work history are the chief sources of such information. Obviously, the clinician must carefully select those historical data most relevant for inclusion in such a brief summary. The general principle is that the most significant history is that which is directly relevant to explaining or aiding in the understanding of the patient's presenting psychopathology or to the formulation of a treatment plan. (For a more elaborate discussion of psychodynamically significant historical data, refer to Chap. 2.)

Key Psychodynamics

Theoretical Considerations

A thorough discussion of the psychodynamics of human behavior is far beyond the scope of this book. Nevertheless, the next few pages will summarize the major theoretical conceptualizations with an expectation that the serious student will want to pursue this material in greater depth elsewhere.

In psychoanalytic theory, human behavior is viewed as the product of hypothetical mental forces, motives, or impulses and of the psychological processes that regulate, inhibit, and control their mode of expression. A person's thoughts, fantasies, and feelings are considered to be central for understanding human behavior. Because these psychological processes are theoretical abstractions, they can only be studied indirectly through inferences about the meaning of the patient's words and acts. Although normal, as well as pathological behavior, can be explained psychodynamically, there are undoubtedly behaviors that are not adequately explained by psychodynamics. Specific learning disabilities or the memory impairment of Alzheimer's disease would be examples, although the patient's emotional reactions to these deficits are of crucial importance.

Psychodynamics explains "how" key psychological processes operate. Nevertheless, many issues pertain to "why" certain mental events take place that are not well understood as yet. Examples would be why the child identifies with particular aspects of each parent and not with other aspects, or why the patient develops a particular set of symptoms. The psychodynamic explanation better accounts for the unconscious significance of the symptoms in the context of the patient's core conflicts and why the patient became ill at this particular time.

Certain aspects of psychoanalytic theory that may be most useful for students will now be categorized.

THE MODEL OF CONFLICT

At the core of Freud's structural hypothesis is the concept of the mind in conflict. He postulated a tripartite model of the mind, consisting of the id, ego, and superego. Each of these agencies has the potential to enter into conflict with one or both of the other agencies. This hypothesis provides the foundation upon which the formulation is constructed. No attempt is made to do justice to such an elegant and complex hypothesis in this book.

THE ID

The term *id* refers to the biologically based drives and motives that determine much of human behavior. In classical psychoanalytic theory, these motives are called instincts or drives, and they are the sexual and the aggressive drives.

Instinctual derivatives are also attributed to the id. An example of a drive derivative would be the need for power and status that is derived from both the sexual and the aggressive drives.

THE EGO

The *ego* is the executive apparatus of the mind; it mediates between the biologically determined motives (the id), the socially determined values and behaviors (the superego), and the external demands of reality. All ego functions enable the organism to adapt to the environment, thereby ensuring survival while allowing for the gratification of basic needs. The ego has a biological substrate, which includes the basic neurophysiological processes of perception, concentration, motor behavior, memory, cognition, learning, language and stimulus control, as well as the capacity of the brain to integrate all of those functions. The infant's biologically developing ego processes blend and interact with the psychological processes mediated by the infant's experience with an attentive and responsive caretaker and significant other humans.

Contemporary psychoanalytic research has focused upon the enviromental factors that influence ego development. Direct observation of infants has provided data to suggest that both the gratification and the frustration of the basic drives during the early months of life have a profound impact on later ego development. The overgratification or overstimulation of the drives causes serious developmental problems, as does undergratification or understimulation of the drives. Because the ego develops through the infant's interaction with the mothering person or persons, a natural connection has developed between ego psychology and object relations theory.

Ego Functions. Let us now consider, in greater detail, how the ego functions, and how one assesses these functions in the clinical situation.

Table 6-1 provides a schematic representation of ego function according to hierarchical principles. It becomes readily apparent that any attempt to organize ego functions into a hierarchical table is misleading because these functions overlap, and because many of the ego functions are at different levels of abstraction and therefore would require a three-dimensional table. For example, perception and memory are relatively simple functions that are understandable in both physiological and psychological terms. However, the more complex functions—such as the synthetic—integrative function, reality testing, and the defensive functions—do not easily lend themselves to study by the neurobiologist and are difficult to measure directly either clinically or by psychological testing.

One alternative system would be to organize ego functions according to the ego's relationships with other mental structures and to the external environment. Such a system could classify functions according to the ego's

1. Relationship to the id or drives,
2. Relationship to the superego and ego ideal,
3. Relationship to external reality, and
4. Relationship to inner reality and representational world.

Numerous other systems are possible, each with its own advantages and disadvantages. The emphasis in this section is not on psychoanalytic the-

TABLE 6-1. **Organization of Ego Functions**

Ego Function	Principle

Defense formation	Conflict resolution
	    Defenses successfully mediate between demands of id, superego, and reality, providing adequate gratification
	    Defenses mediate unsuccessfully leading to inhibitions, symptoms, or pathologic character traits
	Specific defenses
	    Primitive defenses, including denial, projection, introjection, splitting, dissociation, isolation, regression, avoidance; these defneses can occur with less primitive manifestations
	    Later defenses, including repression, rationalization, displacement, identification, symbolization, reaction formation, and undoing; must function in service of sublimation
	Balance of defenses
	    Stability and flexibility of defenses; balance between earlier and later defenses

Regulation and control of drives, affects, and impulses	Appropriate control of direct discharge, allowing adequate fulfillment of pleasure (sublimatory capacity) Postponement of gratification, with ability to tolerate tension and frustration
Relationship to others	Depth of relationships; empathic capacity Stability and duration of relationships Capacity for subordination of narcissistic or symbiotic choices, fusions of good and bad images; others experienced as separate and whole Capacity to mourn losses and establish new relationships
Self-representation	Actual competence regarding active mastery of environment as seen by others and contrasted with individual's self-perception of competence Relationship of self-image to idealized self-image or ego ideal Capacity to fuse good and bad self-images
Stimulus regulation	Passive threshold for regulation of excessive external or internal stimuli (neurophysiological substrate of the ego)

TABLE 6-1. *(Continued)*

Ego Function	Principle
	Active management of excess stimulation (includes selective attention)
	Maintenance of adequate stimulus–nutrient (tonic homeostasis)
Adaptive relaxation in service of ego gratification	Capacity to relax perceptual and cognitive acuity, necessary for emotional enjoyment of sex, music, art, food, literature, theater, sleep, creative imagery, falling in love
	Openness to new experience in these areas
Reality testing and sense of reality	Perception of whether stimulus originates from inside or outside the organism
	Accuracy of perception—prevalence of objectivity over wishful perception
	Selective attention to maintain contact with reality
	Inner reality testing; reflective awareness knowing one's self, openness of self
	Sense of reality, depends on clarity of boundaries between self and world (depersonalization or derealization)
Synthetic integration	Thinking, memory, language, visual and motor functions, concentration, attention
	Anticipation and learning, includes cognitive or planning aspect of fantasy
	Judgment: requires analytic and synthetic use of the above components
	Capacity to integrate new experience with reconciliation of inconsistencies
	Executive interaction with environment; requires utilization of all the above components, with resulting ability to select, control, and integrate systems of mental activity designed to gratify needs and assure security while adapting to outer world

ory, but on its practical application in the clinical evaluation of the ego strength of the patient.

All too frequently the psychodynamic formulation provides a clearly theoretical statement concerning the core psychological conflicts of the patient without addressing the healthy or adaptive capacities of the patient. As a result, two patients with quite different personalities, but with the same symptoms, sound essentially the same because they have similar core psychodynamic conflicts. The following discussion of ego functions is designed to enable the inexperienced clinician to make a more comprehensive evaluation of the patient and his condition.

Defense Formation. The term *defense mechanism* refers to a theoretical construct involving a particular model of the mind as evolved by Freud and later psychoanalysts. Very briefly, Freud stated that the term *defense* should be used "for all the techniques which the ego makes use of in conflicts which may lead to neurosis." He later broadened the concept of defense mechanism to apply to normal as well as pathological situations in which a special method of defense protects the ego against instinctual demands. Defense mechanisms are essentially unconscious in nature.

Defense mechanisms evolve as the ego struggles to mediate between the instinctual demands of the id and the pressures of external and internal reality. Each developmental phase involves its own newly developed characteristic defense mechanisms. Nevertheless, defense mechanisms from earlier periods remain side by side with defense mechanisms from later phases of development. It has been traditional to consider those defenses that develop first as immature defenses and those that develop later as mature defenses. For example, a patient whose predominant defense mechanisms are from the pregenital phase of development appears more infantile as an adult.

Nevertheless, this older, traditional view of mature and immature defenses has been challenged. Willich (1983) states that the maturity of the total ego organization is a more useful concept than which defenses predominate. So-called immature defenses are found in higher functioning people and so-called mature defenses can be found in psychotic patients. The pervasiveness of defensive behavior, its flexibility, and its effectiveness in enabling the ego to adapt to inner and outer demands while providing gratification, is far more important than identifying the developmental stage in which a specific defense originated.

Repression, the most basic and universal defense, is often insufficient to ward off the anxiety created by the ego's conflict with the other agencies of the mind and with reality. When repression fails or is only partially successful, other defense mechanisms come into operation.

Wallerstein distinguishes between defense mechanisms and defensive behavior. He states, "Defense mechanisms are constructs or conceptual abstractions while defensive behaviors are observable phenomena. A defense mechanism denotes a way of functioning of the mind, invoked to explain how behaviors, affects, and ideas serve to avert or modulate unwanted impulse discharge." For example, exaggerated generosity may serve as a defense against selfishness. The postulated mental mechanism by which this transformation occurs is called reaction-formation—a defense mechanism. Brenner (1981) stated, "There are no special ego functions used for defense and defense alone—the ego can use defensively whatever lies at hand that is useful for the purpose. It can use any ego attitude, any perception, or any alteration of attention or awareness—the ego can use for defense anything that comes under the heading of normal ego functioning or defense. Models of defense are as diverse as psychic life itself. All aspects of ego functioning are all purpose. They can as well be used to further the gratification of a drive derivative or to enforce an aspect of superego functioning as to prevent or minimize the unpleasure associated with either."

A clinical assessment of the effectiveness of the patient's defenses should include the following:

Conflict resolution. Successful defenses resolve intrapsychic conflict between the instinctual wishes of the id and the demands of the superego; they permit some measure of instinctual gratification with freedom from the dysphoric affects of fear, guilt, anger, anxiety, and depression while protecting other ego functions. Unsuccessful defenses lead to inhibition or restrictions of function, specific symptoms, or pathological character traits.

Specific defenses. As stated above, psychoanalysts are rethinking the traditional views concerning mature and immature defenses. Nevertheless, certain defenses appear developmentally at an earlier period, whereas other defenses with more subtle potential for sublimatory gratification appear later. The so-called mature defenses include repression, rationalization, displacement, identification, symbolization, reaction formation, and undoing. For a defense to be considered mature, it must serve a sublimatory function. The so-called primitive defenses include denial, projection, introjection, splitting, dissociation, isolation, regression, conversion, and avoidance. Those defenses can occur in mild or attenuated forms in mature persons.

As stated earlier, it is impossible to create a complete list of defense mechanisms, because the ego can utilize practically anything in the service of defense. The preponderance of primitive defenses over mature defenses is still a reflection of ego weakness.

Balance of defenses. The stability and flexibility of defenses is revealed by the patient's resilience under stress and his ability not to regress to more immature levels of defense organization. It is the overall effectiveness of the patient's defenses that measures his degree of successful or impaired adaption.

Defenses must be distinguished from the relatively autonomous character traits that may have originated as defense, but that through the process of secondary autonomy now operate outside of the sphere of conflict as character traits. Examples include conscientiousness and kindliness that evolved through reaction formation. However, reaction formation does not account for all instances of conscientiousness and kindliness, because those traits can also occur through the process of identification. Some theorists would claim that identification is always used to alleviate anxiety, and therefore the process is always defensive. When the concept is used in this sense, one must realize that a normal process is being described and that defense formation does not only mean a pathological process.

Regulation and Control of Drives, Affects, and Impulses. Ego strength is present when the person is capable of postponing gratification of drives while tolerating the resulting sense of frustration and tension. Ego weakness is indicated by low frustration tolerance and the need for immediate gratification. The appropriate control of the direct discharge of drives, affects, and impulses while maintaining adequate supplies of pleasure is a sign of ego strength. It is facilitated by the ego's capacity to maintain gratification through the mechanism of sublimation. Patients with ego weakness show poor impulse control, and their aggressive and sexual drives are expressed directly and often inappropriately. Pathologically impulsive expression of instinctual wishes without regard for reality or the responses of others is a sign of ego weakness.

In the healthy ego, many primitive impulses must be repressed. A mature person has both effective defense mechanisms and effective delay mechanisms. The dysphoric affects of frustration and rage indicate impairment of that function when it is correlated with poor impulse control and inability to postpone the gratification of needs. In the compulsive character, the defense mechanisms of emotional isolation and reaction formation can lead to hypertrophied abilities to postpone the gratification of needs. This is not a sign of ego strength, because the basic need for pleasure has been sacrificed.

Relationship to Others. The patient's relationship to others is referred to by the concept of *capacity for object relations*, which is an important ego function. The current interest in narcissistic and borderline character structures has resulted in a great deal of attention being paid to this area. Ego strength is indicated by the patient's capacity to fuse good and bad mental images of the important people in his past and present life and to experience others as whole people and as separate from himself.

The capacity for deep relationships with others, manifested by mutual love, sharing, and empathy, is another sign of ego strength. The ability to maintain stable relationships over sustained periods of time is an indication of maturity, particularly when that ability is coupled with the ability to tolerate the normal frustrations and anger evoked within the relationship, and the frustrations caused by separation from that person. Finally, the capacity to mourn the loss of a loved one and the ability to form new and lasting relations are examples of ego strength.

Ego weakness is indicated by the patient usually placing his own needs before those of others, his predilection for symbiotic attachments, his inability to relate to others except in a primitive and infantile manner, as well as his using others for the need to feel unique and superior. Sadomasochistic relationships with the accompanying primitive aggression are another example of ego weakness.

Self-Representation. Ego strength is indicated by the patient's overall competence in his functioning in the external world. That competence includes not only the successful mastery of the environment as perceived by others, but the patient's subjective sense of competence or self-confidence. The person is self-confident when he perceives himself as able to obtain gratification of his needs, to have reasonable control of his life, and to ensure his survival.

In addition to his self-representation or mental image of what he is actually like, each person has an image of what he would like to be, or what he thinks he ought to be—his ego ideal. The closeness of approximation of his ego ideal and his actual self-image determines his sense of self-esteem. Both high self-confidence and high self-esteem are an indication of a strong ego. This, of course, must be differentiated from narcissistic grandiosity. Finally, a healthy self-representation must fuse the patient's good and bad self-images into a cohesive unit with adequate self-confidence or self-esteem. Ego weakness is evidenced by fluctuations in the patient's sense of self-worth or alternations between experiencing himself as all good or all bad.

Stimulus Regulation. At birth, the stimulus barrier function is initially a passive, neurophysiological mechanism that protects the infant from excessive stimulation. In early development, the mother plays a vital role in protecting the child from excessive stimulation. At about the age of 4 weeks to 8 weeks, the infant begins to be capable of using active measures to ward off excessive stimulation.

The patient's capacity to read and concentrate in noisy surroundings is an example of the use of selective attention as an organizing ego function to adapt to a disorganizing environment. The person who reads or employs fantasy in an unpleasant environment uses the process of active accommodation to whatever disturbs him as a means of blocking out the unwanted stimuli.

A patient with the symptoms of binge eating, stealing food from grocery stores, and anxiety attacks stated, "I'm afraid to go out of the apartment. All those people, the overstimulation—too damn many people. I feel swept along in a current, overwhelmed. I feel like I haven't got much structure, like my body's a wisp in the ocean, like nothing, like I'm struggling to assert myself, struggling through the crowd—a few blocks is a million miles; seems like you'll never get there—all the distraction—too many stores— too many possibilities." She described similar situations in school where the "flood of information" caused her to panic.

On a different occasion, the patient craved excitement and the stimulation of being around other people. She felt "alive again" and rejuvenated, until at some unpredictable moment she once again felt overwhelmed. In addition to the failure of the stimulus regulation function, she illustrated a weakness of the synthetic integrative function, the drive regulation function, the defense formation function, and judgment plus other impairments implied but not described in the vignette.

The healthy ego also must not block out too many sensory stimuli; the person must receive adequate stimulus nutriment. Sensory deprivation experiments demonstrate the need for stimulus nutriment. Adequate sensory stimulation requires intact functioning of the perceptual and motor apparatuses. The integrative function allows the patient to shift back and forth from external to internal supplies of stimulation as his needs dictate, maintaining what Holt (1965) refers to as "tonic support."

Adaptive Relaxation in the Service of the Ego. Adaptive relaxation in the service of the ego requires the capacity to relax perceptual and cognitive attention and other ego controls to allow the ego to experience preconscious or unconscious material. This function is necessary to fall in love, to be creative, and to enjoy fully sex, music, art, literature, and theater, as well as to fall asleep. Ego strength is indicated by the degree of capacity for pleasurable functioning that the patient shows in those areas. Flexibility of ego organization implies a capacity to allow for new experiences in those areas that add to the overall adaptive pleasure balance. There is some controversy whether this phenomenon actually involves the process of regression, or more the relaxation of other ego functions. We prefer the latter concept.

Reality Testing and Sense of Reality. The reality-testing function of the ego depends on the perceptual apparatus, as well as the ability to discriminate whether a given stimulus originates from inside or outside the organism. Perception is not merely the passive registration of data, as with a tape recorder. Perception and selective attention to a particular stimulus or experience also serve an organizing function for the ego. The strength of the patient's ego is reflected in the accuracy of his perception. Patients with delusions or hallucinations reveal gross impairments of reality testing. An example of a more subtle impairment of reality testing is the man who erroneously believes that his wife's lack of orderliness is deliberately aimed at provoking him. A more severe example of impaired reality testing would be a paranoid delusion.

Reflective awareness refers to the awareness of being aware and the ability to differentiate varieties of conscious experiences, to distinguish dreams, fantasy, memory, and percepts. In other words, reflective awareness is the person's realization that he is the thinker of a thought (Schafer, 1968). When a patient loses his ability to distinguish between a thought and the concrete reality from which it arises, there is an impairment of reality testing, and thus ego weakness.

Reality testing can be impaired through mechanisms that relate primarily to the id, to other ego functions, or to the superego. An example of the first is a perception distorted by an unconscious libidinal wish, as in the case of a young woman who believed that her poetry professor was in love with her because he selected her poem to read to the class. The second is exemplified by a defensive denial that an event occurred, and the third is illustrated by a situation misperceived as the result of excessive guilt with the anticipation of blame or punishment. That phenomenon is exemplified by the patient who felt that his acting teacher spoke to him sharply because he did not like the patient's performance in class, when in reality the teacher was only in a bad mood. Inner reality testing refers to the patient's perception of himself and of how he is viewed by others. Inner reality testing is similar to the concepts contained in the term *insight,* coupled with an accurate appraisal of his inner mental state.

The sense of reality refers to the patient's ability to sense routine events as familiar. Experiences of derealization reveal an ego defect of this function. When the patient's sense of familiarity with his own body and its parts or with his own behavior as belonging to himself is impaired, he experiences feelings of depersonalization. Such a patient might say, "My body does not feel like it belongs to me. My hands don't look familiar and I feel numb." The patient with derealization would report, "Nothing seems real or familiar, everything looks new, strange, or unnatural." Finally, the sense of reality requires that the patient be able to accurately differentiate between self and others (intact ego boundaries). This function overlaps somewhat with the functions titled *relationship to others* and *self-representation.* A subtle example of impairment of ego boundaries is the patient who feels that he need not report details of his personal experiences to his doctor "because the doctor knows me so well he can tell what I'm thinking." A more obvious example is the patient who states, "I feel like I'm my mother."

Synthetic Integrative Functioning. The synthetic integrative function is probably the most complex of the ego functions. A number of more basic ego functions must be intact for synthesis to take place. Those functions include the capacities for thought, memory, language, visual and motor functions, attention, and concentration. In progressing upward in the development of the ego, one encounters the more complex functions of anticipation and learning, including the cognitive or planning aspect of fantasy. Next in complexity is judgment, which requires the analytic and synthetic use of all the above components, coordinated with reality testing and a capacity for self-reflection.

Stress tolerance is one measurement of the synthetic integrative function. The patient who can integrate new experiences and use that knowledge appropriately shows ego strength, as does the patient who is able to reconcile his own inconsistencies or contradictory values, feelings, or attitudes. Likewise, the ability to tolerate inconsistency in others is a measure of the strength of the synthetic function of the ego.

Finally, the ego's executive interaction with the environment uses all of the above functions. Through that function, the organism knows which mental system to select at any given time to assure security and to provide for need gratification while adapting to both inner and outer worlds.

Autonomous Ego Functions. Hartmann (1950) added to the understanding of ego functioning with his emphasis on the autonomy of certain operations of the ego. He described a primary autonomy for the ego functions of perception, intention, object comprehension, thinking, language, recall-phenomena, productivity, motor development, and the maturation and learning process implicit in all of these. By the phrase *primary autonomy*, Hartmann meant that those functions evolve outside of the sphere of conflict and are not dependent upon the drives. In other words, they represent the ego's primary autonomy from the id. Hartmann further postulated a secondary autonomy when a behavior that developed originally as a derivative of an instinctual drive in the course of time becomes self-sustaining, and is no longer dependent upon that drive but operates in a conflict-free area of ego functioning. Rapaport (1960) extended the concept of autonomy to the autonomy of the ego from external reality. By this, he meant that behavior can be autonomous from regulation by external stimuli. He indicated further that this autonomy was a "relative freedom at best."

Later developments in ego psychology state that autonomous functioning describes a process and not a separate function. The term *autonomous functioning* is used as an adjective to describe a property of other ego functions that can operate independent of psychological conflict.

Ego Strength.   No single function of the ego can provide an accurate measurement of ego strength. It is the balance of all ego functions and their effectiveness in promoting the adaptation of the organism to the environment that creates the broad picture of ego strength or weakness. Glover (1958) stated, "Ego strength depends on the quality and stability of the emotional ties to others, on the elastic adaptation to instinctual demands and on optimum freedom from the reactive affects of anxiety and guilt."

In the clinical assessment of a patient, the psychiatrist finds ego strength when the functions of primary autonomy—language, motor function, conceptualization, memory, concentration, attention—show no impairment and have remained free from the influence of psychological conflict. A further indication of ego strength is the freedom from psychological impairment of more complex autonomous patterns such as work routines, hobbies, interest, learned complex skills, or any adaptive patterns. Impairment in any of those areas indicates ego weakness. Ego functions must be viewed in terms of the interrelationship between the defensive functions and the synthetic or organizing functions. Ego function is best understood in terms of adaptation, a concept that is broader than defense formation and includes all of the coping mechanisms necessary for health and survival.

In summary, ego strength means good capacities that are well developed and unimpaired by conflict. Developmental failures may lead to ego weakness even in the absence of current conflict. Such problems are not treatable by dynamic psychotherapy.

Developmental Aspects of Ego Functioning.   Mahler (1967, 1975) described the infant's initial bond to the mother as a state of absolute primary narcissism, in which the infant has no awareness of the mother as a separate person. By the third month, the infant develops a vague realization that gratification is associated with the mothering person. Growing up means that the child must separate himself from this omnipotent symbiosis. This separation–individuation process is augmented by the maturation of the biological aspects of the developing ego (*i.e.*, autonomous functions). This early symbiosis, which must be relinquished for growth, contributes heavily to the infant's experience of each new step towards independence as having lost the maternal object. The separation–individuation process, as described by Mahler, begins in the fourth or fifth month and continues through the second year. The child gradually moves out of a symbiotic relationship with the mother through a process called *hatching.* Concomitant with this process is the child's development of what Sandler (1960, 1962, 1963) called the representational world. Briefly, it is the representation in the child's developing mind of concepts and feelings about himself, his own body, the other significant humans, his possessions, and his living environment.

The child's representational world is based on his sensory experiences, his emotional experiences, his drives, and the interaction of all of these forces. The significance of his mental representations is constantly changing with varying admixtures of reality and fantasy.

In other words, the child reacts not to his real mother and father as perceived by others, but to his own internal representations of each (object representation), which always contain distortions. Nevertheless, it is only by comprehending the inner reality of the patient that his illness becomes understandable.

The supraordinate term for the process of developing a representational world is *internalization*. It begins with imitation and incorporation, and then progresses to introjection and identification as the child matures biologically and psychologically.

Imitation. The capacity for imitation is a property of the neurobiological apparatus of all higher forms of life, and it constitutes the basis of the earliest form of learning. The infant imitates the behaviors of its caretakers at a very early age. Imitative learning continues through life, particularly when one encounters a new situation in the presence of a person who is respected as having greater mastery of that situation. The use of imitation by the more mature person is situation-dependent, in contrast to the more global imitative behavior in immature persons. Situation-dependent imitation is found in the medical student who imitates the behavior of a respected teacher performing a physical examination. The mature student will not imitate other behaviors and attitudes of this teacher that have no relevance to medical skills. Through the process of identification, the student may acquire some of the basic medical values of the teacher.

Identification. Imitation is a precursor of identification, which requires some emotional attachment to the object. Identification has occurred when some attitude, belief, and value of the object has become part of the self. Thus, imitation facilitates the acquisition of specific knowledge or skills, whereas identification facilitates the acquisition of broader and deeper values and attitudes. Identification is a mechanism of personality development, largely unconscious in nature, stemming from the wish to become like the object. In the developing child it is the process by which the self-representation becomes similar to some specific aspect or aspects of the object as it is perceived by the child. Identification is an expression of the ego's synthetic capacity, in which aspects of a model are assimilated, whether they are derived from introjects or real objects, and subsequently integrated into the structure of the ego (Nunberg, 1948).

Incorporation. The most primitive fantasy through which significant others are taken to the body is oral incorporation. This basic urge to possess the gratifying or frustrating object is present in every infant. The prototypic adult derivative of this wish is found in the cannibal who believed that eating one's adversaries led to a possession of their strength. A more common derivative is found in the fantasies of the male homosexual who swallows the semen of a male viewed as more powerful than himself. Incorporation is a global process of internalization whereby the object loses its functions as an object. Primitive incorporative fantasies are found in severely regressed psychotic conditions. Significant differences of opinion exist among psychoanalytic theoreticians concerning incorporation. A further discussion of these points can be found in Meissner's book *Internalization in Psychoanalysis* (1981).

Introjection. Through a process called introjection, the child maintains a connection with the mothering person during the separation–individuation phase. This mechanism enables the child to internalize qualities of the significant other, and thereby enables the child to feel the continued presence of the gratifying person as a part of himself. Introjection is the basic process through which object representations develop. A good introject is based upon the gratifying object representation, whereas a bad introject is based upon the frustrating object representation. The child develops good and bad self-representations based upon how its parents perceived and responded to it. As the normal child's ego develops, it fuses the good and bad self and object representation into composite representations, as described earlier in the chapter. Thus, the introject is the inner presence of a once external object. Sandler believes that an object representation is not necessarily an introject, but that it becomes an introject when it receives a special authority or status it did not previously possess. He views introjection as pertaining to superego formation, and identification as pertaining to ego formation. The more common view is that all object representations are the result of introjection.

Early introjections tend to be more harsh than the parents' actual attitudes would justify, which suggests that this process is important in the child's efforts to regulate and control his aggressive and sexual drives. This point will be clarified later in the discussion of projection.

In the development of bad introjects, the child maintains attachment to the object, even one that gave inadequate gratification of his need to be loved. Negative self-representations also function defensively to maintain the child's attachment to the object. It is as though the child tells himself, "It is my own fault my mother treated me badly; she is not a bad mother, it is I who am a bad child." The child thereby maintains the hope of future gratification if only he can be good enough.

Projection. Projection is the term for a process that is the reciprocal of introjection. It is defined as "the tendency to project onto the external world one's instinctual wishes, conflicts, needs, and ways of thinking" (Moore and Fine, 1967).

As Meissner (1981) points out, projection is a type of externalization. The elements projected onto the external object are derived from specific introjects. It is an unconscious process, so that the person lacks awareness that his experience of the object is actually a projection of an introject. It is the projection of the harsh parental introject that causes the child to perceive the parent as more disapproving or severe than is actually the case. Projection is the core mechanism in the formation of paranoid beliefs, whereas externalization would be the mechanism found in phobic patients.

THE SUPEREGO

The *superego* is a term that involves those psychological functions pertaining to standards of right and wrong, together with the evaluation and judgment of the self in terms of these standards. It also includes the ego ideal, which is the psychological representation of what a person wishes to be—his ideal self. The superego was originally considered a portion of the ego, but it has been found to operate independent of and often at odds with the ego, particularly in conflict situations and pathologic conditions. It develops out of the young child's relationship with his parents, who initially provide him with external judgments, criticism, and praise for his behavior.

The superego is also influenced by parental surrogates such as teachers, peers, and society at large. This is even more true of the ego ideal, which at the age of latency is often concretely symbolized by popular cultural heroes.

As stated earlier, introjection is the predominant mental mechanism involved in creating this dynamically significant mental agency that carries on those functions that formerly belonged to the parents.

The superego is the last of the structural components to evolve. It is incomplete until the first attempted resolution of the Oedipus complex before latency. The boy's striving towards masculinity strengthens his identification with his father, whereas the girl's striving for femininity strengthens her identification with her mother. It is through this mechanism, and the growing displacement of Oedipal attractions towards nonfamily members, that the Oedipal object is relinquished. Typically, the superego precipitates of both parental introjects leads to a structure that resembles the superego of one or both parents.

The earlier concept of superego has been modified in later developments in object relations theory. Current concepts describe a new structure called the *ego ideal,* which is composed of idealized representations of the self and idealized representations of objects. The ego ideal is derived from good object introjects, and it maintains the person's self-esteem by the internal provision of praise. The more critical aspects of superego are derived from the bad object introjects that are associated with parental disapproval. This mechanism is augmented by the projection of the child's own sadistic drives onto the parents. The latter mechanism is especially prominent in the formation of the obsessive character. Object relations theorists consider introjection and projection the core mechanisms in the formation of all character structure. The superego becomes noticeable when a state of tension arises between it and the ego. When positive identification with a good introject has occurred, the superego functions autonomously and almost invisibly.

Practical Considerations

The psychodynamics section of the written case formulation is undoubtedly the most difficult to prepare. Developmental psychodynamics require an understanding of the various phases that characterize human development. Without formal training in normal human development from a psychodynamic frame of reference, it is not possible to construct this section successfully. This, together with a thorough history, organized chronologically, is essential to understand how the patient entered each of the various major developmental phases, as well as to comprehend the patient's success or lack of success in passing from one phase to the next. Developmental psychodynamics formulate a longitudinal view of the patient's psychological development as well as provide insight into his various conflicts, fixation points, and circumstances of regression. A psychologist interprets psychological tests that present a different organization of psychodynamics based upon a cross-sectional review of the various aspects of the patient's psychic apparatus at one point in time, including prominent mechanisms of defense and their degree of success in warding off anxiety or depression.

Typically, the beginner prepares a formulation that suffers from one of two excesses. The first excess is a repetition of the history with little or no attempt to apply psychodynamics to these data and to develop a model of the unfolding of the patient's intrapsychic conflicts. The second excess is an entirely theoretical discussion with little indication of how it applies to the special historical data of this patient. A formulation of this type appears as if

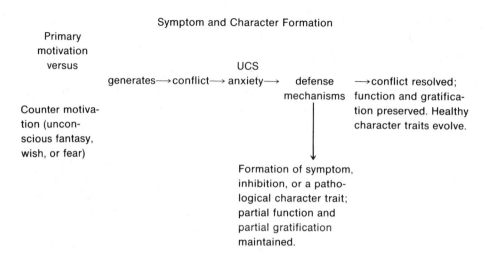

Symptom and Character Formation

FIG. 6-1. This is a currently popular model explaining formation of symptoms and character traits. It is not the only model. Although it explains the content of many symptoms, both neurotic and psychotic, it does not explain the occurrence of psychotic symptoms. In other words, the content of a delusional system can be explained by this formulation, but not the fact that the patient is delusional.

it were copied from a textbook in that it lacks specificity for the individual. The task is a formidable one: to use the relevant historical data from the previous section to explain the patient's presenting illness, his major character traits, his assets, and his failures in adaptation—all in two pages! Of necessity, even the best formulation will be a compromise that focuses on a central theme that is the patient's dominant psychodynamic conflict at the present time.

A MODEL OF SYMPTOM FORMATION

To construct a psychodynamic formulation based on psychoanalytic theories, it is essential to have some fundamental understanding of how symptoms and character traits are formed. The process is represented schematically in Figure 6-1.

The Role of Defense. Conflicting motives, impulses, drives, or aims generate signal (unconscious) anxiety, which is dealt with through the ego's mechanisms of defense. Defenses that occur in the context of healthier overall ego organization favor conflict resolution, providing some measures of instinctual gratification while preserving essential ego aims. In other instances defense mechanisms function less effectively and overall ego functions are impaired. Some gratification of wishes or impulses is maintained, but at the serious cost to the individual of impaired object relations. An example would be a perversion. In such a disorder, less mature defense mechanisms predominate over healthier defenses, and symptoms or pathological character traits appear. This process involves some compromise, so that the ego obtains only partial gratification but preserves partial functioning as well. (A more detailed discussion of the role of defenses may be found earlier in this chapter.)

The Central Conflicts. Using the formula in Figure 6-1 as a template, one can then review the major developmental phases, examining the typical drives, impulses, wishes, and anxieties of each period. These would constitute the primary motives of a normal child: to be fed, to be loved, to gain mastery over one's body and one's environment, and the like, along with the major fears such as separation, castration, guilt, and so forth. Parental control soon leads to conflicting motives, for example, the child wishes to play with a toy when the parent wants the child to take a nap. If a struggle ensues, the child may be punished or scolded. The child's desire to please the parent and to avoid punishment creates a counter-motive and a conflict results in the child's mind.

The power struggle just described is characteristic of the so-called anal sadistic period when the child sets his will against that of the parents. This dynamic conflict would bear significantly upon the later development of a compulsive character. In this instance, one would expect pathological power struggles to characterize each succeeding phase until that conflict becomes resolved.

On the other hand, a superficially similar struggle could develop at an earlier age over the child's attempts to separate from the mother. Here, the mother might be so anxious and overly protective that the child is unable to develop a separate identity. A formulation involving such a patient would follow the continuing efforts of the child to establish a separate identity as he enters each successive developmental phase. In a third situation, a parent might attempt to avoid conflict with the child by not making demands on the child. Such attitudes may foster the development of deficit disorder symptoms or character traits. (This is discussed in more detail later in this chapter.)

If the student carries this model through the patient's major developmental periods, he will encounter each of the patient's original areas of conflict formation. A major psychological conflict carried over into successive phases places continued stress on the child, who is deprived of the security of successfully coping with each developmental challenge before undertaking the next one. The reader is referred to a standard text for a detailed consideration of a contemporary model of developmental psychodynamics that integrates object relations theory into the more classical psychoanalytic framework. This allows the student to consider the patient's development of internalized self and object representations as the child progresses through oral, anal, phallic, latency, and genital development. As stated earlier, the emphasis should be placed on those developmental issues most clearly related to the major adaptive problems of the patient. Issues of object constancy, separation–individuation, and pathological splitting would be more important in a patient with borderline personality organization. In a higher functioning patient, castration anxiety and an unresolved Oedipus complex would provide more help in understanding the patient's psychopathology.

Having now identified the patient's symptoms and the principal conflicts involved in each symptom, the next step is to organize the data. Each of the patient's major symptoms or maladaptive behaviors is related to certain significant early developmental events or experiences. As one decides which symptoms or character traits may best be understood in relation to which event, one has the skeletal framework of the formulation. Some character traits can have significant hereditary determinants.

Next, attempt to identify the conflict that was partially resolved in the formation of each symptom. This constitutes the primary gain of the symptom that allows partial gratification of a forbidden wish or impulse, while the resulting partial loss or impairment of healthy function represents the primary loss. Some symptoms, such as hysterical symptoms or traits, provide substantial secondary gain, such as extra attention, dependent gratification, or freedom from responsibility. The opposite side of the secondary gain is the secondary loss aspect of the symptom. This can best be explained as the price the patient pays for the gratification of the secondary gain. In the example given above, the price or secondary loss would be a lack of self-confidence as an independent adult. The primary gain of the hysterical symptom might be the patient's avoidance of Oedipal anxiety with the threat of incurring maternal wrath.

Next, consider the particular defense mechanisms involved in the resolution of each major conflict. The evaluator can now begin a discursive section starting with the beginning of the patient's life and chronologically tracing each of the major conflicts with the evolving symptoms and character traits and defenses through to the present.

Inexperienced psychiatric residents have considerable difficulty in conceptualizing this complex task. In part, this confusion stems from the fact that the older classical psychoanalytic model views all symptoms as the product of intrapsychic conflict that therefore can be understood in terms of unconscious wishes and defenses against them. That model readily lends itself to explaining neurotic symptoms such as phobias, obsessions, paranoia, and hysterical conversion or dissociation. All of those symptoms also can occur in the context of psychosis. Although the nonpsychotic aspects of such a patient's personality can be explained by a psychoanalytic model, few psychoanalysts today would believe that the psychodynamic conflicts accounted for most psychoses.

Developmental Deficits. Contemporary psychoanalysis has broadened and enriched the earlier concept of symptom formation in explaining a group of psychological disturbances that might be called deficit-determined symptoms rather than conflict-determined symptoms. By the term *deficit symptoms*, we refer to psychological disturbances that originate from a relative deficiency of some important human experience during the early formative years that leads to an arrest or deviation in the development of psychological structures. Although the lack of essential experiences is environmental, the deficit is intrapsychic. Examples would be the early loss of a mother, or a "not good enough" mother, or the lack of a father with whom a little boy could identify or from whom a little girl could develop a sense of being attractive to men. In some instances the experiential lack may give rise to conflict-based symptoms in addition to the direct impact of the deficit. Constitutional and biological deficits also would be mentioned here, along with their psychological impact on the patient and the resulting shifts in constellations of defenses.

Symptoms such as low self-esteem, inability to trust, narcissism, sociopathy, temper tantrums, identity disorders, affective instability, feelings of emptiness, hypersensitivity to rejection, and lack of self-confidence are more easily understood in a deficit framework rather than in a simple wish–defense conceptual model.

The concepts of object constancy, basic trust, separation–individuation, introjection, identification, and good and bad self and object representations help explain the latter group of symptoms.

The same format can be used for both groups of symptoms. In the case of a deficit disorder symptom, one would mention the specific absence or relative deprivation and age of the patient at that time. Then, one would mention the resulting ego or superego deficit that the clinician believes is responsible for the symptom. Next, one would consider what defense mechanisms have been brought into play as the ego attempts to compensate for the deficit.

As the clinician's knowledge and experience increases, it will become clear that the discussion is even more complex than suggested above. This is because even deficit-induced behaviors or inhibitions can become secondarily involved in unconscious conflicts. Furthermore, symptoms that originated in intrapsychic conflict can persist after the conflict has become resolved, due to what Hartmann called a *secondary autonomy*. To avoid hopeless confusion, the inexperienced clinician is advised not to attempt to carry out the psychodynamic formulation to that degree of complexity.

Another confusing concept is that of identification. Although identification is a normal developmental process, it also serves as a defense mechanism to ward off pathological unconscious anxiety generated by intrapsychic conflict. The argument that all healthy character formation and all identification is based upon measures designed to cope with the infant's anxiety seems to be confusing for inexperienced clinicians who are attempting to understand the differences between normal and pathological identifications. Each child has multiple identifications with both parents, which, as the ego matures, become fused or synthesized into a coherent sense of self. Under certain circumstances this synthesis cannot take place, and the child grows up without ever having a sense of wholeness or a consolidated sense of identity necessary for the more mature levels of psychological development. Fragmented and conflicting identifications are important in understanding borderline psychopathology.

These theories are complex, but useful, if the student is willing to spend the time necessary to learn how to apply them.

Diagnostic Classification

In the section on diagnostic classification, the clinician should use the classification of psychiatric disorders provided by the American Psychiatric Association's Diagnostic and Statistical Manual (DSM III). The principles outlined at the beginning of this chapter should be followed. The diagnosis must be consistent with the psychopathology, the psychodynamics, and the initial description of the patient.

Transference–Countertransference

Transference includes all of the patient's conscious and unconscious attitudes, impulses, expectations, fears, and wishes toward the therapist, which are based upon the repetition of the patient's most significant early relationships. Transferences color the patient's reactions, and each personality type will develop certain predictable transference responses during the different phases of treatment.

This can usually be ascertained from an understanding of the developmental history of the patient. In describing the initial transference, the clinician can make reference to the specific relationship from the patient's past that is likely to be repeated in the initial phase of treatment.

An additional statement can be provided with regard to the expected countertransference responses to be experienced by the treating clinician whether or not analytically oriented psychotherapy is recommended. Countertransference is difficult for the novice therapist to predict because it involves unconscious feelings towards the patient. Nevertheless, all therapists have inappropriate reactions and attitudes to their patients, and it is important that the clinician learn about such responses in himself, regardless of the particular treatment modality. In fact, such responses may even influence which therapeutic modality he selects.

Therapeutic Formulation

Goals of Treatment

The clinician begins the section on goals of treatment by providing a concise statement of the goals, and of the form of treatment judged most effective in achieving these goals. Specific goals are based on correcting or modifying failures of adaptation. To imply that the goal of treatment is to get the patient well is inadequate. To state that the patient must be made aware of his unconscious motives or that the patient must get to know himself better is a means to an end, not an end in itself. The goal of relieving the patient's symptoms does not imply that the specific modality of treatment is behavior modification. Psychodynamically oriented interpretations may also be directed toward the ultimate removal of the patient's symptoms, although the therapeutic mechanism of action differs.

Occasionally, in formulating a successful treatment plan, there are certain specific problems for which the patient can be treated without regard for other aspects of personality and psychopathology. Examples would be the patient with an airplane phobia who can be treated by deconditioning techniques, or the patient whose anxiety can be managed by relaxation therapy and a minor tranquilizer. Nevertheless, in some clinical situations, these more superficial therapies are contraindicated, or they may have already been tried without success. In some situations, the clinician recognizes that the patient's presenting symptom is only a surface manifestation of a more complex problem. An example is the 29-year-old man with a chief complaint of low-grade depression and feelings of emptiness. He asked for medication to help him feel better. The psychiatrist learned that the man still lived at home with his parents, was supported by them, and had held a variety of odd jobs after dropping out of college. This patient must be motivated to seek independence and a goal in life if he is to feel better for any sustained period. Another example is the patient who for the first time became phobic and depressed shortly after getting married. It is likely that the therapy will have to explore the patient's marital problems for the patient to get over the phobia and depression.

Motivation

A statement should be made concerning the practical availability (including financial capacity) of the type of treatment the patient requires, as well as the indications for adjunctive therapies such as vocational, occupational, or recreational therapies. One should consider the setting in which the necessary treatment is best obtained (*i.e.*, inpatient/outpatient, or partial hospitalization). Indications for group or family interventions as well as the specific objectives of such interventions are to be described here. The therapeutic formulation must specifically discuss the nature of the patient's motivation. Treatment will not progress satisfactorily unless the patient is motivated to be helped with the same issues that the therapist plans to address. The more complex conceptualizations of psychotherapeutic strategies are beyond this text and require further psychodynamic teaching in a setting of supervised psychotherapy. Nevertheless, in many instances the initial therapeutic strategy must involve strengthening the patient's motivation to face a particular issue in order to enable the patient to accept a referral for treatment.

The Psychodynamic Life Narrative

Viederman has described the *psychodynamic life narrative* as a psychotherapeutic maneuver used during the first few sessions of a consultation to treat a patient in a crisis situation. In describing the narrative he states, "By establishing a powerful bond between physician and patient, it offers the possibility of a rapid relief of dysphoric symptoms. In some situations, it may be useful in mobilizing a recalcitrant patient to accept psychotherapy, or, in the case of the physically ill, to accept diagnostic procedures and treatments previously refused. It is most effective in patients whose general adaptation has been stable, and whose psychological homeostasis has been disrupted by a life event of real and symbolic significance."

Viederman continues, "The narrative is a statement made to the patient that gives his or her current emotional reaction meaning in the context of life history, and shows it to be a logical and inevitable product of previous life experience. It addresses three characteristics of crisis, particularly evident in physical illness: (1) psychic disequilibrium of chaos and confusion, (2) regression with intensification of strong transference wishes, and (3) the inclination to examine the trajectory of one's life as it relates to self perception, to past accomplishments, and to future hopes and aspirations. Note that the narrative is presented in a vigorous and non-neutral fashion in order to engage the patient and is constructed to be egosyntonic, rather than interpretive of unconscious conflict."

Viederman presented a case illustration involving an intractable depression in a young married woman following the stillbirth of her first child. At the end of the first interview she was told the following:

It's very clear why you are having so much difficulty with your loss. You are your father's superwoman. Everything had to be done perfectly, particularly to please him. You carry this off extremely well, though at considerable cost. You handled the pregnancy in your characteristic way. You would not allow yourself to show any anxiety, to feel slowed up in any way and you were planning confidently to present a perfect child to your father. How would it be possible for you not to be depressed and upset after the delivery, when for the first time in your life you had been entirely unable to control something that was of great importance to him and to yourself and something that you did not carry off successfully.

Viederman then explained:

The tension was quite diminished by the second session, and certain other concerns began to clarify themselves—namely, a reluctance to accept support from her husband and her preoccupation with the idea that her body had rejected the pregnancy. It was suggested that the latter issue become a focus for brief psychotherapy. By the third session, the patient indicated that she was feeling infinitely better than she had felt before and she had had the best weekend since the stillbirth. She had dealt much more comfortably with her husband, her brother, and the numerous friends who had been intensely involved in this pregnancy but whom she had recently avoided. She had been able to tolerate looking at young babies in the street, something that she had been unable to do since the stillbirth. She attributed the greater comfort to the fact that she had a person to talk to. This explanation was consistent with her need to maintain the view that she was not dependent on help and understanding coming from outside and made it easier for her to accept referral for psychotherapy.

The above case vignette is an excellent illustration of a technique the clinician may use to engage the patient in a psychotherapeutic endeavor. In those settings where psychotherapy is not available for the patient, such a formulation presented to the patient may in itself have a substantial therapeutic benefit.

Prognosis

In the prognosis section, the expected modifications of the patient's problems are detailed. Physicians are accustomed to assessing a patient's prognosis as good, fair, or poor. However, in psychiatry *prognosis* refers specifically to those therapeutic goals mutually established by the patient and the therapist. As described in the goals of treatment section, if the prognosis is not reasonably optimistic, the therapist has probably set goals that are too ambitious for the patient. In such a circumstance, it is recommended that the therapist rethink the treatment plan and goals section in order to achieve a more favorable prognosis. Because prognosis must be considered in terms of specific treatment goals, it is not sufficient to say that the prognosis is, in general, good. The prognosis may be good for several goals, fair for other goals, and poor for a final group of goals.

As the treatment progresses, new historical and transferential data may require the therapist to revise each section of the formulation. The therapist's initial case formulation provides only a tentative plan, which should never be fixed in the therapist's mind as though it were carved in stone.

SUGGESTED READING

Brenner C: An Elementary Textbook of Psychoanalysis. New York, International Universities Press, 1955

Brenner C: The Mind in Conflict. New York, International Universities Press, 1982

Fenichel O: Ego strength and ego weakness. In Collected Papers, Series 2, p 70. New York, WW Norton, 1984

Freud A: The Ego and the Mechanisms of Defence. New York, International Universities Press, 1946

Gediman HK: The concept of the stimulus barrier: Its review and reformulation as an adaptive ego function. Int J Psychoanal 52:243, 1971

Glover E: Ego distortion. Int J Psychoanal 39:260, 1958

Hartmann H: Psychoanalytic theory of the ego. Psychoanal Study Child 5:93, 1950

Hartmann H: Ego Psychology and the Problem of Adaptation. New York, International Universities Press, 1949

Hartmann H: Essays on Ego Psychology. New York, International Universities Press, 1964

Hartmann H, Kris E, Loewenstein R: Comments on the formation of psychic structure. Psychoanal Study Child 2:11, 1946

Herron WG: The assessment of ego strength. J Psychol Stud 13:173, 1962

Hollingshead AB, Redlich FC: Social Class and Mental Illness. New York, John Wiley & Sons, 1958

Holt RH: Ego autonomy revisited. Int J Psychoanal 46:151, 1965

Hurvich M: On the concept of reality testing. Int J Psychoanal 51:299, 1970

Hurvich M, Bellak L: Ego function patterns in schizophrenics. Psychol Rep 22:29, 1968

Karush A: Ego strength: An unsolved problem in ego psychology. In Masserman JH (ed): Science and Psychoanalysis, Vol 11, p 103. New York, Grune & Stratton, 1967

Karush A, Esser B, Cooper A et al: The evaluation of ego strength: I. A profile of adaptive balance. J Nerv Ment Dis 139:322, 1964

Kernberg O: Borderline personality organization. J Am Psychoanal Assoc 15:641, 1967

Kernberg O: A psychoanalytic classification of character pathology. J Am Psychoanal Assoc 18:800, 1970

Mahler MM, Pine F, Bergman A: The Psychological Birth of the Human Infant. New York, Basic Books, 1975

Menninger K: Regulatory devices of the ego under major stress. Int J Psychoanal 35:412, 1954

Messiner WA: Internalization in Psychoanalysis. New York, International Universities Press, 1981

Moore B, Fine B: A Glossary of Psychoanalytic Terms and Concepts. Washington, DC, The American Psychoanalytic Association, 1967

Mosak HH: Early recollections as a projective technique. J Proj Tech 22:302, 1958

Nunberg H: Ego strength and ego weakness. Am Imago 111:19, 1984

Prelinger E, Zimet C: An Ego Psychological Approach to Character Assessment. New York, The Free Press (Macmillan), 1964

Rapaport D: Structure of Psychoanalytic Theory: A Systematization Attempt. New York, International Universities Press, 1960

Rapaport D: The Collected Papers of David Rapaport. MM Gill, ed. New York, Basic Books, 1967

Rapaport D, Gill M, Schafer R: Diagnostic Psychological Testing, Vols 1 and 2. Chicago, Year Book Medical Publishers, 1946

Roessler R, Greenfield M, Alexander A: Ego strength and response stereotype. Psychophysiology 1:142, 1961

Sandler J, et al: On the concept of superego. Psychoanal Study Child 15:128, 1960

Sandler J, Holder A, Meers D: The ego ideal and the ideal self. Psychoanal Study Child 18:139, 1963

Sandler J, Rosenblatt B: The concept of the representational world. Psychoanal Study Child 17, 1962

Schafer R: Aspects of Internalization. New York, International Universities Press, 1968

Schafer R: An overview of Hartmann's contributions. Int J Psychoanal 51:425, 1970

Viederman M: The psychoanalytic life narrative: A psychotherapeutic intervention useful in crisis intervention. Psychiatry 1, No. 46:236, 1983

Wallerstein RS: Defenses, defense mechanisms, and the structure of the mind. J Am Psychoanal Assoc 31:201, 1983

Weiner H: Some thoughts on the concept of primary autonomous ego functions. In Lowenstein R, Neuman L, Schur M, et al (eds): Psychoanalysis—A General Psychology: Essays in Honor of Heinz Hartmann, p 583. New York, International Universities Press, 1966

Willick M: On the concept of primitive defenses. J Am Psychoanal Assoc (Suppl, International Universities Press) 31:175, 1983

APPENDIX 6-1. CASE FORMULATION

Description

Ms. E., a 22-year-old, single woman of mixed Jewish and Irish-Catholic backgrounds, is studying for a master's degree in Russian literature and rents a room in another woman's apartment. She was referred to the clinic in January, 1985 after a gynecologist found her crying in his examining room. Her chief complaints were "depression, anxiety, and not belonging anywhere," precipitated by breaking up with her boyfriend 2 months prior to her referral.

Ms. E. is a slender, young woman, 5 feet, 4 inches tall, with short, permanented, blonde hair encircling her fair-complexioned roundish face. She has blue eyes rimmed by large, round, pink-tinted eyeglasses, delicate features, freckles, and a small, quick smile. Her clothes are neat and well-coordinated with a casual student or country flair, and are often topped with a bright scarf or elaborate dangling earrings. Arriving up to 30 or 40 minutes early for her sessions, she carries a coat or denim jacket, a green book bag, and the *New York Times*. As I greet her in the hallway, she often has the look of a little girl who is lost but dutifully awaiting the arrival of her mother. She walks with small, measured steps and speaks in a soft, clear voice. She begins each new topic or association with a smile, which often quickly melts to tearfulness and a look of helplessness. She experiences silences as a burden for herself, and tentatively looks to me for a response. She listens raptly to each comment that I make with an expectant, hopeful look. When I indicate that it is the end of the session, she quickly gathers up her belongings, and slips out without a word.

Present Illness

Ms. E.'s first feeling of depression began the fall semester of her junior year at an Ivy League college after plans by both her parents to move to distant states gave her the feeling that she no longer had a home (they had been separated for 1 year). She felt sad and had frequent "crying fits." She felt that she did not fit in with the other students, that she was from a poorer background and was less well educated than they. She worried about finances, and did not enjoy joining in group collegiate activities. She often had difficulty falling asleep, and occasionally woke very early in the morning to find her muscles tensed, teeth clenched, and stomach "tied in knots." She felt tired, "hypersensitive and prone to falling apart over little things." Nevertheless, she received high grades, "never handed in one paper late," and maintained one or two part-time jobs.

Her depressed mood increased the winter that she broke up with her boyfriend, and she began short-term psychotherapy at the university infirmary. She felt "unburdened" but not significantly better, and left treatment after 2 months. Her parents' divorce was finalized that year.

By her senior year, she felt slightly better, made some friends and found her courses more rewarding. Nevertheless, 1 year ago she experienced an intensification of her symptoms after leaving a job she had loved (working with inner-city children). She found herself ruminating, "Where will I go, where will my stuff go after I graduate?" She had thoughts that it wouldn't matter if she lived or died, and she envisioned herself being killed by a car while carelessly crossing a busy street. The fantasy included the thoughts that "It would hurt my parents, because it would disappoint them," and that "What I want is my mother to be my mother . . . to take care of me." She did not reveal these thoughts to friends or family, but made frequent tearful calls to her parents. To bypass a waiting list for individual psychotherapy, she temporarily joined a group. She then revealed her suicidal thoughts and was changed to individual treatment. Again feeling unburdened but that she had received no "feedback," she left treatment after several months.

Her symptoms continued during a difficult graduation weekend and during the past summer, which she spent at her mother's new apartment in the Southeast. She felt relieved with the beginning of a new romance in June, but her symptoms began to reappear when she moved to Manhattan in September to begin graduate school.

Frustrated by a long wait to see a gynecologist for a yeast infection at the university infirmary, Ms. E. burst into tears and was found sobbing by the doctor. She was referred to the university mental health service so that she could "talk to someone," and from there was referred to the clinic.

Psychopathology

DEPRESSED SYMPTOMS

Depressed symptoms are described in the previous section.

GENERALIZED ANXIETY

Ms. E. complains of a feeling of apprehension accompanied by sweaty palms, tremulousness, and tightness of all her muscles. These episodes are most noticeable when she is about to recite in class. Sometimes she becomes so anxious that she loses the thread of what she was saying. She has no structured phobias and at no time has she contemplated avoiding the situations that make her anxious.

OBSESSIVE-COMPULSIVE SYMPTOMS

Obsessive fears. Ms. E. has intrusive obsessive thoughts. She worries about everything, often despite contradictory realities. She worries about money and how to live without spending it (even walking to school in the coldest weather because buses are too expensive), despite having adequate although limited resources. She worries about her weight even though she has never been fat. She worries that she might not do well in school, although she is first in her class. She also worries about decisions, most recently whether to take a leave of absence from school next year to live and work in the Southeast or to return to New York to complete her program after a summer near her mother.

Ms. E. ruminates about her body. She considers herself inadequate and unattractive—her breasts are too small, her rear end too flabby, many other features are ugly. She is very fearful about revealing her body. She cannot wear tight clothing, almost never wears shorts in public, and feels "mortified" at attention paid to her in public.

Rigid and perfectionistic behaviors. Ms. E. traces her "rigid" behavior back to her early childhood. For example, as a child she broke her leg, and 10 minutes of exercises each day was prescribed. She therefore set an alarm to get up exactly 10 minutes early, so that she could exercise without disturbing her regular activities, which included going to bed exactly at the same time each night. Although able to relax her routines while on vacation, she is compelled to run a set distance twice each day during the semester. She carefully watches her weight and food selection, and completes all of her school assignments early. "There's a lot of room between A and an A+," she states, and "Any grade less than an A+ is failure."

HISTRIONIC SYMPTOMS

Irrational angry outbursts or tantrums. When feeling in need of attention or assistance, Ms. E. resorts to having temper tantrums, replete with "yelling and screaming" and much crying. She speaks of these episodes with reluctance, but feels that they are the only possible way to get what she wants or needs, especially tuition money from her father or attention from her mother.

Self-dramatization. Ms. E. portrays herself as helpless and victimized by others. An enactment of this role was in a "practical joke" on her friend P. Late one night she lay down on the sidewalk outside her apartment building, pretending to be injured, while another friend called up to P. She came frantically rushing down. Ms. E. could not understand P.'s anger when the "joke" was revealed.

Manipulative interpersonal relationships. Throughout her life, Ms. E.'s relationships with her family, friends, and lovers have been intense and unstable. She uses people in a manipulative way. If they object to her behavior, she becomes furious and threatens to terminate the relationship. She often storms out in a "huff" and then waits for the other person to make a peace offering. If that does not occur, she becomes contrite, solicitous, and apologetic. Another example occurs each time her tuition is due when she creates "a scene" in order to manipulate her father into paying the bill.

SOMATIZATION

Ms. E. tells me tearfully about the yeast infections that she develops (at times before a visit with her boyfriend). She has had weeklong bouts of diarrhea, and often feels her stomach is "tied up in knots." She reports that frequent colds accompany her depressed mood, and has had several over the past 6 months.

IDENTITY DISTURBANCE

Ms. E. has never had a sense of belonging to any group in which she found herself. She lacks familial, academic, ethnic, social, religious, or career sense of identity. She has difficulty knowing her own views on any subject, feels that she is a chameleon, and states she subscribes to the opinion of any person to whom she is speaking.

Developmental Data

Ms. E.'s mother is a 44-year-old social worker from an Irish-Catholic background. The patient describes her as ill-tempered and always angry. She frequently screamed at the children and readily practiced character assassination. On other occasions she was excessively indulgent, particularly if the children were hurt or ill. Mealtimes were erratic, and her mother hated to cook.

Her father, a 48-year-old professor of history, is of Russian-Jewish background. He had been incarcerated in a Russian prison camp. Following the war, he immigrated to the United States, where he met the patient's mother while they were in college together. He is known for his liberal political views, and is also totally involved in his academic work and his reading. He was strict, aloof, demanding, and never spoke of his parents who were killed during the war. Since his divorce from the patient's mother 1 year ago, he dates younger women and drives a sports car.

Ms. E.'s younger sister P. spent much of her childhood fighting with the patient, whose room she shared. They had drawn a line down the middle of the double bed, which they shared until the patient was 11 years old and was given her own room. P. was a dramatic and creative child who frequently got into mischief. She was labeled as cute. Like the patient, she was often ill during her childhood. Unlike the patient, she had the father's dark hair and brown eyes. This increased the patient's feeling of alienation from the family. P. is now a college student and lives with the mother.

Ms. E. was born in a northwestern city in 1963. Her mother told her that she was "surprised" by becoming pregnant with the patient. The couple had only chosen a boy's name, so the patient remained "Baby E" for 3 months. They brought her home to an apartment that did not allow children, and they were constantly trying to control her crying. After 6 months they moved to the rural town where the patient's sister was born. Ms. E. reports feeling closer to her mother's family despite the fact that her mother's family would have nothing to do with them. Her mother's family objected to her marrying a Jew and refused to attend the wedding. The patient was raised with no religious affiliation. Jewish holidays were not recognized and neither parent showed any interest in their respective ethnicity.

Her earliest memory is being left in a stroller outside the supermarket and screaming for her mother who had disappeared inside. She also remembers her father playing ball with her when she was age 5.

When the patient was 3 years old, the family moved to a large Northeastern city. The patient cried for several weeks at night for her playmates, whom she never saw again. Her father had a low-ranking academic appointment in a small university.

She was admitted to a progressive private school on a scholarship and she learned that success came from being good and excelling in school.

At age 9, her mother gave her a book on menstruation that confused her. At age 11 she reached menarche, and recalled only that she was treated as though she were sick and perhaps dirty. Her periods have always been irregular, and she usually has to stay in bed the first day because of severe cramps and heavy bleeding.

When she was 11 years old, the family fortunes improved. The mother inherited a modest amount from her grandmother, and her father obtained an associate professorship at a large Eastern university. They moved to an upper middle class neighborhood. Again, the patient felt she did not belong, but managed to have several friends. She was in a tomboy phase during these years and participated in boys' athletics until her breast development led to sexual teasing. At this time (age 14) she withdrew from her male "buddies" and tried without success to be accepted by girls. When she was 16 and began to date, her parents remained strict about curfews, which led to a number of scenes where the patient would be called a "little whore" by her mother. Finally, in the patient's last year of high school, the parents extended her curfew whereupon the patient began having regular sex with her boyfriend and smoking pot. She preferred oral sex to intercourse, which was painful.

The patient attended an Ivy League university in New England, where she felt out of place and envied the "preppies" who had nicer clothes and better manners. Her father promised to send money, but it was usually necessary for her to have a temper tantrum before it was sent. During her college years the parents fought incessantly, and the patient was too ashamed to bring any of her college friends home.

She had three affairs during college, but in each instance she was abandoned by the man after a few months of stormy courtship. They resented her bad temper and rejection whenever she had to study for exams.

Ms. E. met her current boyfriend, D., 1 month prior to her moving to New York City. He is a 30-year-old lawyer who works for a large company in the city where her mother lives. He is described as an attractive, successful young man, who works with inner-city youths in his spare time.

Ms. E. (as stated earlier) is confused about her career goals but wants to do something to help the poor. However, she also recognizes that she wants a more materially comfortable life.

Key Psychodynamics

Ms. E. was born into a home where considerable tension already existed between her Jewish father and her Irish-Catholic mother. This tension was aggravated by the mother's family disapproving of the marriage. Both parents wanted a boy and were disappointed in their new baby girl, not naming her for 3 months.

The mother's short temper and lack of nurturing feelings impaired the early infant–mother bond with the result that the patient has felt a lifelong sense of disconnection from others, depression, feelings of worthlessness, and identity impairment.

The rage she felt towards her angry mother was repressed. She unconsciously attempted to maintain a good object image of her mother by blaming herself for her mother's outbursts. This led to a bad self-representation.

For additional love, she turned to her father, who enjoyed her intelligence and found her to be cute. She learned to manipulate him with temper tantrums whenever she found him too absorbed in his own affairs. The tantrums also represented both an early identification with the angry mother, and served as a means to discharge her own angry feeling through the mechanism of displacement. As a result of her perfectionistic academic performance and by being sick or hurt, she succeeded in winning some maternal love. Thus, in her physical symptoms and masochistic behavior, we see her partially successful attempts to maintain maternal nurturance.

When Ms. E. was 13, her younger sister was born and replaced her in the role of cute baby. Her father preferred the younger girl, who bore his own features, and this contributed to the patient's feelings of ugliness. She has unconsciously experienced her mother's controlling behavior and not letting her grow up as a castration, which adds further to her feeling of physical defectiveness. Her belief that she is ugly is also due to her guilt over her sexual attraction to her father.

Her relationship with her sister and with all female contemporaries has been excessively competitive. The wish to compete with the sister probably led to her tomboy behavior out of a wish to win the father's and mother's love by becoming the long-desired son. Also, the role of the tomboy represented a compromise formation to resolve partially her guilty fear over her Oedipal strivings. Nevertheless, this was a transient and partial identification, because shortly after puberty the patient abandoned that role in favor of a sexualized feminine role. Now able to displace her Oedipal attraction to boys her own age, she obtained acceptance and approval from them by using her sexuality as payment. However, she still feared her punitive mother, with whom she could only partially identify and whose love she continued to need. Thus, she utilized sex to obtain gratification of her frustrated dependency needs in her relationships with boys. Furthermore, her manipulative use of the sick or injured role provided additional dependent gratification while protecting her from the dangers of the adult female role.

She used her choice of career (Russian history) to strengthen her partial identification with her father and to maintain closeness to him without challenging her mother. However, the lack of a consolidated sense of identity makes it impossible for her to decide how to use her education in pursuit of a career or whether or not to progress towards marriage and a family. Her wish to work with underpriviledged people strengthens her own identification with the oppressed. To do otherwise strengthens her identification with the aggressor mother and increases her guilt and her fear of competition with a powerful rival. This hypothesis is supported by the patient's performance anxiety when confronted by the competitive classroom situation. She views her academic success as defeating her sister and her mother for her father's love. Thus, even her attempt to maintain her connection to her father through her career is fraught with danger.

Lacking a positive identification with the mother, Ms. E. has instead introjected a bad mother image that is critical, angry, and rejecting except when she is sick or masochistically defeated. By constantly criticizing and attacking herself, she both maintains the masochistic connection to her mother and neutralizes the intensity of her murderous competitive wishes. The parents' divorce made the Oedipal object more available, and consequently, the patient became even more frightened of competing with the mother. Her guilty feeling that she had caused the parents' divorce resulted in an increased depression. In addition, the parents both moving after their recent divorce intensified the patient's feeling of having been abandoned. This coupled with rejection by her boyfriend precipitated the patient's acute depressive illness. Her more chronic depression has other roots, as described earlier.

In summary, Ms. E.'s core conflicts are neurotic, based on an unresolved Oedipal conflict with pre-Oedipal aspects resulting from fixation at an oral dependent level. This has led to faulty identification as a woman and a lack of fusion of good and bad self and object representations. She utilized depressive, masochistic, obsessive, and hysterical defenses in warding off aggressive and sexual wishes. Her principal strengths are her intelligence, obsessive defenses, and academic success.

Diagnosis

Axis I: Generalized anxiety disorder, 300.02
Dysthymic disorder, 300.40

Axis II: Mixed personality disorder, and compulsive histrionic and masochistic features, 301.89

Axis III: Vaginal infections, gastrointestinal distress, and upper respiratory infections

Axis IV: Moderate (move to New York City, beginning graduate school, beginning serious romantic relationship)

Axis V: Good

Transference–Countertransference

It is expected that Ms. E. will first develop a maternal transference by obediently submitting to the therapist in order to win love, and by playing the role of the good patient. She will arrive early, pay on time, and never miss sessions. Quick insights and enthusiastic acceptance of the role of patient will prevail for a time. She will use her depression and her physical complaints to elicit sympathy and to dramatize her feeling of damage. It is expected that as she develops a feeling of intimacy and trust, a more competitive transference will emerge with her perhaps perceiving me as her more successful sister. Countertransference was manifested in my identification with the patient and my desire to give her advice and win her approval. I anticipate feeling threatened when her more assertive, competitive feelings emerge, although I recognize they will represent progress for us both.

Therapeutic Formulation

The treatment of choice for Ms. E. is analytically oriented psychotherapy twice a week on an outpatient basis. If her depression deepens to the degree of a major depressive episode, I will consider one of the tricyclic antidepressants.

I plan to devote the first few months to eliciting a careful history. I will look for opportunities to demonstrate the patient's fear of competition with other women, while at the same time I will highlight her ability to compete successfully in certain areas, although at a price. Initially, I will attempt to show her that her own efforts do count but that she is fearful of the adult female role, seeking safety in regressive childlike behavior in her relationships with men and women alike. As her self-esteem improves, I will begin to interpret her depression and masochism as a function of the loss of self-approval resulting from the strength of her repressed anger. I realize that my interpretation of her anger must proceed slowly so that she does not become more depressed.

Prognosis

The possibility of her overcoming her performance anxiety is good, and I anticipate that the psychophysiological symptoms will remit as well.

The goal of enabling her to find a suitable career will probably take more time to achieve. Her depression will improve as she builds better relationships with her family and finds a new boyfriend. Her infantile and histrionic behaviors have good prognoses. The pre-Oedipal problems are more serious, and her capacity for deeper object relations with the relinquishment of pathological introjects cannot be predicted at this time.

APPENDIX 6-2.   CASE FORMULATION

Description

Mr. F. is a 42-year-old, black, Protestant, married, male, city government administrator who lives with his wife, 10-year-old son, and 7-year-old daughter in a three-bedroom apartment in the Bronx. He came to the clinic in July, 1984 with anxiety, panic attacks, fears of homosexuality, and difficulties in his interpersonal relations.

Mr. F. is a handsome, pleasant man, 6 feet tall, of medium build, and light brown complexion. His curly black hair and neat moustache set off his hazel-colored eyes. He dresses casually, wearing tightly fitting slacks and shirts that emphasize his lean athletic build, with the top button of his shirt undone and his tie loosened and pulled down several inches.

He avoids eye contact, plays with his fingers, and chain smokes cigarettes. His voice is soft and sometimes monotonous, and he often laughs nervously. Mr. F.'s language is rather stilted, he selects passive verb forms in his choice of phrases.

Present Illness

Six months ago the patient became extremely anxious after seeing a movie about male homosexuality. He experienced tremulousness, diaphoresis, and palpitations lasting for a few hours. During the attack, he feared becoming a homosexual, or at some time "going crazy" or even dying. After the second attack, 3 months ago, he consulted his general practitioner, who gave him diazepam and reassurance. The medication helped at first, but 2 months ago he experienced a third attack of "panic." This occurred in the subway when he saw two men embracing. He stopped riding the subway and began to take buses, although at considerable inconvenience. The fourth and most recent episode of panic occurred when he was at home watching a movie on TV with his wife and children. It was a war movie in which the hero is gripped with fear in the presence of the enemy.

He felt better after several hours of comforting by his wife, but the diazepam was ineffective in this attack, and he decided to seek psychiatric advice. He called his physician, who recommended the clinic. Although he has no conscious homosexual wishes, and he has had no adult homosexual experience, he is plagued by a recurring fear that he "will turn into a fairy." Related to this fear is his belief that his penis is too small, a conviction he has maintained despite reassurance from several physicians.

During his initial evaluation session he also indicated his awareness of the following problems.

Psychopathology

PHOBIAS

In addition to the mild phobia of entering the subway (see Present Illness), Mr. F. recalls a period in his 20s when he was afraid to enter elevators. He would become tremulous and dizzy and have to leave the elevator. He gradually mastered this problem through "will power."

GENERALIZED ANXIETY

Mr. F. frequently feels anxious and upset, particularly when approaching a male protagonist whom he views as powerful and successful. He also feels anxious when he and his wife are on bad terms or when he has to speak before a group. He has decided that this feeling is a way of life and states, "I never travel without my Tums."

OBSESSIVE-COMPULSIVE FEATURES

Mr. F. carries a small overnight bag about which he states, "My life is in this bag: my budgets, my important papers. I figure out everything to the penny. I like to be organized, I have this compulsion to write everything down and make lists."

He is also very concerned with cleanliness and orderliness at home. "There's shit all over the floor, it drives me crazy." He often cleans rather than spending time talking or making love with his wife. He insists that others clean on his schedule and in his way. "I want it done now, and not later!"

He is parsimonious, passive-aggressive, and obstinate. He pays his household bills late and then fights over late finance charges. He is often indecisive and ruminates about decisions for days. At times, he ruminates about his transient impotence (see below).

PARANOID FEATURES

Mr. F. states, "I take offense easily. I don't like anyone speaking to me nastily or putting their hands on me." He describes himself as constantly testing people, "seeing if they cross the line. I'd do anything to avenge a wrong done to me; I never forget."

He has a black belt in karate and keeps in peak physical condition in order to be able to defend himself if attacked. Nevertheless, he has not actually been in a fight during his adult years. He generally feels disliked, and constantly wonders if people are making fun of him or talking about him behind his back.

NARCISSISTIC FEATURES

Grandiose Features. Mr. F. has multiple grandiose fantasies. He dreams of "traveling the world and sampling different pussy every night;" of "leading a double life—having a family and home but also a bachelor pad and orgies; working at a job but also being a secret agent." He also imagines himself as a race car driver winning the world championships.

He watches for every opportunity to get something for nothing and feels a sense of entitlement. That he actually has to work for his salary and pay his bills he feels is clearly unjust. At work he does the minimum, only when pressed, and then with resentment. Mr. F. is also painfully aware of his low self-esteem and feelings of helplessness.

Mr. F. takes pleasure in being admired by women in his brief bathing suit at poolside, and by being told how young and attractive he is. He lurks in the shadows of a disco, in fear of being discovered as old and undesirable when the bright lights come on and people could realize that he is not 28 years old.

Disturbed Interpersonal Relations. Mr. F.'s relationships with women have been dependent, exploitative, and sadistic. "When I was younger, in my 20s, I just used broads and did not try to please them." He has never been monogamous in a relationship, and feels that he is special and needs more than one woman.

He has trouble in his relationship with his wife, whom he feels does not take good care of him and puts the needs of the children before his own. They fight over money, her "untidiness," and how to spend their leisure time. He also has trouble with his two children, from whom he demands excessive obedience and the subordination of their interests for his. At the same time, he feels hurt and unloved if they do not constantly appreciate him.

Developmental Data

The patient was born in a middle class, black neighborhood in a large Midwestern city. The patient describes his mother as "the strongest woman I ever met." She is of light complexion like the patient. She was possessive, controlling, and punished him harshly if he misbehaved. Her methods involved whipping with a belt, scolding, and humiliating him in front of others. She worked as a registered nurse and usually held two jobs. His mother took only 1 week off from work when the patient was born, and left him with her mother, who died when the patient was 2 years of age. After that time, he was left with neighbors or with a baby-sitter when his mother worked. He describes his father as a tall, powerful, dark-skinned man who worked "off and on" in an automotive repair shop. His father was frequently intoxicated and absent from the home and his job for several days at a time. The patient has an early memory of seeing his father "on the street" with another woman and a little girl. His father left for good when the patient was 5 years old, and the patient has seen him only sporadically since then. Another early memory is his father catching him playing with his penis in the bath and threatening to "cut the little thing off if he didn't quit." As a result, the patient masturbated infrequently during his childhood and adolescence.

The patient has a brother, 2 years younger, of dark complexion, a sister 3 years younger, light skinned like himself, and a half brother 6 years younger, also dark skinned. The patient recalls James, the man who fathered the half brother, as tall, athletic, kindly, and generous. James lived with the family intermittently for the next 8 years, and finally moved away when the patient was 13 years old. Both his brothers were more athletic and less intellectual than Mr. F., but it was the brother closest to his own age with whom there was a constant struggle for dominance. That brother has become a schoolteacher and the younger half brother works as a garage mechanic. His sister, with whom he has been quite close, is a nurse and is married with two children. He recalls being caught "playing sex games" with her when he was 9 years old and being beaten for this by his mother. Because he was the oldest, his mother insisted that he take care of his "baby brothers," fix meals, clean up, and change diapers when she was on the evening shift.

When he was 12 years old, his mother was hospitalized for a hysterectomy. He was "terrified" and recalls leaning against a school fence and crying for hours. A year later his "stepfather" disappeared for good. During his adolescence he withdrew from physical competition with his younger brother, who then was able to pin him. He concentrated on his schoolwork and became one of the top students in his class. At the age of 13 years, he allowed an older boy to perform fellatio on him, and he found the experience disgusting. At 15 years of age, he first became afraid of being homosexual while reading a magazine article on that subject. In his early teen years he felt shy and uncomfortable with girls, but when he was 16 years old an older girl in the neighborhood seduced him. In retrospect, he realizes that he ejaculated very quickly, but he had no difficulty becoming erect. It was around that time that he first experienced a recurring dream of being in a gun battle with other males and using a gun that doesn't shoot straight or that has ineffective bullets.

Upon graduation from high school, he refused two scholarships from good colleges to join the Air Force "to become a man and to see the world." It was then that he learned karate, and earned a black belt by the time of his discharge 4 years later. He began dating more frequently while he was in the Air Force, and had affairs with numerous white women prior to meeting his wife. It was during this period that his masculine self-confidence rose significantly, yet, for reasons he could not understand, he would occasionally be unable to "achieve" an erection.

Following his discharge, he enrolled in a full-time college program, which was partially financed by a scholarship and partially by his two part-time jobs in a restaurant. Four years later he obtained a degree in government administration. In his last year of college, he met C., an attractive, light-skinned, sharp-tongued, ambitious classmate. They were married a year later at her insistence. She is employed as a grade-school teacher. They have frequent arguments in which he insults her intelligence, and she criticizes his masculinity and his sexual performance. He feels enraged, but there has been no physical violence. Instead, he has had numerous affairs, usually short-lived, and invariably with white women. He derives only transient satisfaction from these relationships other than proving his attractiveness to women. His description of these encounters emphasizes the success of his conquests as opposed to his enjoyment.

His career advancement has been sporadic. He obtained a job with the city government shortly after being graduated from college, but episodic conflicts with superiors has retarded his advancement. He rationalizes that these arguments are the result of his boss being threatened by his higher intelligence. Actually, he seduced his boss's secretary and then told him about the fact.

Two years ago, Mr. F.'s mother died suddenly of a stroke. The patient was grief stricken and "cried for days on end" for approximately a year.

During the past year, his sexual activities have been markedly curtailed because of his involvement with his new high-performance car, which he takes around the drag race circuit. "At 120 miles per hour, I feel like all that power is part of me." In spite of his new passion, he continues to dream of finding the ideal woman: "warm, passionate, beautiful, and intelligent." In his career he feels stymied, but lacks a plan for what he would like to do next. He states that he is dissatisfied with his job because he feels it is no challenge.

Key Psychodynamics

The patient's core conflicts center around homosexual fears, wishes and accompanying feelings of dependency; anal conflicts involving obedience and defiance; and narcissistic conflicts with feelings of helplessness and unworthiness alternating with compensatory feelings of entitlement and grandiosity. His predominant defense mechanisms include denial, reaction formation, phobic and counterphobic mechanisms, projection, isolation, displacement, and splitting.

The patient's dependency problems began in his infancy with a mother who was more involved with her job than with him, as evidenced by her turning his early care over to her mother, who died when the patient was 2 years old. The patient experienced this early loss as an abandonment and reacted with depression and feelings of being to blame. He turned more to his father at that time and developed a strong negative Oedipal tie. This relationship was threatened by the repeated disappearances of the father, and his ultimate abandonment when the patient was 5 years old.

The birth of a sister when he was 3 years old further added to the patient's sense of deprivation and loss. When he turned 6 years old, a new father figure arrived on the scene. The patient was both threatened by the new rival for his mother's love and relieved that she was no longer available, which reduced his guilt that he had successfully driven off his biologic father. He dealt with the new competition through submission and ingratiation and a partial identification with this man, who was somewhat stronger than the patient's biological father. Once again, a new sibling arrived, one who had the advantage of a biological connection to the "new father." Once again, profound feelings of inferiority were triggered. The youngest brother identified more strongly with his biological father and pursued more "manly" interests. The patient reacted by strengthening his identification with his mother, and created the foundation for later fears of homosexuality. His castration anxiety can be traced both to the prohibiting biological father and the rejecting stepfather who created guilt over his sexual feelings toward his mother.

Mr. F.'s partial feminine identification and his continuing negative Oedipal wishes further added to his fear and unconscious wish for a homosexual solution. Also, through homosexual submission, he avoids competition with the father and retains his love while warding off castration. Although he blames his mother for forcing him into the female role of caring for the younger siblings, this may also represent some defensive rationalization on the patient's part, because the mother also criticized him for not being more aggressive and masculine. The patient further identifies with the mother, because he experienced her as the more powerful and more constant figure.

Mr. F.'s high intelligence and academic success fed into a developing secondary narcissism, which was designed to repair his feelings of helplessness and dependency. The disappearance of his stepfather at age 13 years again reinforced his sense of omnipotence and grandiosity at having defeated another Oedipal rival. It was at this age that the patient experimented sexually with an older boy out of the dual motivation described above. His sense of masculinity was sufficiently adequate that he consciously rejected the homosexual solution, and abandoned physical contact with other males to reduce his temptation to submit "homosexually."

He concentrated on building his intellectual power, felt boosted by grandiose fantasies, and beginning at age 16, by some success with girls. At this point, he chose the Air Force over college in an attempt to counterphobically master his homosexual conflict and feminine identification. There he learned karate, earned a black belt, and achieved some "success" at chasing women. These activities only partially strengthened his masculine identification, as is evidenced by the continuing grandiose fantasies. Nevertheless, his improved self-representation allowed him to resume an intellectual and occupational career, a development that was only partially successful as the patient developed an inhibition of competition. The collapse of his defensive organization began 2 years ago when his mother died, re-enacting his multiple abandonments.

The patient's current inability to establish an affectionate relationship with his wife stems from his fears of castration and engulfment by a powerful black woman—who is like his mother. His choice of white women as sexual partners is determined by the relative safety of women who are different from his mother, as well as the opportunity this behavior provides for symbolic competitive victory over white males. His current preoccupation with drag racing is another vicarious attempt to repair his low masculine self-esteem. He equates his inhibition of assertion and excessive dependency with a feminine identification, and this leads to homosexual anxiety, which, in turn, precipitates his panic attacks, phobias, and activates paranoid character traits. The compulsive and narcissistic traits have a reparative value in his present character organization.

Diagnosis

Axis I: Panic disorder, 300.01
Axis II: Mixed personality disorder, 301.89, with paranoid, compulsive, narcissistic, and aggressive features
Axis III: None
Axis IV: Psychosocial stressors minimal; attended a homosexual movie
Axis V: Fair; occupational inhibitions, marital discord

Transference–Countertransference

The patient will probably initially develop an unconsciously competitive transference toward a younger, white male therapist. Mr. F. will perceive the therapist as a potentially powerful male to whom he must behave in a passive-submissive fashion in order to defeat. On the other hand, he hopes he cannot defeat me and that I will be the powerful father with whom he can identify. Next, he will fear my abandoning him as other fathers have in the past. I predict that my first vacation will activate such fears. After this initial phase, the patient will probably develop a maternal transference with fears of castration and engulfment. The maternal transference will probably be acted out outside the transference with his wife or perhaps a female figure of authority at work.

Countertransferentially, I will probably enjoy the role of father/protector and will be tempted to give him advice and perhaps even to view his wife as an adversary. I might not recognize the unconscious resentment over his submissive and compliant role. Although ignorance is not countertransference, there are many issues about being a black person with which I am unfamiliar. The opportunity to learn more about the black culture is interesting, and furthermore, I could be entertained by his macho exploits, which could represent an unconscious seduction on the part of the patient.

Therapeutic Formulation

I recommend twice a week analytically oriented psychotherapy for the patient's characterological problems, and I will prescribe imipramine to control his panic attacks.

Initially, I plan to take a more detailed history, and I will look for material that will clarify the circumstances that precipitate panic or a fear of panic. I suspect these have some unconscious homosexual significance, which can be interpreted. I will then try to link the patient's inhibition of competition in his job, to his fear of the white establishment as related to his homosexual anxiety and its attempted resolution through his adopting a passive-submissive stance of not competing, but symbolically expressing his rage through passive-aggressive techniques and seducing white women. I expect his fear of black women will emerge, which can be interpreted both in pre-Oedipal and Oedipal dynamics.

If my beginner's status initially elicits a negative transference, I will interpret that he is angry or disappointed that I am not the powerful male he wishes could treat him.

Prognosis

The prognosis for the relief of his panic attacks is excellent. The prognosis for enabling him to become more assertive and to be more successful in his job is good. He is very intelligent, ambitious, and seems insightful. The prognosis for improving the marriage is more guarded, because he has chosen a woman who fits in with his psychopathology. His relationships with his children should improve significantly as he develops a more realistic attitude to them. His obsessive-compulsive traits and his narcissistic features will probably be the most difficult to change, because those traits are quite egosyntonic.

APPENDIX 6-3.   CASE FORMULATION

Description

Dr. G. is a 63-year-old married college physics professor of Italian-American heritage who lives with his wife in a modest home in a small Midwestern town. His four children are all married. He was admitted to an inpatient neuropsychiatric service of a university-affiliated general hospital in May, 1985 with depressed mood, impaired memory, inability to concentrate or to make decisions, fatigue, insomnia, and decreased appetite with a 23-pound weight loss over the previous 6 months.

Dr. G. is slender, 5 feet 7 inches tall, has thinning, straight black hair, dark eyes, and a swarthy complexion. His brown tweed jacket and gray slacks fit loosely, and he is wearing no tie although the top button on his neatly pressed white oxford-cloth shirt is buttoned. Accompanying him to the inpatient unit is his wife, who carries the patient's leather briefcase bulging with term papers and scientific journals. Dr. G. repeatedly rolls into a tight cylinder and unrolls a copy of *Science* magazine. He sits forward in his chair with his shoulders slumped and stares at his feet while responding to questions. He listens intently to the psychiatrist and makes some effort to respond with accuracy. He is mannerly and communicates his professional respect for the psychiatrist.

Present Illness

For the past 2 years, Dr. G. has noticed increasing difficulty in remembering the names of new students. He also complains of difficulty recalling the names of former students whom he no longer has occasion to think about regularly. He states, "The face is familiar, but the name just won't come to mind." Because of his problem remembering names, he has been embarrassed in several public meetings and has begun to avoid people. For the past year he has, in addition, experienced difficulty understanding articles in technical journals. In May, Dr. G.'s schedule of professional obligations, which is perennially full, becomes even more demanding. He is responsible for reading and grading final examinations in the advanced undergraduate courses that he teaches; for reviewing and making critical comments related to Ph.D. theses that are submitted in May; and for putting the "final touches" on his own scholarly reports and seminars. During this month, he became aware that even the mathematics involved in Ph.D. theses he was reviewing—which he felt was relatively straightforward—had become difficult for him to handle. He also noted that his ability to concentrate on his own research was poor and that he was, uncharacteristically, making "careless" errors in his calculations. When he met personally with his students and colleagues, he was indecisive and unsure of himself. Important deadlines for returning students' papers and for the submission of articles were delayed. Although he felt fatigued, Dr. G.'s response to his increasing work load was to drive himself even harder and to blame himself for work that was not being completed. He rejected the advice of his experienced secretary that he request his department chairman to transfer a junior staff member to assist him with his work. He believed that such a request would be excessive and indulgent, particularly in light of what he felt to be his present state of ineffectiveness. Instead, Dr. G. became increasingly dependent upon his secretary at work and his wife at home to remind him of things or to wait on him constantly. On two occasions, when he was confronted by students regarding delays in the completion of his critique of their doctoral theses, Dr. G. lost his temper and raised his voice in obvious irritation. He recalls saying at one point, "You will just have to wait. If you aren't happy with the job I am doing, get another faculty advisor." The complaints of students ultimately came to the attention of the chairman of the physics department, who was surprised to discover the disarray of Dr. G.'s academic obligations. The chairman met with Dr. G., who attributed his problem to persistent insomnia for the past couple of months. A pattern had developed in which Dr. G. would go to bed at 12 midnight, fall asleep at approximately 2 AM, and awaken at 5 AM unable to fall back to sleep. Dr. G. found that he no longer derived pleasure from his favorite hobby, working with his personal computer, nor did he enjoy reading technical journals, which was his other favorite pastime. As his symptoms progressed, Dr. G. began to blame himself for his decreased productivity at work. His mood was increasingly depressed, with pervasive pessimism and negativistic ruminations. He felt that food no longer tasted good, lost his appetite, and often skipped meals. With the encouragement of his wife and children, Dr. G. sought outpatient psychiatric care. His psychiatrist diagnosed him as depressed, and initiated twice a week psychotherapy, which did not result in improvement of Dr. G.'s symptoms. After 6 months of treatment, Dr. G. was referred for inpatient diagnostic evaluation, to include the consideration of an antidepressant medication, and for electroconvulsive therapy.

Psychopathology

DEPRESSION

Symptoms of depression are described in the discussion of present illness.

COGNITIVE AND MEMORY DISTURBANCES

Cognitive and memory disturbances are discussed in the section on present illness.

PASSIVE-DEPENDENT TRAITS

Dr. G. is overly dependent both upon his wife and his secretary. For example, he assumes very little responsibility for the family finances. His wife pays all the bills, balances the checking account, and prepares the tax information for the accountant. On several occasions when Dr. G. had forgotten to take to work the lunch his wife perennially prepares and packs for him, he did not have sufficient money in his wallet to buy his lunch in the university cafeteria. He also assumes little initiative for family recreational activities. His wife complains that he will not participate in the choice of a restaurant for dinner, or the selection of a movie, or even the planning of a vacation. She states that his response is usually, "Whatever you like will be fine with me, dear." He makes few efforts to cultivate friendships, so that his social relationships are almost exclusively derivative of friendships established by his wife and children. He also is passive related to his own medical care. He neglected going to the dentist for many years with the result that extensive periodontal surgery was required to prevent him from losing many of his teeth.

At work, Dr. G. is highly dependent upon his secretary. He insists that she take her vacation on precisely those dates that he takes his own, because he does not feel that he could function professionally without her. On one occasion when she was hospitalized for 4 weeks with a sudden surgical illness, Dr. G.'s professional life almost ground to a halt. Not knowing the filing system in his office, he was unable to locate the outlines of his lectures or to find information crucial for his research. He relies on his secretary to remember the birthdays of his wife and children and even his own anniversary date. It is his secretary who buys the presents on these occasions; she does his Christmas shopping, and takes care of other personal matters (such as picking up his medicine at the pharmacy) as well.

Somatization

Dr. G. suffers both from migraines and from "acid stomach." Typically, his migraines occur on the weekends or after he has completed difficult projects at work. From the time the patient completed graduate school, he has suffered from what he terms "acid stomach." This symptom is also worse during times of stress and work pressure. At age 36 years, Dr. G. had an episode of "tarry stools" and anemia secondary to gastrointestinal bleeding.

Developmental Data

Dr. G. was born in a small, working-class "steel mill town" adjacent to a large Midwestern city. Both of his parents were of Italian-Catholic backgrounds and were also born in that same city. All four grandparents were born in Italy and immigrated to this country around the turn of the century. His maternal grandparents lived with the patient, his parents, his three older brothers and two younger sisters in a small three-bedroom home in a run-down residential area. During the patient's childhood, he shared a bedroom with his three older brothers (2, 5, and 7 years older than he). His two sisters shared the second bedroom, and his grandparents occupied the remaining and largest bedroom. Dr. G.'s parents slept in the small livingroom on a couch that converted into a double bed. The patient describes his mother as very warm and loving but somewhat overprotective and indulgent. She spent many hours with him teaching him to read and to play the piano. The patient recalls the feeling that his mother hovered over him too much, and when he became older, he avoided her by studying in the library after school. His father was a union laborer at the giant steel mill located several blocks from their home. He described his father as a "fiercely religious Catholic, a hard worker, and a strict disciplinarian." The patient's father was a tall and muscular individual who took great pride in his physical strength and capacity to do hard work, both in his job in the steel mill and at a second job that he worked at nights and on weekends. The patient states that his brothers, who were all taller, stronger, and more athletic than he, "took after" their father, while he resembled the mother, who had a slight frame and was more intellectual. The patient recalls feeling that his father was disappointed that he was not as aggressive as his brothers. Two of the patient's brothers received football scholarships to a large state university, and the third brother quit high school in his senior year to take a job working in the steel mill where his father was employed. The patient recalls being picked on by all three of his brothers, but particularly being constantly harassed by the brother who was 2 years older than he. The patient was protective of his two younger sisters and recalls them following him around and eager to wait on him. The patient's academic achievements gradually won him a measure of respect from his father and brothers.

When he was 13 years of age, his father's left arm was mangled in an accident at the steel mill. The father, thereafter, was retired from the steel mill "on disability," and having only the skills of a manual laborer, was unable to obtain employment elsewhere. The father became despondent, increasingly irritable, and began to drink excessively. On numerous occasions, Dr. G. had to intervene when his father had become drunk and was being physically abusive with his mother.

From the time of grade school, the patient's principal source of self-esteem was his excellence in school. With his gift both for mathematics and for languages, the patient was perennially the top student in his class. He had few close friends among his peers, but became captain of the debating team. He never dated in high school; rather, his closest relationships were with his mathematics and science teachers. Upon the advice of his high school principal, the patient applied for and received a full (tuition, room, and board) scholarship to an excellent Eastern university.

In college, Dr. G. continued his pattern of hard work without "interference" from such outside diversions as sports, dating, or other forms of recreation. He supplemented his scholarship by tutoring underclassmen in mathematics. In the spring semester of his junior year, he tutored a freshman whom, following her initiative and persistence, he began to date. Approximately 30 pounds overweight, Jane was the first female whom Dr. G. had dated more than twice. He had no prior sexual experience, nor was it his practice to masturbate, which he felt to be dirty and an act of weakness. He gradually became acquainted with Jane's family and was soon taken under the wing of her father, who took increasing interest in the patient's career. Jane's father advised Dr. G., who did not receive less than an A during college, to attend graduate school in physics in order to pursue a career as a college professor. He had previously considered a career as a high-school mathematics teacher or applying for work in the accounting department of a large steel company.

Jane and Dr. G. were married during the summer that he completed graduate school. The patient recalls felling ashamed of his one-armed father, his boisterous brothers, and other relatives at the wedding ceremonies. The couple were married by a Protestant minister after the patient had converted to that faith. On one occasion prior to his marriage, he overheard his prospective father-in-law saying to a friend, "Wait till you meet Jane's new boyfriend. He is a Phi Beta Kappa and a real gentleman. I'm not losing a daughter, I'm gaining a son." Nevertheless, the patient believed that his father-in-law was troubled with his daughter's choice of a husband.

On the patient's wedding night and during his honeymoon, he was unable to achieve an erection and consummate his marriage. The problem persisted for the first 2 months of his marriage, and the patient, at Jane's advice, sought advice from her gynecologist. This specialist referred Dr. G. to a urologist, who assured him that he had no medical problems and that the problem would "take care of itself if he would relax and not worry about it so much." Gradually, Dr. G. was able to achieve erections and a pattern emerged of 2-minute sex without foreplay, which persisted through their marriage. With the birth of their children, three girls and 1 boy, Jane, who continued to gain weight, assumed almost complete responsibility for managing the household and the lives of the children. Unlike the patient, Jane is warm, vivacious, and has many friends. She also has labile emotions and frequently loses her temper with the patient. Dr. G. rarely fights back, but urges her to be more reasonable. He feels closer to his daughters than to his son, although he is not inclined to be overtly affectionate to any of his children. Dr. G.'s son was a hyperactive child and rebellious in grade school. Dr. G. felt "uncomfortable" in most of his interactions with his son and was "frustrated" by his son's lack of discipline. Unlike his sisters, Dr. G.'s son did poorly academically, and barely was graduated from high school. He is now employed in a factory as a blue-collar worker and recently married a kindergarten teacher. The patient's daughters all completed college. The oldest daughter is a physician, the next is a lawyer, and the youngest is a marine biologist. All are married, and the older two have young children. Dr. G. has never been particularly interested in his grandchildren, but his wife sees them frequently and enjoys them.

With regard to the patient's career, Dr. G. joined the faculty of a small but prestigious Midwestern university, where he ultimately rose to the rank of tenured professor. He conceived and developed a well-regarded subspecialty division of the physics department.

Key Psychodynamics

Dr. G. was born into a home where there was tension between his strict and punitive father and his warm and indulgent mother. The mother was disappointed when her fourth child, the patient, was also born a boy, but she was pleased with his more delicate physique, placid temperament, and more intellectual proclivities.

The patient experienced himself as the mother's favorite, a position he enjoyed until the birth of his sister. At that time, when the patient was 5 years old, the mother's attention turned to the new daughter. The patient felt betrayed, but soon found that he could win the favor of his school-teachers by being better behaved and more conscientious than his class-mates. Thus, he shifted his role from being his mother's pet to being the teacher's pet.

The patient maintained a favorite position with his mother through his intelligence and his sensitivity to her moods. This favorite position made the patient fearful of the envious responses of his father and brothers, who picked on him. The patient's observations of his father punishing his older and more powerful brothers frightened him. Nevertheless, he envied the acclaim his brothers received for their sports activities and attempted to compensate for this through academic achievement. He disliked their rough and tumble ways, but at the same time, felt less manly than they were. The patient did not fight back against his brothers or father, but adopted a pas-sive-submissive mode to reduce his castration fear. Therefore, he was only partially able to identify with his powerful father. His incomplete paternal identification led to the development of an impaired sense of masculinity, which is later expressed in his impotence. His strongest masculine identifi-cation is with the father's capacity for discipline and hard work. His re-pressed anger towards more powerful men led him to experience guilt fol-lowing the father's loss of his right arm. He was unconsciously glad, but frightened by the consequent humiliation of his father, who was no longer able to be gainfully employed.

The intimate relationship that the patient maintained with his mother was inherently seductive, leading to guilt feelings and castration anxiety for having defeated his father and brothers in the quest for his mother's love. He warded off this Oedipal anxiety by remaining passive and allowing women to wait on him and to protect him from his father and brothers. This accounts for the late development of the interest in girls and for his waiting to be chosen by a woman who wanted to marry him, thereby providing him both a wife and a substitute mother. His passive role in his relationship to the maternalized wife further accounts for his impotence. The support and encouragement of his idealized father-in-law may have strengthened his shaky masculine identification and allowed him to function sexually in a limited fashion as well as to pursue a successful career.

The major change in his status quo occurred when memory, cognitive, and intellectual impairments reduced his capacity to function at work at his previous high level. These changes preceded his change in affect. The patient denied his illness because of threats to the main area of his masculine pride—his work. Unconsciously, his brain had come to symbolize his phallus, and he reacted to the threat of its impairment by attempts to compensate by heightened effort, and later, when that failed, with depression.

Mental status revealed that the patient experienced impaired memory, intellectual changes including problems with mathematic and technical concepts, and a mild anomic aphasia. It is likely that these symptoms contributed to his depression. These changes were confirmed later on neuropsychological testing, which showed moderately diminished performance on visual–perceptual–motor tasks, reduced capacities to use arithmetic, with decreased forward and reverse digit spans. Measurement of his memory showed an impaired capacity to remember newly acquired facts and difficulty with abstract and conceptual thought. The patient's physical examination and neurological examination were normal. Measurement of blood chemistries and evaluation of the patient's cerebral spinal fluid (including pressure) were also within normal ranges. Electroencephalogram showed diffuse slowing and increased amplitude of brain waves. Brain CT scan showed generalized, scattered atrophy, which was manifested by widened sulci and ventricular enlargement. There was also an increase in the patient's ventricles-to-brain ratio (VBR). Magnetic resonance imaging (MRI or NMR) confirmed abnormal findings of the CT scan as well as showing higher spin density values for all brain white matter. All other laboratory values were within normal limits.

In the case of Dr. G., a persuasive argument for a DSM III Axis I diagnosis of Major Depressive Episode can be made, arguing that depressive symptomatologies were an emotional reaction to the situational incapacities brought on by Alzheimer's disease. Clearly, the patient meets all DSM III diagnostic criteria for Major Depressive Episode except criteria E, which states that the illness is "not due to any organic mental disorder." However, the scientific evidence is persuasive that affective changes are inherent features of Alzheimer's disease, and in the case of Dr. G., would therefore indicate an Axis I diagnosis of organic affective syndrome and dementia.

Diagnosis

Axis I: Organic affective syndrome, 293.83
                Dementia, 294.10
Axis II: Dependent personality disorder, 301.60
Axis III: Alzheimer's disease
Axis IV: Psychosocial stressors—onset of a seriously disabling illness in the context of high-pressure work responsibilities: 5, severe
Axis V: Highest level of adaptive functioning over the past year: 4, fair

Transference–Countertransference

The patient will probably initially view me as the omnipotent physician–mother with unlimited power to understand and to treat both his organic and functional illnesses. Therefore, it is likely that he will experience the role of patient as being passive, dependent, and gratifying. After this initial phase the patient may feel competitive with me as a younger male with an academic career. He could also become envious of my youth and nonsenile brain. If his physical condition should deteriorate secondary to Alzheimer's disease, it is likely that the patient will experience intensified anger towards and suspicion of me as the ineffective caretaker.

Countertransferentially, I might have difficulty accepting the gradual deterioration that is inherent in his illness. It would be easier for me to see this nice father figure as depressed rather than demented, and I might tend to conceptualize his dysfunction more as the result of a serious depression than as a product of Alzheimer's disease. I may become discouraged or bored if the patient fails to respond to my efforts, or tend to be overprotective or overdirective if his dementia worsens.

Therapeutic Formulation

The patient will receive inpatient psychiatric care involving multiple therapeutic modalities, which will include daily brief psychotherapy, for approximately 3 weeks. Attempts will first be made to treat the patient's depression with antidepressant agents with low anticholigeric properties. Blood levels will be utilized to ensure that therapeutic levels of the drug are achieved. Should the patient be unable to tolerate the side-effects of antidepressant agents, electroconvulsive therapy (ECT) will be considered.

Once the patient's depression is adequately treated, he will be discharged and followed in once per week supportive psychotherapy. With the patient's permission, I will meet with his wife and family to gain additional history, to apprise them of the treatment plan, and to prepare them for the long-term prognosis. The family will be both supported and advised regarding methods of helping the patient with his memory and orientation problems without making him overly dependent. They will be encouraged to allow Dr. G. to do as much as he can for himself within the realistic range of his limitations and will be advised not to wait on him or to treat him as an invalid. In his individual treatment, the patient will also be encouraged to be more self-reliant and not to "give up" as his Alzheimer's disease progresses. The patient's antidepressant agent will be tapered slowly if no depressive symptomatology recurs for 6 months. Should depressive symptomatology re-emerge with the tapering of the antidepressant agents, the medication will be returned to its treatment dose and plasma level.

Prognosis

It must be noted that in the living patient, the diagnosis of Alzheimer's disease can be established only by observing the patient's clinical course over time. Even abnormal values on computed tomography and magnetic resonance imaging as described for Dr. G. are nonconclusive: a number of authors have shown the occurrence of these changes in nondemented elderly individuals. In the case of Dr. G., if cognitive, intellectual, and memory changes remain after treating his depression with either therapeutic doses of antidepressant agents and/or ECT, the diagnosis of dementia of the Alzheimer's type would be more likely.

The goal of successfully treating the symptoms of the patient's depression is realistic, and there is an excellent chance that this will be accomplished within a 4-week hospital stay. The goal of enabling the patient to function better interpersonally with improvement in his relationships with his family and in his business life will be more difficult to achieve. The patient's progress in psychiatric treatment is also dependent upon the course of his Alzheimer's disease, which cannot be predicted.

SUGGESTED READING

DeMyer MK, Hendrie HC, Gilmor RL et al: Magnetic resonance imaging in psychiatry. Psychiatr Annals, 15, No. 4:262, 1985

Hall RC, Beresford TP: Handbook of Psychiatric Diagnostic Procedures, Vol I. New York, Spectrum Publications, 1984

Hall RC, Beresford TP: Handbook of Psychiatric Diagnostic Procedures, Vol II. New York, Spectrum Publications, 1985

Solomon S: Clinical Neurology and Pathophysiology. Comprehensive Textbook of Psychiatry IV. Vol I, 131–145. Baltimore, Williams & Wilkins, 1985

Index

Numbers followed by an *f* indicate a figure; *t* following a page number indicates tabular material.

abstraction test, 159
abstract thinking, 66
acetaminophen (Tylenol), 107, 107t
acetylsalicylic acid, blood level
    data for, 107, 107t
adaptive functioning, rating, 218
adaptive relaxation in service of
    ego, 227t, 232
adulthood, patient history of, 54–57
affect, 69–71
  blunted, 70
  flat, 70
  inappropriate, 70–71
  regulation of, 226t, 230
  restricted, 70
  shallow, 70
affective disorder
  brain changes in, 113–116
  in frontal lobe injury, 126
  mental status examination in,
    81–84
  Schedule for Affective Disorders
    and Schizophrenia, 171–176,
    172f-175f

  in temporal lobe impairment,
    135
  written psychodynamic case for-
    mulation in, 267–275
affective display, as resistance
    mechanism, 15
aggression, and Overt Aggression
    Scale, 169–170, 203–206
agoraphobia, 5
alcohol, blood level data for, 107,
    108t
alcoholism, 106
  brain changes in, 117
  diagnosis of, 175f-176f
alertness, 71, 73
alpha rhythm, 110
Alzheimer's disease, 267–275
aminophylline, blood level data for,
    107t
amitriptyline (Elavil), 101, 103
  blood level data for, 107t
amnesia, 136
amphetamine, blood level data for,
    106, 107t

anal-sadistic period, 241
anamnesis. *See* psychiatric history
anarthria, 130
anomic aphasia, 132–133, 134t
anosognosia, 137
  visual, 138
antidepressants, tricyclic
  blood level measurements of,
    101–104
  laboratory testing before treat-
    ment with, 101–102
antipsychotic medication, blood
    level measurements of, 104–
    105
antisocial personality, 49
Anton's syndrome, 138
anxiety, 250–259. *See also* panic
    disorder
  generalized, 252
  Hamilton Anxiety Rating Scale,
    176, 195–196
  managing in interview, 27
aphasia, 129–135, 159, 164
  Boston Aphasia Battery, 159
  clinical types of, 130–135, 134t
  fluent, 129–130, 134t
  Halstead-Wepman Aphasia
    Screening Test, 164
  nonfluent, 129, 134t
  questions used in diagnosis of,
    133t
aphonia, 130
appearance of patient, 61–63
  patient concerns about, 252
appropriateness of emotional re-
    sponses, 70–71
arsenic, blood level data for, 107t
attitude of patient, 61–63
auditory testing, 161–164
autonomy
  primary, 234
  secondary, 234, 244
Aventyl. *See* nortriptyline
awareness, reflective, 233

barbiturates, blood level data for,
    106, 107t
BDI. *See* Beck Depression Inven-
    tory
BEAM technique, 112
Beck Depression Inventory (BDI),
    167, 190–192
behavior, 61–63
  assessment of, 179f-181f
  disturbance of, 221
    in frontal lobe injury, 125–126
  perfectionist, 252–253
  rigid, 252–253
Benadryl (diphenhydramine), blood
    level data for, 108t
Bender visual-motor gestalt test,
    158–159, 158f
benzodiazepines, 107
beta activity, 110
blocking, 64
blood flow, cerebral, 117, 128
boredom, 65
Boston Aphasia Battery, 159
Boston Naming Test, 160
brain
  architectonic areas of, 124t
  blood flow in, 117, 128
  computed tomography of, 112–
    114, 128
  dysfunction of, 157–159
    minimal, 53, 73, 137
  function of, assessment of, 160–
    165
  imaging techniques for, 112–119
  injury to, 124
  magnetic resonance imaging of,
    114–115, 115f
  organic disease of, substance-in-
    duced, 105–110
  positron emission tomography of,
    115–116, 128
brain electrical activity and map-
    ping (BEAM) technique, 112
Brief Symptom Inventory, 167
Broca's aphasia, 130–131, 134t

cannabis, 106
capacity for object relations, 230–231
Capgras' syndrome, 137
carbamazepine (Tegretol), blood level data for, 105, 107t
cardiovascular system
    lithium treatment and, 97–98, 100t
    tricyclic antidepressants and, 101–102
case formulation. *See* written psychodynamic case formulation
catatonia, 71
character traits, 61
    formation of, 240f
chief complaint, 43–44, 182f
childhood, patient history of, 50–53, 222
Children's Behavior Inventory, 170
chloral hydrate (Noctec), blood level data for, 107t
chlordiazepoxide (Librium), blood level data for, 108t
chlorpromazine (Thorazine), blood level data for, 104, 108t
circumstantiality, 64
cocaine, blood level data for, 106, 108t
cognitive function, 66–67
    in elderly, assessment of, 159–160, 162t-163t
    impairment of, 138, 221, 268–269
    in parietal lobe injury, 137
computed tomography (CT), of brain, 112–114, 128
conation, 62
concentration, 66–67
conduction aphasia, 132, 134t
confabulation, 136
confidentiality, 20–21, 31–32
conflict
    central, in symptom formation, 241–243

model of, 224
    resolution of, 229
consciousness, 71
    alterations of, 39
    clouding of, 71
coordination, testing of, 159
cortex, architectonic areas of, 124t
cortical impairment
    diffuse, 138–142
    evaluation of, 123–142
countertransference, 17–18, 244–245
CT. *See* computed tomography
cultural history of patient, 54
curiosity, of patient about himself, 24–25

Darvon (propoxyphene), blood level data for, 109t
data, interview. *See* interview, data of
daydreams, 48
defense
    balance of, 229–230
    immature, 228–229
    mature, 228–229
    primitive, 229
    in symptom formation, 240–241
defense formation, 226t, 228–230
defense mechanism, 228–230, 242–244
defensive behavior, 228–229
deficit symptoms, 243–244
deja vu phenomenon, 135
Delayed Recognition Span Test, 160
delirium, 138–139, 162t
delta activity, 110
delusions, 61, 65–67
dementia, 138–140, 141t
    Alzheimer's disease, 267–275

dementia *(continued)*
  brain changes in, 114, 117
  categories of, 139–140
  clinical features of, 141t
  cognitive functioning in, 163t
  Dementia Rating Scale, 160
  written psychodynamic case for-
    mulation in, 267–275
Dementia Rating Scale, 160
Demerol (meperidine), blood level
    data for, 108t
depersonalization, 68–69, 233
depression, 39, 69, 86, 268–269
  Beck Depression Inventory, 167,
    190–192
  brain changes in, 117
  case formulation of, 250–259
  cognitive impairment in, 140–
    142, 141t, 163t
  dexamethasone suppression test
    in, 88–91, 88t, 89f
  Hamilton Rating Scale for, 170–
    171, 197–200
  mental status examination in,
    78–81
  sleep patterns in, 112
  stuporous, 71
  thyroid function tests in, 92–96,
    94t
  thyrotropin-releasing hormone
    test in, 91–92, 91t
derealization, 69, 233. *See also* real-
    ity
desipramine (Norpramin), 140
  blood level data for, 108t
desmethylimipramine, blood level
    measurements of, 101–104
developmental data, 222–223
developmental deficits, 243–244
dexamethasone suppression test,
    87–91, 88t, 89f
diabetes insipidus, lithium treat-
    ment and, 98
Diagnostic and Statistical Manual.
    See DSM-III diagnosis

diagnostic interview, 4–5
diagnostic labels, 29
diazepam (Valium), blood level data
    for, 108t
digoxin, blood level data for, 108t
Dilantin (phenytoin), blood level
    data for, 109t
diphenhydramine (Benadryl), blood
    level data for, 108t
disorientation, 66–67
dissociative disorder, 142
distractibility, 64–65
Dolophine (methadone), blood level
    data for, 108t
Doriden (glutethimide), blood level
    data for, 108t
doxepin (Sinequan), blood level
    data for, 108t
Draw-A-Family Test, 155
Draw-A-Person Test, 154
drawings, projective, 154–155
dreams, 47–48, 65
  in childhood, 52–53
dream state, 71
drives, 224
  regulation of, 226t, 230
drugs. *See* medication
drug screen, 107
DSM III diagnosis, 212–219. *See
    also specific diagnoses*
  Axis I, 215
  Axis II, 215–216
  Axis III, 217
  Axis IV, 217–218
  Axis V, 218
  multiple diagnoses with Axis I
    and II, 216–217
  in written psychodynamic case
    formulation. *See* written psy-
    chodynamic case formula-
    tion
dysarthria, 130
dyslexia, 137
dysphasia, 130, 159
dysphonia, 130

echolalia, 62
echopraxia, 62
ECT. *See* electroconvulsive therapy
educational history of patient, 54–55
EEG. *See* electroencephalogram
ego, 224–238
ego functions, 59, 225–234
    autonomous, 234
    developmental aspects of, 235–238
    organization of, 226t-227t
ego ideal, 239
ego strength, 59, 235
ego weakness, 49, 59
Elavil. *See* amitriptyline
elderly, cognitive function in, assessment of, 159–160, 162t-163t
electrical diagnosis, 110–112
electroconvulsive therapy (ECT), 129, 140
    pretreatment evaluation for, 102
electroencephalogram (EEG), 110–112
    during sleep, 111
emotional disturbance, 221
emotional needs, unmet, 51
emotional regulation, 69–71
emotions, uncovering in interview, 21–22
empathy, of interviewer, 3, 5–6
epilepsy, 111
ethanol. *See* alcohol
euphoria, 86
evaluation, multiaxial. *See* DSM III diagnosis
expressive aphasia, 130
externalization, 238

family history, 57

family member, interview of, 31–33
fantasy, 48, 234, 261
    in childhood, 52–53
fear, obsessive, 252
feelings. *See* emotional *entries;* emotions
Finger Oscillation Test, 161
finger-tapping test, 159
flight of ideas, 64
free thyroxine index, 93, 97
frontal lobes, evaluation of function of, 125–129
frustration tolerance, 74–75, 230
fugue, 71

Ganser's syndrome, 142
garrulousness, as resistance mechanism, 14–15
GAS. *See* Global Assessment Scale
generalization, as resistance mechanism, 14
global aphasia, 130, 134t
Global Assessment Scale (GAS), 176, 192–195
glutethimide (Doriden), blood level data for, 108t
Grip Test, 161
guilt, 21

Haldol. *See* haloperidol
hallucinations, 39, 61, 67–68, 139
hallucinogens, 106
hallucinosis, 68
haloperidol (Haldol), blood level data for, 105, 108t
Halstead Category Test, 161
Halstead-Reitan neuropsychological battery, 159–164
Halstead-Wepman Aphasia Screening Test, 164

HAMD. *See* Hamilton Rating Scale for Depression
Hamilton Anxiety Rating Scale (HARS), 176, 195–196
Hamilton Rating Scale for Depression (HAMD), 170–171, 197–200
HARS. *See* Hamilton Anxiety Rating Scale
hatching process, 235
hematologic system
    lithium treatment and, 97–98, 100t
    tricyclic antidepressants and, 101–102
history
    personal. *See* personal history
    psychiatric. *See* psychiatric history
histrionic symptoms, 253
homosexuality, 56
    fears concerning, 259–267
House-Tree-Person Test, 154–155
hypothyroidism, 86, 92–96, 94t–95t

id, 224
ideas, flight of, 64
identification, 236–237, 244
identity disturbance, 253
illness
    present, 220
        history of, 182f
        impact of, 46–47
        onset of, 45–46
    previous psychiatric, 48
illusions, 68
imipramine (Tofranil), blood level data for, 101–104, 108t
imitation, 236
impulse control, 74–75, 226t, 230
incorporation, 237

Inderal (propranolol), blood level data for, 109t
information, status of patient's, 75
insight, 76, 233
insomnia, 47
instinct, 224
integration, synthetic, 227t, 234
intellectual change, in frontal lobe injury, 126–128
intellectualization, as resistance mechanism, 14
intelligence, 75
    testing of, 148–151, 158. *See also specific tests*
intelligence quotient (IQ), 150
interest, of interviewer in patient, 20
internalization, 236
interpersonal relationships
    disturbed, 261–262
    manipulative, 253
interpretation, by interviewer, 7–8
interview, 1–33. *See also* interviewer
    closing phase of, 27–30
    content of, 10
    data of
        inspective, 11
        introspective, 11
        patient, 11–18
        systems of classification of, 10–11
    diagnostic versus therapeutic, 4–5
    middle phase of, 22–27
    note taking during, 10
    opening phase of, 19–22
    pre-interview considerations in, 18–19
    process of, 11
    with relatives of patient, 31–33
    with significant others, 31–33
    space considerations in, 9–10
    subsequent, 30–31
    time factors in, 8–9

interviewer, 15–18. *See also* interview
  as authority figure, 3
  building patient's self-esteem by, 7
  empathy toward patient, 3, 5–6
  greeting of patient by, 19–20
  inexperienced, 16–17
  interest in patient, 20
  interpretation by, 7–8
  limit setting by, 6–7
  patient's attitude toward, 62–63
  pre-interview expectations of, 18–19
  reassurance of patient by, 5–6
  suggestions by, 6–7
  understanding of patient by, 5–6, 20
intoxication, 139
introjection, 237–238
IQ, 150

jargon, 131
jokes, 65
judgment, 76, 234
  testing of, 158

laboratory testing
  in frontal lobe injury, 128
  risk-benefit ratio of, 86–87, 117–119
  sensitivity of, 86–87
  specificity of, 87
language
  disturbance of. *See also* aphasia
  in schizophrenia, 132
  in temporal lobe impairment, 129–135
  testing of, 159
lead, blood level data for, 108t
learning disability, 53, 137
Librium (chlordiazepoxide), blood level data for, 108t
life narrative, psychodynamic, 246–247
limit setting, by interviewer, 6–7
lithium
  blood level data for, 96–101, 100t, 108t
  laboratory tests before treatment with, 96–98, 100t
  side-effects of, 96–97
liver, effect of tricyclic antidepressants on, 101–102
LSD, blood level data for, 108t
Luria-Nebraska neuropsychological battery, 159, 164–165

magnetic resonance imaging (MRI), of brain, 114–115, 115f
malingering, 142
mania, 66
manic-depressive illness, lithium treatment of, 96–101
Manic-State Rating Scale, 170
manic syndrome, screening for, 173f-174f
manipulative relationships, 253
marital history, 56
masturbatory history, 54
medication
  blood level measurements of, 96–104
  side-effects of, evaluation of, 105–110, 107t-109t
  toxicity of, evaluation of, 105–110, 107t-109t

Mellaril (thioridazine), blood level
　　data for, 109t
memory, 73
　　impairment of, 66–67, 268–269
　　in temporal lobe impairment,
　　　135–137
　　remote, 136
　　short-term, 136
　　tests of, 157–158
　　Wechsler Memory Scale, 136,
　　　157–158, 160, 206–211
mental status examination, 36–40,
　　38t, 58–77, 200–203
　　affect, 69–71
　　in affective disorder, 81–84
　　appearance of patient, 61–63
　　attitude of patient, 61–63
　　behavior of patient, 61–63
　　consciousness, 71
　　in depression, 78–81
　　emotional regulation, 69–71
　　frustration tolerance, 74–75
　　impulse control, 74–75
　　information, 75
　　insight, 76
　　intelligence, 75
　　judgment, 76
　　memory, 73
　　mood, 69–71
　　organization of data in, 61–78
　　orientation, 72
　　perception, 67–69
　　sample report of, 78–84
　　in schizophrenia, 81–84
　　thought process, 64–69
Mental Status Examination Record
　　(MSER), 176
Mental Status Questionnaire, 160
Mental Status Schedule (MSS), 176
meperidine (Demerol), blood level
　　data for, 108t
meprobamate, blood level data for,
　　108t
mercury, blood level data for, 108t
metal, heavy, toxicity of, 106

methadone (Dolophine), blood level
　　data for, 108t
methamphetamine, blood level
　　data for, 108t
methanol, blood level data for, 107,
　　109t
methaqualone (Quaalude), blood
　　level data for, 109t
methohexital, 111
methylphenidate (Ritalin), blood
　　level data for, 109t
Metrazol (pentylenetetrazol), 111
military history of patient, 57
Mini-Mental State Examination,
　　200–203
Minnesota Multiphasic Personality
　　Inventory (MMPI), 155–157,
　　161, 167
mixed aphasia, 134t
MMPI. *See* Minnesota Multiphasic
　　Personality Inventory
mood, 69–71
mood swings, 69
moral background of patient, 54
morphine, blood level data for, 109t
motivation, 246
MRI. *See* magnetic resonance imag-
　　ing
MSER, 176
MSS, 176
multiaxial evaluation. *See* DSM III
　　diagnosis
multiple sclerosis, 86
Mysoline (primidone), blood level
　　data for, 109t

narcissism, 261–262
neologism, 131
neuroendocrine testing, 87–96
neurological change, in frontal lobe
　　injury, 128

neuropsychological tests and assessment, 157–159
neutrality, 12
technical, 12
Noctec (chloral hydrate), blood level data for, 107t
Norpramin. *See* desipramine
nortriptyline (Aventyl)
blood level data for, 101–104, 109t
therapeutic window for, 103
NOSIE-30, 167–168
note taking, during interview, 10
Nurses' Observation Scale for Inpatient Evaluation (NOSIE-30), 167–168

OAS. *See* Overt Aggression Scale
object relations, capacity for, 230–231
obsessive-compulsive personality, 49, 252–253, 260–261
criteria for, 185f-186f
occipital lobe, evaluation of function of, 138
occupational history, 54–55
opiates, 106–107
orientation, disorders of, 72
outbursts, irrational angry, 253
Overt Aggression Scale (OAS), 169–170, 203–206
oxycodone (Percodan), blood level data for, 109t

PADL, 170
panic disorder, 39
criteria for, 183f-184f

written psychodynamic case formulation in, 259–267
paraldehyde, blood level data for, 109t
parallel history technique, 46
paranoia, 86, 261
paraphasia, 131
parietal lobe, evaluation of function of, 137
passive-dependent traits, 268–270
past, exploring in interview, 24
patient
concealing data from interviewer, 3
description of, 219–220
history of. *See* personal history; psychiatric history
interview of. *See* interview
pre-interview expectations of, 18
payment for treatment, 21
PCP (phencyclidine), 106–107
PDE. *See* Personality Disorder Examination
pentazocine (Talwin), blood level data for, 109t
pentylenetetrazol (Metrazol) 111
perception, 67–69
impairment of
in parietal lobe injury, 137
in temporal lobe impairment, 135
testing of, 158
perceptual motor capacity, testing of, 158
Percodan (oxycodone), blood level data for, 109t
perfectionist behavior, 252–253
Performance Test of Activities of Daily Living (PADL), 170
perphenazine (Trilafon), blood level data for, 109t
personal description, of patient, 45
personal history, 48–57
adulthood, 54–57
childhood, 50–53

personal history *(continued)*
  cultural, 54
  family, 57
  moral, 54
  prenatal, 50
  psychosexual, 53–54
  religious, 54
personality, 23–24
  types of, 55
Personality Disorder Examination
  (PDE), 176–177, 178f-181f
personality testing, 151–157. *See
  also specific tests*
  nonprojective, 155–157
  projective, 151–155
PET. *See* positron emission tomography
phencyclidine (PCP), 106–107
phenobarbital, blood level data for,
  107t
phenytoin (Dilantin), blood level
  data for, 109t
phobias, 260. *See also fear; panic
  disorder; specific phobias*
physical symptoms, emotional disturbances and, 39, 47–48
physiological disturbances, 217,
  221
play, 52
positron emission tomography
  (PET), of brain, 115–116, 128
pre-interview consideration, 18–19
prenatal history, 50
preoccupation, 65, 69
press, Murray's theory of, 154
primidone (Mysoline), blood level
  data for, 109t
privacy, 20–21
process of interview, 11
prognosis, 30, 248
projection, 238
projective drawings, 154–155
propoxyphene (Darvon), blood level
  data for, 109t

propranolol (Inderal), blood level
  data for, 109t
proverbs, 66, 127
pseudodementia, 140–142, 141t
PSS, 176
psychiatric history, 36–40, 37t
  history of present illness in, 45–
    47
  organization of data in, 43–58
  personal history in, 48–57
  preliminary identification in, 43–
    45
  previous illness in, 48
  of psychotic patient, 43
  purpose of, 40–41
  by questionnaire, 42
  techniques of, 41–42
psychiatric interview. *See* interview
psychiatric review of systems, 47–
  48
Psychiatric Status Schedule (PSS),
  176
psychodynamic case formulation.
  See written psychodynamic
  case formulation
psychodynamic life narrative, 246–
  247
psychodynamics
  practical considerations in, 239–
    244
  theoretical considerations in,
    223–239
psychological assessment, 147
psychological change, in frontal
  lobe injury, 125
psychological testing, 146–148
  clinical applications of, 159–165
  reliability of, 147–148
  standardization of, 147
  validity of, 148
psychomotor activity, 62
psychopathology, 220–222. *See also
  specific disorders*
psychosexual history, 53–54

psychosomatic disorder, 39
psychotic patient, psychiatric history from, 43
puberty, onset of, 54
Purdue Pegboard test, 159

Quaalude (methaqualone), blood level data for, 109t
questions
   open-ended, in interview, 25–26
   of patient, answering in interview, 27–28
   of relatives of patient, 33
quinidine, blood level data for, 109t
quinine, blood level data for, 109t

rapid eye movement (REM) sleep, 111–112
rapport, between interviewer and patient, 5, 20–22
rating scale, psychiatric, 146–148, 165–187. *See also specific scales*
   naturalistic, 167
   self-report questionnaires, 166–167
reaction-formation, 229–230
reality, sense of, 227t, 232–233. *See also* disrealization
reality testing, 227t, 232–233
reasoning, 127
reassurance
   of patient by interviewer, 5–6, 24
   of relatives of patient, 33
recall, 73, 136. *See also* memory
referentiality, 65–66
registration, 73, 135–136. *See also* memory

relationship to others, 226t, 230–231, 233
relatives. *See* family *entries*
relaxation, adaptive, in service of ego, 227t, 232
reliability of psychological testing, 147–148
religious history of patient, 54
REM sleep, 111–112
renal function, monitoring of, 96–97, 100t
representational world, child's, 235–236
resin T_3 uptake test, 94t
resistance, 14–15
retention, 73, 136–137. *See also* memory
review of systems, psychiatric, 47–48
Rhythm Test, 161
rigid behavior, 252–253
Ritalin (methylphenidate), blood level data for, 109t
Rorschach Personality Test, 151–153, 153f

sadness, 69
SADS. *See* Schedule for Affective Disorders and Schizophrenia
salicylate. *See* acetylsalicylic acid
Schedule for Affective Disorders and Schizophrenia (SADS), 171–176, 172f-175f
   lifetime version, 172
   for measuring change, 172
schizophrenia, 66, 70–71
   brain changes in, 113–117, 128
   electroencephalogram patterns in, 112
   language disturbance in, 132

schizophrenia *(continued)*
  mental status examination in, 81–84
  personality testing in, 152
  Schedule for Affective Disorders and Schizophrenia, 171–176, 172f-175f
Schneiderian symptoms, 84
SCID. *See* Structured Clinical Interview for DSM-III-R
SCL-90-R. *See* Self-Report Symptom Inventory-Revised
self-confidence, 231
self-dramatization, 253
self-esteem, 7, 231
self-report questionnaire, for psychiatric rating, 166–167
Self-Report Symptom Inventory-Revised (SCL-90-R), 166–167, 168f
self-representation, 226t, 231, 233
sensitive topics, in interview, 26
sensory aphasia, 134t
sensory capacity
  impairment of, in parietal lobe injury, 137
  testing of, 159
Sensory-Perceptual examination, 161
separation-individuation process, 235–236
sexuality
  adult, 55–56
  psychosexual history, 53–54
shame, 21
sibling rivalry, 51–52
significant others, interview of, 31–33
silence, as resistance mechanism, 15
Sinequan (doxepin), blood level data for, 108t
SKID-UP study, 181
sleep
  disturbance of, 47

stages of, 111
slips of tongue, 65
social capacity, testing of, 158
social relationships
  adult, 55–57
  changes in frontal lobe injury, 125–126
somatic disturbance, 221
somatization, 270
space consideration, in interview, 9–10
speech, 63
Speech-Sounds Perception Test, 161
speed, testing of, 159
standardization, of psychological testing, 147
Stanford-Binet test, 127
Stelazine (trifluoperazine), blood level data for, 109t
stimulus regulation, 226t-227t, 231–232
Strength of Grip Test, 161
stress, precipitating, 44, 46, 217–218
stressing of patient, in interview, 26–27
stress tolerance, 234
stroke, 124
Structured Clinical Interview for DSM-III-R (SCID), 177–187, 182f-186f
  Nonpatient Version, 181
  Patient Version, 181
substance-use disorder, 105–106
suggestion(s), by interviewer, 6–7
suicide, 69, 81
  by poisoning, 105
superego, 49, 75, 238–239
sympathy, of interviewer, 3
symptoms
  formation of, 240–244, 240f
  primary gain of, 242
  primary loss of, 242

secondary gain of, 46–47, 242
secondary loss of, 46–47, 242
synthetic integrative functioning, 227t, 234
systems, psychiatric review of, 47–48

tact, in interview, 26
Tactile Finger Localization Test, 164
Tactile Form Recognition Test, 164
Tactile Performance test, 159, 161
tactile testing, 161–164
Talwin (pentazocine), blood level data for, 109t
tantrums, 253
TAT. *See* Thematic Apperception Test
Tegretol. *See* carbamazepine
temporal lobe, evaluation of function of, 129–137
Thematic Apperception Test (TAT), 153–154, 155f
theophylline. *See* aminophylline
therapeutic interview, 4–5
theta activity, 110
thioridazine (Mellaril), blood level data for, 109t
Thorazine. *See* chlorpromazine
thought
    abstract, 66
    concrete, 66
    content of, 65–66
    continuity of, 64–65
    process of, 64–69
    production of, 64
thought disorder, 64
thyroid-binding globulin, 93, 94t
thyroid function
    effect of lithium on, 97, 100t
    tests of, 92–96, 94t
thyroid scan, 94t

thyroid stimulating hormone (TSH) test, 94t, 95t, 97
thyrotropin-releasing hormone (TRH) test, 91–92, 91t
thyroxine assay, 93, 94t, 97
time factor, in interview, 8–9
Tofranil. *See* imipramine
toilet training, 51
Token Test, 159
tonic support, 232
Trail Making Test, 161
transcortical motor aphasia, 134t
transference, 12–14, 244–245
    competitive, 14
    negative, 13
    omnipotent, 13–14
    positive, 12–13
transition, abrupt, in interview, 22–23
treatment
    duration of, 30
    goals of, 245–246
    plan of, 28–30
TRH test. *See* thyrotropin-releasing hormone test
trifluoperazine (Stelazine), blood level data for, 109t
triiodothyronine assay, 94t, 97
Trilafon (perphenazine), blood level data for, 109t
TSH test. *See* thyroid stimulating hormone test
Tylenol. *See* acetaminophen

understanding, of patient by interviewer, 5–6, 20
unreality, 68–69. *See also* reality

validity of psychological testing, 148

Valium (diazepam), blood level data for, 108t
Vineland Social Maturity Scale, 158
vision disturbance in occipital lobe injury, 138
visual testing, 161–164

WAIS-R. *See* Wechsler Adult Intelligence Scale-Revised
wakefulness, 71
Wechsler Adult Intelligence Scale-Revised (WAIS-R), 126–127, 149–150, 158, 160
Wechsler Intelligence Scale for Children-Revised (WISC-R), 151
Wechsler Memory Scale (WMS), 136, 157–158, 160, 206–211
Wechsler Preschool and Primary Scale of Intelligence (WPPSI), 151
Wernicke's aphasia, 131–133, 134t
WISC-R, 151
WMS. *See* Wechsler Memory Scale

words, patient's, repeating in interview, 25
WPPSI, 151
written psychodynamic case formulation, 51, 219–248
in affective disorder, 267–275
developmental data in, 222–223
in dementia, 267–275
in depression, 250–259
description of patient in, 219–220
diagnostic classification in, 244
formulation of, therapeutic, 245–247
in panic disorder, 259–267
present illness section of, 220
psychodynamics section of, 223–244
psychopathology section of, 220–222
transference-countertransference in, 244–245

Zung Self-Rating Scale, 167